# 50% OFF Online TEAS Prep Course!

By Mometrix University

Dear Customer,

We consider it an honor and a privilege that you chose our TEAS Study Guide. As a way of showing our appreciation and to help us better serve you, we are offering **50% off our online TEAS Prep Course.** Many TEAS courses cost hundreds of dollars and don't deliver enough value. With our course, you get access to the best TEAS prep material, and **you only pay half price**.

**We have structured our online course to perfectly complement your printed study guide**. The TEAS Prep Course contains **over 60 lessons** that cover all the most important topics, **70 video reviews** that explain difficult concepts, over **1,800 practice questions** to ensure you feel prepared, over **500 digital flashcards** for studying on the go, and even an **audio mode**, so you can listen to lessons as you do other things.

*Online TEAS Prep Course*

**Topics Covered:**

- Reading
  - *Key Ideas and Details*
  - *Craft and Structure*
  - *Integration of Knowledge & Ideas*
- English & Language Usage
  - *Conventions of Standard English*
  - *Knowledge of Language*
  - *Vocabulary Acquisition*
- Science
  - *Human Anatomy & Physiology*
  - *Life & Physical Sciences*
  - *Scientific Reasoning*
- Math
  - *Numbers & Algebra*
  - *Measurement & Data*

**Course Features:**

- TEAS Study Guide
  - Get content that complements our best-selling study guide.
- 8 Full-Length Practice Tests
  - With over 1,800 practice questions, you can test yourself again and again.
- Mobile Friendly
  - If you need to study on the go, the course is easily accessible from your mobile device.
- TEAS Flashcards
  - Our course includes a flashcard mode consisting of over 500 content cards to help you study.
- Audio Mode
  - Every lesson in our course has an audio mode, allowing you to listen to the lessons.

To receive this discount, simply head to our website: mometrix.com/university/courses/teas and add the course to your cart. At the checkout page, enter the discount code: **teas50**

If you have any questions or concerns, please don't hesitate to contact us at universityhelp@mometrix.com.

Sincerely,

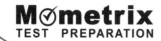

# ATI TEAS®

# SECRETS

## Study Guide
### Your Key to Exam Success

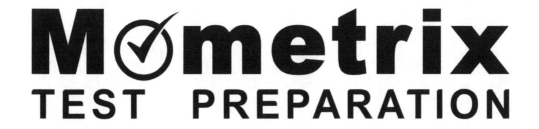

Written and edited by the Mometrix Nursing School Admissions Test Team

Mometrix offers volume discount pricing to institutions. For more information or a price quote, please contact our sales department at sales@mometrix.com or 888-248-1219.

ATI TEAS® is a registered trademark of the Assessment Technologies Institute®, which was not involved in the production of, and does not endorse, this product.

Paperback
ISBN 13: 978-1-5167-0383-8
ISBN 10: 1-5167-0383-9

Ebook
ISBN 13: 978-1-5167-0732-4
ISBN 10: 1-5167-0732-X

Hardback
ISBN 13: 978-1-5167-1415-5
ISBN 10: 1-5167-1415-6

# DEAR FUTURE EXAM SUCCESS STORY

First of all, **THANK YOU** for purchasing Mometrix study materials!

Second, congratulations! You are one of the few determined test-takers who are committed to doing whatever it takes to excel on your exam. **You have come to the right place.** We developed these study materials with one goal in mind: to deliver you the information you need in a format that's concise and easy to use.

In addition to optimizing your guide for the content of the test, we've outlined our recommended steps for breaking down the preparation process into small, attainable goals so you can make sure you stay on track.

We've also analyzed the entire test-taking process, identifying the most common pitfalls and showing how you can overcome them and be ready for any curveball the test throws you.

Standardized testing is one of the biggest obstacles on your road to success, which only increases the importance of doing well in the high-pressure, high-stakes environment of test day. Your results on this test could have a significant impact on your future, and this guide provides the information and practical advice to help you achieve your full potential on test day.

### Your success is our success

**We would love to hear from you!** If you would like to share the story of your exam success or if you have any questions or comments in regard to our products, please contact us at **800-673-8175** or **support@mometrix.com**.

Thanks again for your business and we wish you continued success!

Sincerely,
The Mometrix Test Preparation Team

> **Need more help? Check out our flashcards at:**
> **http://MometrixFlashcards.com/TEAS**

# TABLE OF CONTENTS

# Introduction

**Thank you for purchasing this resource!** You have made the choice to prepare yourself for a test that could have a huge impact on your future, and this guide is designed to help you be fully ready for test day. Obviously, it's important to have a solid understanding of the test material, but you also need to be prepared for the unique environment and stressors of the test, so that you can perform to the best of your abilities.

For this purpose, the first section that appears in this guide is the **Secret Keys**. We've devoted countless hours to meticulously researching what works and what doesn't, and we've boiled down our findings to the five most impactful steps you can take to improve your performance on the test. We start at the beginning with study planning and move through the preparation process, all the way to the testing strategies that will help you get the most out of what you know when you're finally sitting in front of the test.

We recommend that you start preparing for your test as far in advance as possible. However, if you've bought this guide as a last-minute study resource and only have a few days before your test, we recommend that you skip over the first two Secret Keys since they address a long-term study plan.

If you struggle with **test anxiety**, we strongly encourage you to check out our recommendations for how you can overcome it. Test anxiety is a formidable foe, but it can be beaten, and we want to make sure you have the tools you need to defeat it.

# Secret Key #1 – Plan Big, Study Small

There's a lot riding on your performance. If you want to ace this test, you're going to need to keep your skills sharp and the material fresh in your mind. You need a plan that lets you review everything you need to know while still fitting in your schedule. We'll break this strategy down into three categories.

## Information Organization

Start with the information you already have: the official test outline. From this, you can make a complete list of all the concepts you need to cover before the test. Organize these concepts into groups that can be studied together, and create a list of any related vocabulary you need to learn so you can brush up on any difficult terms. You'll want to keep this vocabulary list handy once you actually start studying since you may need to add to it along the way.

## Time Management

Once you have your set of study concepts, decide how to spread them out over the time you have left before the test. Break your study plan into small, clear goals so you have a manageable task for each day and know exactly what you're doing. Then just focus on one small step at a time. When you manage your time this way, you don't need to spend hours at a time studying. Studying a small block of content for a short period each day helps you retain information better and avoid stressing over how much you have left to do. You can relax knowing that you have a plan to cover everything in time. In order for this strategy to be effective though, you have to start studying early and stick to your schedule. Avoid the exhaustion and futility that comes from last-minute cramming!

## Study Environment

The environment you study in has a big impact on your learning. Studying in a coffee shop, while probably more enjoyable, is not likely to be as fruitful as studying in a quiet room. It's important to keep distractions to a minimum. You're only planning to study for a short block of time, so make the most of it. Don't pause to check your phone or get up to find a snack. It's also important to **avoid multitasking**. Research has consistently shown that multitasking will make your studying dramatically less effective. Your study area should also be comfortable and well-lit so you don't have the distraction of straining your eyes or sitting on an uncomfortable chair.

The time of day you study is also important. You want to be rested and alert. Don't wait until just before bedtime. Study when you'll be most likely to comprehend and remember. Even better, if you know what time of day your test will be, set that time aside for study. That way your brain will be used to working on that subject at that specific time and you'll have a better chance of recalling information.

Finally, it can be helpful to team up with others who are studying for the same test. Your actual studying should be done in as isolated an environment as possible, but the work of organizing the information and setting up the study plan can be divided up. In between study sessions, you can discuss with your teammates the concepts that you're all studying and quiz each other on the details. Just be sure that your teammates are as serious about the test as you are. If you find that your study time is being replaced with social time, you might need to find a new team.

# Secret Key #2 – Make Your Studying Count

You're devoting a lot of time and effort to preparing for this test, so you want to be absolutely certain it will pay off. This means doing more than just reading the content and hoping you can remember it on test day. It's important to make every minute of study count. There are two main areas you can focus on to make your studying count:

## Retention

It doesn't matter how much time you study if you can't remember the material. You need to make sure you are retaining the concepts. To check your retention of the information you're learning, try recalling it at later times with minimal prompting. Try carrying around flashcards and glance at one or two from time to time or ask a friend who's also studying for the test to quiz you.

To enhance your retention, look for ways to put the information into practice so that you can apply it rather than simply recalling it. If you're using the information in practical ways, it will be much easier to remember. Similarly, it helps to solidify a concept in your mind if you're not only reading it to yourself but also explaining it to someone else. Ask a friend to let you teach them about a concept you're a little shaky on (or speak aloud to an imaginary audience if necessary). As you try to summarize, define, give examples, and answer your friend's questions, you'll understand the concepts better and they will stay with you longer. Finally, step back for a big picture view and ask yourself how each piece of information fits with the whole subject. When you link the different concepts together and see them working together as a whole, it's easier to remember the individual components.

Finally, practice showing your work on any multi-step problems, even if you're just studying. Writing out each step you take to solve a problem will help solidify the process in your mind, and you'll be more likely to remember it during the test.

## Modality

*Modality* simply refers to the means or method by which you study. Choosing a study modality that fits your own individual learning style is crucial. No two people learn best in exactly the same way, so it's important to know your strengths and use them to your advantage.

For example, if you learn best by visualization, focus on visualizing a concept in your mind and draw an image or a diagram. Try color-coding your notes, illustrating them, or creating symbols that will trigger your mind to recall a learned concept. If you learn best by hearing or discussing information, find a study partner who learns the same way or read aloud to yourself. Think about how to put the information in your own words. Imagine that you are giving a lecture on the topic and record yourself so you can listen to it later.

For any learning style, flashcards can be helpful. Organize the information so you can take advantage of spare moments to review. Underline key words or phrases. Use different colors for different categories. Mnemonic devices (such as creating a short list in which every item starts with the same letter) can also help with retention. Find what works best for you and use it to store the information in your mind most effectively and easily.

# Secret Key #3 – Practice the Right Way

Your success on test day depends not only on how many hours you put into preparing, but also on whether you prepared the right way. It's good to check along the way to see if your studying is paying off. One of the most effective ways to do this is by taking practice tests to evaluate your progress. Practice tests are useful because they show exactly where you need to improve. Every time you take a practice test, pay special attention to these three groups of questions:

- The questions you got wrong
- The questions you had to guess on, even if you guessed right
- The questions you found difficult or slow to work through

This will show you exactly what your weak areas are, and where you need to devote more study time. Ask yourself why each of these questions gave you trouble. Was it because you didn't understand the material? Was it because you didn't remember the vocabulary? Do you need more repetitions on this type of question to build speed and confidence? Dig into those questions and figure out how you can strengthen your weak areas as you go back to review the material.

Additionally, many practice tests have a section explaining the answer choices. It can be tempting to read the explanation and think that you now have a good understanding of the concept. However, an explanation likely only covers part of the question's broader context. Even if the explanation makes sense, **go back and investigate** every concept related to the question until you're positive you have a thorough understanding.

As you go along, keep in mind that the practice test is just that: practice. Memorizing these questions and answers will not be very helpful on the actual test because it is unlikely to have any of the same exact questions. If you only know the right answers to the sample questions, you won't be prepared for the real thing. **Study the concepts** until you understand them fully, and then you'll be able to answer any question that shows up on the test.

It's important to wait on the practice tests until you're ready. If you take a test on your first day of study, you may be overwhelmed by the amount of material covered and how much you need to learn. Work up to it gradually.

On test day, you'll need to be prepared for answering questions, managing your time, and using the test-taking strategies you've learned. It's a lot to balance, like a mental marathon that will have a big impact on your future. Like training for a marathon, you'll need to start slowly and work your way up. When test day arrives, you'll be ready.

Start with the strategies you've read in the first two Secret Keys—plan your course and study in the way that works best for you. If you have time, consider using multiple study resources to get different approaches to the same concepts. It can be helpful to see difficult concepts from more than one angle. Then find a good source for practice tests. Many times, the test website will suggest potential study resources or provide sample tests.

# Practice Test Strategy

When you're ready to start taking practice tests, follow this strategy:

## Untimed and Open-Book Practice

Take the first test with no time constraints and with your notes and study guide handy. Take your time and focus on applying the strategies you've learned.

## Timed and Open-Book Practice

Take the second practice test open-book as well, but set a timer and practice pacing yourself to finish in time.

## Timed and Closed-Book Practice

Take any other practice tests as if it were test day. Set a timer and put away your study materials. Sit at a table or desk in a quiet room, imagine yourself at the testing center, and answer questions as quickly and accurately as possible.

Keep repeating timed and closed-book tests on a regular basis until you run out of practice tests or it's time for the actual test. Your mind will be ready for the schedule and stress of test day, and you'll be able to focus on recalling the material you've learned.

# Secret Key #4 – Pace Yourself

Once you're fully prepared for the material on the test, your biggest challenge on test day will be managing your time. Just knowing that the clock is ticking can make you panic even if you have plenty of time left. Work on pacing yourself so you can build confidence against the time constraints of the exam. Pacing is a difficult skill to master, especially in a high-pressure environment, so **practice is vital**.

Set time expectations for your pace based on how much time is available. For example, if a section has 60 questions and the time limit is 30 minutes, you know you have to average 30 seconds or less per question in order to answer them all. Although 30 seconds is the hard limit, set 25 seconds per question as your goal, so you reserve extra time to spend on harder questions. When you budget extra time for the harder questions, you no longer have any reason to stress when those questions take longer to answer.

Don't let this time expectation distract you from working through the test at a calm, steady pace, but keep it in mind so you don't spend too much time on any one question. Recognize that taking extra time on one question you don't understand may keep you from answering two that you do understand later in the test. If your time limit for a question is up and you're still not sure of the answer, mark it and move on, and come back to it later if the time and the test format allow. If the testing format doesn't allow you to return to earlier questions, just make an educated guess; then put it out of your mind and move on.

On the easier questions, be careful not to rush. It may seem wise to hurry through them so you have more time for the challenging ones, but it's not worth missing one if you know the concept and just didn't take the time to read the question fully. Work efficiently but make sure you understand the question and have looked at all of the answer choices, since more than one may seem right at first.

Even if you're paying attention to the time, you may find yourself a little behind at some point. You should speed up to get back on track, but do so wisely. Don't panic; just take a few seconds less on each question until you're caught up. Don't guess without thinking, but do look through the answer choices and eliminate any you know are wrong. If you can get down to two choices, it is often worthwhile to guess from those. Once you've chosen an answer, move on and don't dwell on any that you skipped or had to hurry through. If a question was taking too long, chances are it was one of the harder ones, so you weren't as likely to get it right anyway.

On the other hand, if you find yourself getting ahead of schedule, it may be beneficial to slow down a little. The more quickly you work, the more likely you are to make a careless mistake that will affect your score. You've budgeted time for each question, so don't be afraid to spend that time. Practice an efficient but careful pace to get the most out of the time you have.

# Secret Key #5 – Have a Plan for Guessing

When you're taking the test, you may find yourself stuck on a question. Some of the answer choices seem better than others, but you don't see the one answer choice that is obviously correct. What do you do?

The scenario described above is very common, yet most test takers have not effectively prepared for it. Developing and practicing a plan for guessing may be one of the single most effective uses of your time as you get ready for the exam.

In developing your plan for guessing, there are three questions to address:

- When should you start the guessing process?
- How should you narrow down the choices?
- Which answer should you choose?

## When to Start the Guessing Process

Unless your plan for guessing is to select C every time (which, despite its merits, is not what we recommend), you need to leave yourself enough time to apply your answer elimination strategies. Since you have a limited amount of time for each question, that means that if you're going to give yourself the best shot at guessing correctly, you have to decide quickly whether or not you will guess.

Of course, the best-case scenario is that you don't have to guess at all, so first, see if you can answer the question based on your knowledge of the subject and basic reasoning skills. Focus on the key words in the question and try to jog your memory of related topics. Give yourself a chance to bring the knowledge to mind, but once you realize that you don't have (or you can't access) the knowledge you need to answer the question, it's time to start the guessing process.

It's almost always better to start the guessing process too early than too late. It only takes a few seconds to remember something and answer the question from knowledge. Carefully eliminating wrong answer choices takes longer. Plus, going through the process of eliminating answer choices can actually help jog your memory.

**Summary**: Start the guessing process as soon as you decide that you can't answer the question based on your knowledge.

# How to Narrow Down the Choices

The next chapter in this book (**Test-Taking Strategies**) includes a wide range of strategies for how to approach questions and how to look for answer choices to eliminate. You will definitely want to read those carefully, practice them, and figure out which ones work best for you. Here though, we're going to address a mindset rather than a particular strategy.

Your chances of guessing an answer correctly depend on how many options you are choosing from.

| How many choices you have | How likely you are to guess correctly |
| --- | --- |
| 5 | 20% |
| 4 | 25% |
| 3 | 33% |
| 2 | 50% |
| 1 | 100% |

You can see from this chart just how valuable it is to be able to eliminate incorrect answers and make an educated guess, but there are two things that many test takers do that cause them to miss out on the benefits of guessing:

- Accidentally eliminating the correct answer
- Selecting an answer based on an impression

We'll look at the first one here, and the second one in the next section.

To avoid accidentally eliminating the correct answer, we recommend a thought exercise called **the $5 challenge**. In this challenge, you only eliminate an answer choice from contention if you are willing to bet $5 on it being wrong. Why $5? Five dollars is a small but not insignificant amount of money. It's an amount you could afford to lose but wouldn't want to throw away. And while losing $5 once might not hurt too much, doing it twenty times will set you back $100. In the same way, each small decision you make—eliminating a choice here, guessing on a question there—won't by itself impact your score very much, but when you put them all together, they can make a big difference. By holding each answer choice elimination decision to a higher standard, you can reduce the risk of accidentally eliminating the correct answer.

The $5 challenge can also be applied in a positive sense: If you are willing to bet $5 that an answer choice *is* correct, go ahead and mark it as correct.

**Summary**: Only eliminate an answer choice if you are willing to bet $5 that it is wrong.

# Which Answer to Choose

You're taking the test. You've run into a hard question and decided you'll have to guess. You've eliminated all the answer choices you're willing to bet $5 on. Now you have to pick an answer. Why do we even need to talk about this? Why can't you just pick whichever one you feel like when the time comes?

The answer to these questions is that if you don't come into the test with a plan, you'll rely on your impression to select an answer choice, and if you do that, you risk falling into a trap. The test writers know that everyone who takes their test will be guessing on some of the questions, so they intentionally write wrong answer choices to seem plausible. You still have to pick an answer though, and if the wrong answer choices are designed to look right, how can you ever be sure that you're not falling for their trap? The best solution we've found to this dilemma is to take the decision out of your hands entirely. Here is the process we recommend:

**Once you've eliminated any choices that you are confident (willing to bet $5) are wrong, select the first remaining choice as your answer.**

Whether you choose to select the first remaining choice, the second, or the last, the important thing is that you use some preselected standard. Using this approach guarantees that you will not be enticed into selecting an answer choice that looks right, because you are not basing your decision on how the answer choices look.

This is not meant to make you question your knowledge. Instead, it is to help you recognize the difference between your knowledge and your impressions. There's a huge difference between thinking an answer is right because of what you know, and thinking an answer is right because it looks or sounds like it should be right.

**Summary**: To ensure that your selection is appropriately random, make a predetermined selection from among all answer choices you have not eliminated.

# Test-Taking Strategies

This section contains a list of test-taking strategies that you may find helpful as you work through the test. By taking what you know and applying logical thought, you can maximize your chances of answering any question correctly!

It is very important to realize that every question is different and every person is different: no single strategy will work on every question, and no single strategy will work for every person. That's why we've included all of them here, so you can try them out and determine which ones work best for different types of questions and which ones work best for you.

## Question Strategies

### READ CAREFULLY

Read the question and answer choices carefully. Don't miss the question because you misread the terms. You have plenty of time to read each question thoroughly and make sure you understand what is being asked. Yet a happy medium must be attained, so don't waste too much time. You must read carefully, but efficiently.

### CONTEXTUAL CLUES

Look for contextual clues. If the question includes a word you are not familiar with, look at the immediate context for some indication of what the word might mean. Contextual clues can often give you all the information you need to decipher the meaning of an unfamiliar word. Even if you can't determine the meaning, you may be able to narrow down the possibilities enough to make a solid guess at the answer to the question.

### PREFIXES

If you're having trouble with a word in the question or answer choices, try dissecting it. Take advantage of every clue that the word might include. Prefixes and suffixes can be a huge help. Usually they allow you to determine a basic meaning. Pre- means before, post- means after, pro - is positive, de- is negative. From prefixes and suffixes, you can get an idea of the general meaning of the word and try to put it into context.

### HEDGE WORDS

Watch out for critical hedge words, such as *likely, may, can, sometimes, often, almost, mostly, usually, generally, rarely*, and *sometimes*. Question writers insert these hedge phrases to cover every possibility. Often an answer choice will be wrong simply because it leaves no room for exception. Be on guard for answer choices that have definitive words such as *exactly* and *always*.

### SWITCHBACK WORDS

Stay alert for *switchbacks*. These are the words and phrases frequently used to alert you to shifts in thought. The most common switchback words are *but, although*, and *however*. Others include *nevertheless, on the other hand, even though, while, in spite of, despite, regardless of*. Switchback words are important to catch because they can change the direction of the question or an answer choice.

## FACE VALUE

When in doubt, use common sense. Accept the situation in the problem at face value. Don't read too much into it. These problems will not require you to make wild assumptions. If you have to go beyond creativity and warp time or space in order to have an answer choice fit the question, then you should move on and consider the other answer choices. These are normal problems rooted in reality. The applicable relationship or explanation may not be readily apparent, but it is there for you to figure out. Use your common sense to interpret anything that isn't clear.

# Answer Choice Strategies

## ANSWER SELECTION

The most thorough way to pick an answer choice is to identify and eliminate wrong answers until only one is left, then confirm it is the correct answer. Sometimes an answer choice may immediately seem right, but be careful. The test writers will usually put more than one reasonable answer choice on each question, so take a second to read all of them and make sure that the other choices are not equally obvious. As long as you have time left, it is better to read every answer choice than to pick the first one that looks right without checking the others.

## ANSWER CHOICE FAMILIES

An answer choice family consists of two (in rare cases, three) answer choices that are very similar in construction and cannot all be true at the same time. If you see two answer choices that are direct opposites or parallels, one of them is usually the correct answer. For instance, if one answer choice says that quantity $x$ increases and another either says that quantity $x$ decreases (opposite) or says that quantity $y$ increases (parallel), then those answer choices would fall into the same family. An answer choice that doesn't match the construction of the answer choice family is more likely to be incorrect. Most questions will not have answer choice families, but when they do appear, you should be prepared to recognize them.

## ELIMINATE ANSWERS

Eliminate answer choices as soon as you realize they are wrong, but make sure you consider all possibilities. If you are eliminating answer choices and realize that the last one you are left with is also wrong, don't panic. Start over and consider each choice again. There may be something you missed the first time that you will realize on the second pass.

## AVOID FACT TRAPS

Don't be distracted by an answer choice that is factually true but doesn't answer the question. You are looking for the choice that answers the question. Stay focused on what the question is asking for so you don't accidentally pick an answer that is true but incorrect. Always go back to the question and make sure the answer choice you've selected actually answers the question and is not merely a true statement.

## EXTREME STATEMENTS

In general, you should avoid answers that put forth extreme actions as standard practice or proclaim controversial ideas as established fact. An answer choice that states the "process should be used in certain situations, if..." is much more likely to be correct than one that states the "process should be discontinued completely." The first is a calm rational statement and doesn't even make a definitive, uncompromising stance, using a hedge word *if* to provide wiggle room, whereas the second choice is a radical idea and far more extreme.

## BENCHMARK

As you read through the answer choices and you come across one that seems to answer the question well, mentally select that answer choice. This is not your final answer, but it's the one that will help you evaluate the other answer choices. The one that you selected is your benchmark or standard for judging each of the other answer choices. Every other answer choice must be compared to your benchmark. That choice is correct until proven otherwise by another answer choice beating it. If you find a better answer, then that one becomes your new benchmark. Once you've decided that no other choice answers the question as well as your benchmark, you have your final answer.

## PREDICT THE ANSWER

Before you even start looking at the answer choices, it is often best to try to predict the answer. When you come up with the answer on your own, it is easier to avoid distractions and traps because you will know exactly what to look for. The right answer choice is unlikely to be word-for-word what you came up with, but it should be a close match. Even if you are confident that you have the right answer, you should still take the time to read each option before moving on.

# General Strategies

## TOUGH QUESTIONS

If you are stumped on a problem or it appears too hard or too difficult, don't waste time. Move on! Remember though, if you can quickly check for obviously incorrect answer choices, your chances of guessing correctly are greatly improved. Before you completely give up, at least try to knock out a couple of possible answers. Eliminate what you can and then guess at the remaining answer choices before moving on.

## CHECK YOUR WORK

Since you will probably not know every term listed and the answer to every question, it is important that you get credit for the ones that you do know. Don't miss any questions through careless mistakes. If at all possible, try to take a second to look back over your answer selection and make sure you've selected the correct answer choice and haven't made a costly careless mistake (such as marking an answer choice that you didn't mean to mark). This quick double check should more than pay for itself in caught mistakes for the time it costs.

## PACE YOURSELF

It's easy to be overwhelmed when you're looking at a page full of questions; your mind is confused and full of random thoughts, and the clock is ticking down faster than you would like. Calm down and maintain the pace that you have set for yourself. Especially as you get down to the last few minutes of the test, don't let the small numbers on the clock make you panic. As long as you are on track by monitoring your pace, you are guaranteed to have time for each question.

## DON'T RUSH

It is very easy to make errors when you are in a hurry. Maintaining a fast pace in answering questions is pointless if it makes you miss questions that you would have gotten right otherwise. Test writers like to include distracting information and wrong answers that seem right. Taking a little extra time to avoid careless mistakes can make all the difference in your test score. Find a pace that allows you to be confident in the answers that you select.

## KEEP MOVING

Panicking will not help you pass the test, so do your best to stay calm and keep moving. Taking deep breaths and going through the answer elimination steps you practiced can help to break through a stress barrier and keep your pace.

# Final Notes

The combination of a solid foundation of content knowledge and the confidence that comes from practicing your plan for applying that knowledge is the key to maximizing your performance on test day. As your foundation of content knowledge is built up and strengthened, you'll find that the strategies included in this chapter become more and more effective in helping you quickly sift through the distractions and traps of the test to isolate the correct answer.

Now it's time to move on to the test content chapters of this book, but be sure to keep your goal in mind. As you read, think about how you will be able to apply this information on the test. If you've already seen sample questions for the test and you have an idea of the question format and style, try to come up with questions of your own that you can answer based on what you're reading. This will give you valuable practice applying your knowledge in the same ways you can expect to on test day.

**Good luck and good studying!**

# About the TEAS Test

*ATI TEAS Secrets* by Mometrix Test Preparation includes comprehensive review sections on each of the four TEAS test sections. Following those review sections are two complete TEAS practice tests, and a link to an additional **online interactive practice test**.

> **Online Interactive Practice Test**
> Visit mometrix.com/university/teas-bonus-practice-test

The TEAS is an important test, so it is essential that you adequately prepare for your test day. Be sure to set aside enough study time to be able to take each of the practice tests using only the amount of time that is specified. You are encouraged to minimize your external distractions in order to make the practice test conditions as similar to the real test conditions as possible.

Below is a breakdown of the four sections on the exam, including the subcategories, how many questions are in each section, and how much time will be allotted for you to complete that section. Each section of the test contains more questions for you to answer than will actually be scored. Those extra questions are being evaluated by the test makers for future use.

| Content Areas | Time | Test Items | % of Test | Scored Items |
|---|---|---|---|---|
| **Reading** | **64 min** | **53** | **31%** | **47** |
| Key Ideas and Details | | | | 22 |
| Craft and Structure | | | | 14 |
| Integration of Knowledge and Ideas | | | | 11 |
| **Mathematics** | **54 min** | **36** | **21%** | **32** |
| Number and Algebra | | | | 23 |
| Measurement and Data | | | | 9 |
| **Science** | **63 min** | **53** | **31%** | **47** |
| Human Anatomy and Physiology | | | | 32 |
| Life and Physical Sciences | | | | 8 |
| Scientific Reasoning | | | | 7 |
| **English and Language Usage** | **28 min** | **28** | **17%** | **24** |
| Conventions of Standard English | | | | 9 |
| Knowledge of Language | | | | 9 |
| Vocabulary Acquisition | | | | 6 |
| **Total** | **209 min** | **170** | | **150** |

# Reading

## Key Ideas and Details

### SUMMARIZING A COMPLEX TEXT

#### SUMMARIZE

A helpful tool is the ability to **summarize** the information that you have read in a paragraph or passage format. This process is similar to creating an effective outline. First, a summary should accurately define the **main idea** of the passage though the summary does not need to explain this main idea in exhaustive detail. The summary should continue by laying out the most important **supporting details** or arguments from the passage. All of the significant supporting details should be included, and none of the details included should be irrelevant or insignificant. Also, the summary should accurately report all of these details. Too often, the desire for brevity in a summary leads to the sacrifice of clarity or accuracy. Summaries are often difficult to read because they omit all of the graceful language, digressions, and asides that distinguish great writing. However, an effective summary should contain much the same message as the original text.

#### PARAPHRASE

Paraphrasing is another method that the reader can use to aid in comprehension. When paraphrasing, one puts what they have read into their words by **rephrasing** what the author has written, or one "translates" all of what the author shared into their words by including as many details as they can.

> **Review Video: Summarizing Text**
> Visit mometrix.com/academy and enter code: 172903

### IDENTIFYING THE LOGICAL CONCLUSION

Identifying a logical conclusion can help you determine whether you agree with the writer or not. Coming to this conclusion is much like making an inference: the approach requires you to combine the information given by the text with what you already know in order to make a **logical conclusion**. If the author intended the reader to draw a certain conclusion, then you can expect the author's argumentation and detail to be leading in that direction. One way to approach the task of drawing conclusions is to make brief **notes** of all the points made by the author. When the notes are arranged on paper, they may clarify the logical conclusion. Another way to approach conclusions is to consider whether the reasoning of the author raises any **pertinent questions**. Sometimes you will be able to draw several conclusions from a passage. On occasion these will be conclusions that were never imagined by the author. Therefore, be aware that these conclusions must be **supported** directly by the text.

### DIRECTLY STATED INFORMATION

A reader should always be drawing conclusions from the text. Sometimes conclusions are implied from written information, and other times the information is **stated directly** within the passage. One should always aim to draw **conclusions** from information stated within a passage, rather than to draw them from mere implications. At times an author may provide some information and then describe a **counterargument**. Readers should be alert for direct statements that are subsequently rejected or weakened by the author. Furthermore, you should always read through the **entire passage** before drawing conclusions. Many readers are trained to expect the author's conclusions at either the beginning or the end of the passage, but many texts do not adhere to this format.

*INFERENCES*

Readers are often required to understand a text that claims and suggests ideas without stating them directly. An **inference** is a piece of information that is implied but not written outright by the author. For instance, consider the following sentence: *After the final out of the inning, the fans were filled with joy and rushed the field.* From this sentence, a reader can infer that the fans were watching a baseball game and their team won the game. Readers should take great care to avoid using information **beyond the provided passage** before making inferences. As you practice drawing inferences, you will find that they require concentration and attention.

> **Review Video: Inference**
> Visit mometrix.com/academy and enter code: 379203

***Test-taking tip***: While being tested on your ability to make correct inferences, you must look for **contextual clues**. An answer can be *true* but not *correct*. The contextual clues will help you find the answer that is the **best answer** out of the given choices. Be careful in your reading to understand the context in which a phrase is stated. When asked for the implied meaning of a statement made in the passage, you should immediately locate the statement and read the **context** in which the statement was made. Also, look for an answer choice that has a similar phrase to the statement in question.

*IMPLICATIONS*

**Drawing conclusions** from information implied within a passage requires confidence on the part of the reader. **Implications** are things that the author does not state directly, but readers can assume based on what the author does say. Consider the following passage: *I stepped outside and opened my umbrella. By the time I got to work, the cuffs of my pants were soaked.* The author never states that it is raining, but this fact is clearly implied. Conclusions based on implication must be well supported by the text. In order to draw a solid conclusion, readers should have multiple pieces of **evidence**. If readers have only one piece, they must be assured that there is no other possible explanation than their conclusion. A good reader will be able to draw many conclusions from information implied by the text which will be a great help in the exam.

## TOPICS, MAIN IDEAS, AND SUPPORTING DETAILS
### TOPICS AND MAIN IDEAS

One of the most important skills in reading comprehension is the identification of **topics** and **main ideas.** There is a subtle difference between these two features. The topic is the **subject** of a text (i.e., what the text is all about). The main idea, on the other hand, is the **most important point** being made by the author. The topic is usually expressed in a few words at the most while the main idea often needs a full sentence to be completely defined. As an example, a short passage might have the topic of penguins and the main idea could be written as *Penguins are different from other birds in many ways.* In most nonfiction writing, the topic and the main idea will be stated directly and often appear in a sentence at the very beginning or end of the text. When being tested on an understanding of the author's topic, you may be able to skim the passage for the general idea, by reading only the first sentence of each paragraph. A body paragraph's first sentence is often—but not always—the main topic sentence which gives you a summary of the content in the paragraph.

However, there are cases in which the reader must figure out an **unstated** topic or main idea. In these instances, you must read every sentence of the text and try to come up with an overarching idea that is supported by each of those sentences.

> **Review Video: Topics and Main Ideas**
> Visit mometrix.com/academy and enter code: 407801

### SUPPORTING DETAILS

Supporting details provide **evidence** and backing for the main point. In order to show that a main idea is correct, or valid, authors add details that prove their point. All texts contain details, but they are only classified as **supporting details** when they serve to reinforce some larger point. Supporting details are most commonly found in **informative** and **persuasive** texts. In some cases, they will be clearly indicated with terms like *for example* or *for instance*, or they will be enumerated with terms like *first*, *second*, and *last*. However, you need to be prepared for texts that do not contain those indicators. As a reader, you should consider whether the author's supporting details really back up his or her **main point**. Supporting details can be factual and correct, yet they may not be relevant to the author's point. Conversely, supporting details can seem pertinent, but they can be ineffective because they are based on opinion or assertions that cannot be proven.

> **Review Video: Supporting Details**
> Visit mometrix.com/academy and enter code: 396297

### TOPIC AND SUMMARY SENTENCES

Topic and summary sentences are a convenient way to encapsulate the **main idea** of a text. In some textbooks and academic articles, the author will place a **topic** or **summary sentence** at the beginning of each section as a means of preparing the reader for what is to come. Research suggests that the brain is more receptive to new information when it has been prepared by the presentation of the main idea or some key words. The phenomenon is somewhat akin to the primer coat of paint that allows subsequent coats of paint to absorb more easily. A good topic sentence will be **clear** and not contain any **jargon**. When topic or summary sentences are not provided, good readers can jot down their own so that they can find their place in a text and refresh their memory.

### FOLLOWING DIRECTIONS

Technical passages often require the reader to **follow a set of directions**. For many people, especially those who are tactile or visual learners, this can be a difficult process. It is important to approach a set of directions differently than other texts. First, it is a good idea to **scan** the directions to determine whether special equipment or preparations are needed. Sometimes in a recipe, for instance, the author fails to mention that the oven should be preheated first, and then halfway through the process, the cook is supposed to be baking. After briefly reading the directions, the reader should return to the first step. When following directions, it is appropriate to **complete each step** before moving on to the next. If this is not possible, it is useful at least to visualize each step before reading the next.

### INFORMATION FROM PRINTED COMMUNICATION

#### MEMO

A memo (short for *memorandum*) is a common form of written communication. There is a standard format for these documents. It is typical for there to be a **heading** at the top indicating the author, date, and recipient. In some cases, this heading will also include the author's title and the name of his or her institution. Below this information will be the **body** of the memo. These documents are typically written by and for members of the same organization. They usually contain a plan of action, a request for information on a specific topic, or a response to such a request. Memos are considered to be official documents, and so are usually written in a **formal** style. Many memos are organized with numbers or bullet points, which make it easier for the reader to identify key ideas.

## POSTED ANNOUNCEMENT

People post **announcements** for all sorts of occasions. Many people are familiar with notices for lost pets, yard sales, and landscaping services. In order to be effective, these announcements need to *contain all of the information* the reader requires to act on the message. For instance, a lost pet announcement needs to include a good description of the animal and a contact number for the owner. A yard sale notice should include the address, date, and hours of the sale, as well as a brief description of the products that will be available there. When composing an announcement, it is important to consider the perspective of the **audience**—what will they need to know in order to respond to the message? Although a posted announcement can have color and decoration to attract the eye of the passerby, it must also convey the necessary information clearly.

## CLASSIFIED ADVERTISEMENT

Classified advertisements, or **ads**, are used to sell or buy goods, to attract business, to make romantic connections, and to do countless other things. They are an inexpensive, and sometimes free, way to make a brief **pitch**. Classified ads used to be found only in newspapers or special advertising circulars, but there are now online listings as well. The style of these ads has remained basically the same. An ad usually begins with a word or phrase indicating what is being **sold** or **sought**. Then, the listing will give a brief **description** of the product or service. Because space is limited and costly in newspapers, classified ads there will often contain abbreviations for common attributes. For instance, two common abbreviations are *bk* for *black*, and *obo* for *or best offer*. Classified ads will then usually conclude by listing the **price** (or the amount the seeker is willing to pay), followed by **contact information** like a telephone number or email address.

## SCALE READINGS OF STANDARD MEASUREMENT INSTRUMENTS

The scales used on **standard measurement instruments** are fairly easy to read with a little practice. Take the **ruler** as an example. A typical ruler has different units along each long edge. One side measures inches, and the other measures centimeters. The units are specified close to the zero reading for the ruler. Note that the ruler does not begin measuring from its outermost edge. The zero reading is a black line a tiny distance inside of the edge. On the inches side, each inch is indicated with a long black line and a number. Each half-inch is noted with a slightly shorter line. Quarter-inches are noted with still shorter lines, eighth-inches are noted with even shorter lines, and sixteenth-inches are noted with the shortest lines of all. On the centimeter side, the second-largest black lines indicate half-centimeters, and the smaller lines indicate tenths of centimeters, otherwise known as millimeters.

## LEGEND OR KEY OF A MAP

Almost all maps contain a **key**, or **legend**, that defines the **symbols** used on the map for various landmarks. This key is usually placed in a corner of the map. It should contain listings for all of the important symbols on the map. Of course, these symbols will vary depending on the nature of the map. A road map uses different colored lines to indicate roads, highways, and interstates. A legend might also show different dots and squares that are used to indicate towns of various sizes. The legend may contain information about the map's **scale**, though this may be elsewhere on the map. Many legends will contain special symbols, such as a picnic table indicating a campground.

## EVENTS IN A SEQUENCE

Readers must be able to identify a text's **sequence**, or the order in which things happen. Often, when the sequence is very important to the author, the text is indicated with signal words like *first*, *then*, *next*, and *last*. However, a sequence can be merely implied and must be noted by the reader. Consider the sentence: *He walked through the garden and gave water and fertilizer to the plants*. Clearly, the man did not walk through the garden before he collected water and fertilizer for the plants. So, the implied sequence is that he first collected water, then he collected fertilizer, next he walked through the garden, and last he gave water or fertilizer as necessary to the plants. Texts do not always proceed in an **orderly** sequence from first to last. Sometimes they begin at the end and start over at the beginning. As a reader, you can enhance your understanding of the passage by taking brief **notes** to clarify the sequence.

> **Review Video: Sequence**
> Visit mometrix.com/academy and enter code: 489027

# Craft and Structure

## FACT AND OPINION

Readers must always be conscious of the distinction between **fact** and **opinion**. A fact can be subjected to analysis and can be either **proved or disproved**. An opinion, on the other hand, is the author's **personal thoughts or feelings** which may not be alterable by research or evidence. If the author writes that the distance from New York to Boston is about two hundred miles, then he or she is stating a fact. If the author writes that New York is too crowded, then he or she is giving an opinion because there is no objective standard for overpopulation.

An opinion may be indicated by words like *believe*, *think*, or *feel*. Readers must be aware that an **opinion** may be supported by **facts**. For instance, the author might give the population density of New York as evidence of an overcrowded population. An opinion supported by fact tends to be more convincing. On the other hand, when authors support their opinions with other opinions, readers should not be persuaded by the argument to any degree.

> **Review Video: How to Tell the Difference Between Facts and Opinions**
> Visit mometrix.com/academy and enter code: 717670

## BIASES AND STEREOTYPES

Every author has a point-of-view, but authors demonstrate a **bias** when they ignore reasonable counterarguments or distort opposing viewpoints. A bias is evident whenever the author is **unfair** or **inaccurate** in his or her presentation. Bias may be intentional or unintentional, and readers should be skeptical of the author's argument. Remember that a biased author may still be correct; however, the author will be correct in spite of his or her bias, not because of the bias. A **stereotype** is like a bias, yet a stereotype is applied specifically to a **group** or **place**. Stereotyping is considered to be particularly abhorrent because the practice promotes negative generalizations about people. Readers should be very cautious of authors who stereotype in their writing. These faulty assumptions typically reveal the author's ignorance and lack of curiosity.

> **Review Video: Bias and Stereotype**
> Visit mometrix.com/academy and enter code: 644829

## STRUCTURE OF TEXTS

### PROBLEM-SOLUTION TEXT STRUCTURE

Some nonfiction texts are organized to present a **problem** followed by a **solution**. For this type of text, the problem is often explained before the solution is offered. In some cases, as when the problem is well known, the solution may be introduced briefly at the beginning. Other passages may focus on the solution, and the problem will be referenced only occasionally. Some texts will outline *multiple solutions* to a problem, leaving readers to choose among them. If the author has an interest or an allegiance to one solution, he or she may fail to mention or describe accurately some of the other solutions. Readers should be careful of the author's **agenda** when reading a problem-solution text. Only by understanding the author's perspective and interests can one develop a proper judgment of the proposed solution.

### DESCRIPTIVE TEXT

In a sense, almost all writing is descriptive, insofar as an author seeks to describe events, ideas, or people to the reader. Some texts, however, are primarily concerned with **description**. A descriptive text focuses on a particular subject and attempts to depict the subject in a way that will be clear to readers. Descriptive texts contain many adjectives and adverbs (i.e., words that give shades of meaning and create a more detailed mental picture for the reader). A descriptive text fails when it is unclear to the reader. A descriptive text will certainly be informative and may be persuasive and entertaining as well.

> **Review Video: Descriptive Texts**
> Visit mometrix.com/academy and enter code: 174903

### COMPARISON AND CONTRAST

Authors will use different stylistic and writing devices to make their meaning clear for readers. One of those devices is **comparison and contrast**. As mentioned previously, when an author describes the ways in which two things are **alike**, he or she is comparing them. When the author describes the ways in which two things are **different**, he or she is contrasting them. The "compare and contrast" essay is one of the most common forms in nonfiction. These passages are often signaled with certain words: a comparison may have indicating terms such as *both*, *same*, *like*, *too*, and *as well*; while a contrast may have terms like *but*, *however*, *on the other hand*, *instead*, and *yet*. Of course, comparisons and contrasts may be implicit without using any such signaling language. A single sentence may both compare and contrast. Consider the sentence *Brian and Sheila love ice cream, but Brian prefers vanilla and Sheila prefers strawberry*. In one sentence, the author has described both a similarity (love of ice cream) and a difference (favorite flavor).

> **Review Video: Compare and Contrast**
> Visit mometrix.com/academy and enter code: 171799

### CAUSE AND EFFECT

One of the most common text structures is **cause and effect**. A cause is an **act** or **event** that makes something happen, and an effect is the thing that happens as a **result** of the cause. A cause-and-effect relationship is not always explicit, but there are some terms in English that signal causes, such as *since*, *because*, and *due to*. Furthermore, terms that signal effects include *consequently, therefore, this lead(s) to*. As an example, consider this sentence: *Because the sky was clear, Ron did not bring an umbrella*. The cause is the clear sky, and the effect is that Ron did not bring an umbrella. However, readers may find that sometimes the cause-and-effect relationship will not be clearly noted. For instance, the sentence *He was late and missed the meeting* does not contain any signaling words, but the sentence still contains a cause (he was late) and an effect (he missed the meeting).

> **Review Video: Rhetorical Strategy of Cause-and-Effect Analysis**
> Visit mometrix.com/academy and enter code: 725944

### TYPES OF PASSAGES
#### NARRATIVE PASSAGE

A **narrative** passage is a story that can be fiction or nonfiction. However, there are a few elements that a text must have in order to be classified as a narrative. First, the text must have a **plot** (i.e., a series of events). Narratives often proceed in a clear sequence, but this is not a requirement. If the narrative is good, then these events will be interesting to readers. Second, a narrative has **characters**. These characters could be people, animals, or even inanimate objects—so long as they participate in the plot. Third, a narrative passage often contains **figurative language** which is meant to stimulate the imagination of readers by making comparisons and observations. For instance, a *metaphor*, a common piece of figurative language, is a description of one thing in terms of another. *The moon was a frosty snowball* is an example of a metaphor. In the literal sense this is obviously untrue, but the comparison suggests a certain mood for the reader.

## EXPOSITORY PASSAGE

An **expository** passage aims to **inform** and enlighten readers. The passage is nonfiction and usually centers around a simple, easily defined topic. Since the goal of exposition is to teach, such a passage should be as clear as possible. Often, an expository passage contains helpful organizing words, like *first*, *next*, *for example*, and *therefore*. These words keep the reader **oriented** in the text. Although expository passages do not need to feature colorful language and artful writing, they are often more effective with these features. For a reader, the challenge of expository passages is to maintain steady attention. Expository passages are not always about subjects that will naturally interest a reader, so the writer is often more concerned with **clarity** and **comprehensibility** than with engaging the reader. By reading actively, you will ensure a good habit of focus when reading an expository passage.

> **Review Video: Expository Passages**
> Visit mometrix.com/academy and enter code: 256515

## TECHNICAL PASSAGE

A **technical** passage is written to *describe* a complex object or process. Technical writing is common in medical and technological fields, in which complex ideas of mathematics, science, and engineering need to be explained *simply* and *clearly*. To ease comprehension, a technical passage usually proceeds in a very logical order. Technical passages often have clear headings and subheadings, which are used to keep the reader oriented in the text. Additionally, you will find that these passages divide sections up with numbers or letters. Many technical passages look more like an outline than a piece of prose. The amount of **jargon** or difficult vocabulary will vary in a technical passage depending on the intended audience. As much as possible, technical passages try to avoid language that the reader will have to research in order to understand the message, yet readers will find that jargon cannot always be avoided.

> **Review Video: A Technical Passage**
> Visit mometrix.com/academy and enter code: 478923

## PERSUASIVE PASSAGE

A **persuasive** passage is meant to change the mind of readers and lead them into **agreement** with the author. The persuasive intent may be very obvious or quite difficult to discern. In some cases, a persuasive passage will be indistinguishable from one that is informative. Both passages make an assertion and offer supporting details. However, a persuasive passage is more likely to appeal to the reader's **emotions** and to make claims based on **opinion**. Persuasive passages may not describe alternate positions, but when they do, they often display significant **bias**. Readers may find that a persuasive passage is giving the author's viewpoint, or the passage may adopt a seemingly objective tone. A persuasive passage is successful if it can make a convincing argument and win the trust of the reader.

> **Review Video: Persuasive Essay**
> Visit mometrix.com/academy and enter code: 621428

## WORD MEANING FROM CONTEXT

One of the benefits of reading is the expansion of one's vocabulary. In order to obtain this benefit, however, one needs to know how to identify the definition of a **word from its context**. This means defining a word based on the **words around it** and the way it is **used in a sentence**. Consider the following sentence: *The elderly scholar spent his evenings hunched over arcane texts that few other people even knew existed.* The adjective *arcane* is uncommon, but you can obtain significant information about it based on its use in the sentence. The fact that few other people know of their existence allows you to assume that "arcane texts" must be rare and be of interest to few people. Also, the texts are being read by an elderly scholar. So, you can assume that they focus on difficult academic subjects. Sometimes, words can be defined by **what they are not**. Consider the following sentence: *Ron's fealty to his parents was not shared by Karen, who disobeyed their every command.* Someone who disobeys is not demonstrating *fealty*. So, you can infer that the word means something like *obedience* or *respect*.

## FIGURATIVE LANGUAGE

There are many types of language devices that authors use to convey their meaning in a descriptive way. Understanding these concepts will help you understand what you read. These types of devices are called **figurative language** – language that goes beyond the literal meaning of a word or phrase. **Descriptive language** that evokes imagery in the reader's mind is one type of figurative language. **Exaggeration** is another type of figurative language. Also, when you compare two things, you are using figurative language. **Similes** and **metaphors** are ways of comparing things, and both are types of figurative language commonly found in poetry. An example of figurative language (a simile in this case): *The child howled like a coyote when her mother told her to pick up the toys.* In this example, the child's howling is compared to that of a coyote and helps the reader understand the sound being made by the child.

> **Review Video: Figurative Language**
> Visit mometrix.com/academy and enter code: 584902

## METAPHOR

A **metaphor** is a type of figurative language in which the writer equates one thing with a different thing. For instance: *The bird was an arrow arcing through the sky.* In this sentence, the arrow is serving as a metaphor for the bird. The point of a metaphor is to encourage the reader to consider the item being described in a *different way*. Let's continue with this metaphor for a bird: you are asked to envision the bird's flight as being similar to the arc of an arrow. So, you imagine the flight to be swift and bending. Metaphors are a way for the author to describe an item *without being direct and obvious*. This literary device is a lyrical and suggestive way of providing information. Note that the reference for a metaphor will not always be mentioned explicitly by the author. Consider the following description of a forest in winter: *Swaying skeletons reached for the sky and groaned as the wind blew through them.* In this example, the author is using *skeletons* as a metaphor for leafless trees. This metaphor creates a spooky tone while inspiring the reader's imagination.

> **Review Video: Metaphor**
> Visit mometrix.com/academy and enter code: 133295

## SIMILE

A **simile** is a figurative expression that is similar to a metaphor, yet the expression requires the use of the distancing words *like* or *as*. Some examples: *The sun was like an orange*, *eager as a beaver*, and *nimble as a mountain goat*. Because a simile includes *like* or *as*, the device creates a space between the description and the thing being described. If an author says that *a house was like a shoebox*, then the tone is different than the author saying that the house *was* a shoebox. In a simile, authors explicitly indicate that the description is **not** the same thing as the thing being described. In a metaphor, there is no such distinction. The decision of which device to use will be made based on the authors' intended **tone**.

**Review Video: Simile**
Visit mometrix.com/academy and enter code: 642949

## PERSONIFICATION

Another type of figurative language is **personification**. This is the description of a nonhuman thing as if the item were **human**. Literally, the word means the process of making something into a person. The general intent of personification is to describe things in a manner that will be comprehensible to readers. When an author states that a tree *groans* in the wind, he or she does not mean that the tree is emitting a low, pained sound from a mouth. Instead, the author means that the tree is making a noise similar to a human groan. Of course, this personification establishes a tone of sadness or suffering. A different tone would be established if the author said that the tree was *swaying* or *dancing*.

**Review Video: Personification**
Visit mometrix.com/academy and enter code: 260066

## DENOTATIVE AND CONNOTATIVE MEANING OF WORDS

The **denotative** meaning of a word is the literal meaning of the word. The **connotative** meaning goes beyond the denotative meaning to include the **emotional reaction** that a word may invoke. The connotative meaning often takes the denotative meaning a step further due to associations which the reader makes with the denotative meaning. Readers can differentiate between the denotative and connotative meanings by first recognizing how authors use each meaning. Most nonfiction, for example, is fact-based and authors do not use flowery, figurative language. The reader can assume that the writer is using the denotative meaning of words. In fiction, the author may use the connotative meaning. Readers can determine whether the author is using the denotative or connotative meaning of a word by implementing **context clues**.

**Review Video: Denotation and Connotation**
Visit mometrix.com/academy and enter code: 310092

## DICTIONARY ENTRY

Dictionaries can be used to find a word's meaning, to check spelling, and to find out how to say or pronounce a word. **Dictionary entries** are in alphabetical order. **Guide words** are the two words at the top of each page. One word is the first word listed on the page and the other word is the last word listed on the page. Using these guide words will help you use dictionaries more effectively. You may notice that many words have more than one definition. These different definitions are numbered. Also, some words can be used as different **parts of speech**. The definitions for each part of speech are separated. A simple entry might look like this:

WELL: (adverb) 1. in a good way | (noun) 1. a hole drilled into the earth

The correct definition of a word depends on how the word is used in a sentence. To know that you are using the word correctly, you can try to replace the dictionary's definitions for the word in the passage. Then, choose the definition that seems to be the best fit.

## PURPOSE

Usually, identifying the **purpose** of an author is easier than identifying his or her position. In most cases, the author has no interest in hiding his or her purpose. A text that is meant to entertain, for instance, should be written to please the reader. Most narratives, or stories, are written to entertain, though they may also inform or persuade. Informative texts are easy to identify, while the most difficult purpose of a text to identify is persuasion because the author has an interest in making this purpose *hard to detect*. When a reader discovers that the author is trying to persuade, he or she should be skeptical of the argument. For this reason, persuasive texts often try to establish an entertaining tone and hope to amuse the reader into agreement. On the other hand, an informative tone may be implemented to create an appearance of authority and objectivity.

> **Review Video: Purpose**
> Visit mometrix.com/academy and enter code: 511819

An author's purpose is evident often in the **organization** of the text (e.g., section headings in bold font points to an informative text). However, you may not have such organization available to you in your exam. Instead, if the author makes his or her main idea clear from the beginning, then the likely purpose of the text is to **inform**. If the author begins by making a claim and provides various arguments to support that claim, then the purpose is probably to **persuade**. If the author tells a story or seems to want the attention of the reader more than to push a particular point or deliver information, then his or her purpose is most likely to **entertain**. As a reader, you must judge authors on how well they accomplish their purpose. In other words, you need to consider the type of passage (e.g., technical, persuasive, etc.) that the author has written and whether the author has followed the requirements of the passage type.

## PERSUASIVE WRITING

In a persuasive essay, the author is attempting to change the reader's mind or **convince** him or her of something that he or she did not believe previously. There are several identifying characteristics of **persuasive writing**. One is **opinion presented as fact**. When authors attempt to persuade readers, they often present their opinions as if they were fact. Readers must be on guard for statements that sound factual but which cannot be subjected to research, observation, or experiment. Another characteristic of persuasive writing is **emotional language**. An author will often try to play on the emotions of readers by appealing to their sympathy or sense of morality. When an author uses colorful or evocative language with the intent of arousing the reader's passions, then the author may be attempting to persuade. Finally, in many cases, a persuasive text will give an **unfair explanation of opposing positions**, if these positions are mentioned at all.

## INFORMATIVE TEXTS

An **informative text** is written to educate and enlighten readers. Informative texts are almost always nonfiction and are rarely structured as a story. The intention of an informative text is to deliver information in the most comprehensible way. So, look for the structure of the text to be very clear. In an informative text, the thesis statement is one or two sentences that normally appears at the end of the first paragraph. The author may use some colorful language, but he or she is likely to put more emphasis on clarity and precision. Informative essays do not typically appeal to the emotions. They often contain facts and figures and rarely include the opinion of the author; however, readers should remain aware of the possibility for a bias as those facts are presented. Sometimes a persuasive essay can resemble an informative essay, especially if the author maintains an even tone and presents his or her views as if they were established fact.

> **Review Video: Informative Text**
> Visit mometrix.com/academy and enter code: 924964

## ENTERTAINING TEXTS

The success or failure of an author's intent to **entertain** is determined by those who read the author's work. Entertaining texts may be either fiction or nonfiction, and they may describe real or imagined people, places, and events. Entertaining texts are often narratives or poems. A text that is written to entertain is likely to contain **colorful language** that engages the imagination and the emotions. Such writing often features a great deal of figurative language, which typically enlivens the subject matter with images and analogies.

Though an entertaining text is not usually written to persuade or inform, authors may accomplish both of these tasks in their work. An entertaining text may *appeal to the reader's emotions* and cause him or her to think differently about a particular subject. In any case, entertaining texts tend to showcase the personality of the author more than other types of writing.

## EXPRESSION OF FEELINGS

When an author intends to **express feelings,** he or she may use **expressive and bold language**. An author may write with emotion for any number of reasons. Sometimes, authors will express feelings because they are describing a personal situation of great pain or happiness. In other situations, authors will attempt to persuade the reader and will use emotion to stir up the passions. This kind of expression is easy to identify when the writer uses phrases like *I felt* and *I sense*. However, readers may find that the author will simply describe feelings without introducing them. As a reader, you must know the importance of recognizing when an author is expressing emotion and not to become overwhelmed by sympathy or passion. Readers should maintain some **detachment** so that they can still evaluate the strength of the author's argument or the quality of the writing.

> **Review Video: Emotional Language in Literature**
> Visit mometrix.com/academy and enter code: 759390

## IDENTIFYING AN AUTHOR'S POSITION

In order to be an effective reader, one must pay attention to the author's **position** and purpose. Even those texts that seem objective and impartial, like textbooks, have a position and **bias**. Readers need to take these positions into account when considering the author's message. When an author uses emotional language or clearly favors one side of an argument, his or her position is clear. However, the author's position may be evident not only in what he or she writes, but also in what he or she doesn't write. In a normal setting, a reader would want to review some other texts on the same topic in order to develop a view of the author's position. If this was not possible, then you would want to acquire some *background* about the author. However, since you are in the middle of an exam and the only source of information is the text, you should look for *language and argumentation that seems to indicate a particular stance* on the subject.

## TEXT FEATURES

### HEADINGS AND SUBHEADINGS

Many informative texts, especially textbooks, use **headings** and **subheadings** for organization. Headings and subheadings are printed in larger and bolder fonts than the rest of the text. Sometimes, they are in a different color than the main body of the book. Headings are often larger than subheadings. Also, headings and subheadings are not always complete sentences. A heading gives the **topic** that will be addressed in the paragraphs below. Headings are meant to alert you about what is coming next. Subheadings give the **topics of smaller sections**. For example, the heading of a section in a science textbook might be *AMPHIBIANS*. Within that section, you may have subheadings for *Frogs*, *Salamanders*, and *Newts*. Pay close attention to headings and subheadings. They make it easy to go back and find specific details in a book.

### FOOTNOTES AND ENDNOTES

Footnotes and endnotes can also be used in word processing programs. A **footnote** is text that is listed at the *bottom of a page* which lists where facts and figures within that document page were obtained. An **endnote** is similar to a footnote, but differs in the fact that it is listed at the *end of paragraphs and chapters* of a document, instead of the bottom of each page of the document.

### BOLD TEXT AND UNDERLINING

Authors will often incorporate text features like bold text and underlining to communicate meaning to the reader. When text is made **bold**, it is often because the author wants to emphasize the point that is being made. Bold text indicates **importance**. Also, many textbooks place key terms in bold. This not only draws the reader's attention, but also makes it easy to find these terms when reviewing before a test. **Underlining** serves a similar purpose. It is often used to suggest **emphasis**. However, underlining is also used on occasion beneath the **titles** of books, magazines, and works of art. This was more common when people used typewriters, which weren't able to create italics. Now that word processing software is nearly universal, italics are generally used for longer works.

### ITALICS

Italics, like bold text and underlines, are used to **emphasize** important words, phrases, and sentences in a text. However, italics have other uses as well. A word is placed in italics when it is being discussed as a word; that is, when it is being **defined** or its use in a sentence is being **described**. For instance, it is appropriate to use italics when saying that *esoteric* is an unusual adjective. Italics are also used for the titles of long or large works, like books, magazines, long operas, and epic poems. Shorter works are typically placed within **quotation marks**. A reader should note how an author uses italics, as this is a marker of style and tone. Some authors use them frequently, creating a tone of high emotion, while others are more restrained in their use, suggesting calm and reason.

### INDEX

Normally, a nonfiction book will have an **index** at the end. The index is for you to find information about specific topics. An index lists the topics in alphabetical order (i.e., a, b, c, d...). The names of people are listed by last name. For example, *Adams, John* would come before *Washington, George*. To the right of a topic, the page numbers are listed for that topic. When a topic is spread over several pages, the index will connect these pages with a dash. For example, if a topic is said to be on pages 35 to 42 and again on 53, the topic will be labeled as 35–42, 53. Some topics will have **subtopics**. These subtopics are listed below the main topic, indented slightly, and placed in alphabetical order. This is common for subjects that are covered over several pages in the book. For example, if you have a book about Elizabethan drama, William Shakespeare is likely an important topic. Beneath Shakespeare's name in the index, you may find listings for *death of, dramatic works of, life of*, etc. These specific sub-topics help you narrow your search.

### TABLE OF CONTENTS

Most books, magazines, and journals have a **table of contents** at the beginning. The table of contents lists the different **subjects** or **chapter titles** with a page number. This information allows you to find what you need with ease. Normally, the table of contents is found a page or two after the title page in a book or in the first few pages of a magazine. In a book, the table of contents will have the chapters listed on the left side. The page number for each chapter comes on the right side. Many books have a **preface** (i.e., a note that explains the background of the book) or introduction. The preface and introduction come with Roman numerals. The chapters are listed in order from the beginning to the end.

# Integration of Knowledge and Ideas

## PRIMARY SOURCES AND INTERNET SOURCES

### PRIMARY SOURCES

When conducting research, it is important to depend on reputable **primary sources**. A primary source is the **documentary evidence** closest to the subject being studied. For instance, the primary sources for an essay about penguins would be photographs and recordings of the birds, as well as accounts of people who have studied penguins in person. A **secondary source** would be a review of a movie about penguins or a book outlining the observations made by others. A primary source should be credible and, if it is on a subject that is still being explored, recent. One way to assess the credibility of a work is to see how often it is mentioned in other books and articles on the same subject. Just by reading the works cited and bibliographies of other books, one can get a sense of what the reliable sources authorities in the field are.

> **Review Video: Primary and Secondary Sources**
> Visit mometrix.com/academy and enter code: 383328

### INTERNET SOURCES

The Internet was once considered a poor place to find sources for an essay or article, but its credibility has improved greatly over the years. Still, students need to exercise caution when performing research online. The best sources are those affiliated with **established institutions**, such as *universities, public libraries, and think tanks*. Most newspapers are available online, and many of them allow the public to browse their archives. Magazines frequently offer similar services. When obtaining information from an unknown website, however, one must exercise considerably more caution. A website can be considered trustworthy if it is referenced by other sites that are known to be reputable. Also, credible sites tend to be properly maintained and frequently updated. A site is easier to trust when the author provides some information about himself, including some credentials that indicate expertise in the subject matter.

## MAKING PREDICTIONS AND DRAWING CONCLUSIONS

### PREDICTIONS

A prediction is a **guess** about what will happen next. Readers constantly make predictions based on what they have read and what they already know. Consider the following sentence: *Staring at the computer screen in shock, Kim blindly reached over for the brimming glass of water on the shelf to her side.* The sentence suggests that Kim is agitated, and that she is not looking at the glass that she is going to pick up. So, a reader might **predict** that Kim is going to knock over the glass. Of course, not every prediction will be accurate: perhaps Kim will pick the glass up cleanly. Nevertheless, the author has certainly created the expectation that the water might be spilled. Predictions are always subject to revision as the reader acquires more information.

> **Review Video: Predictions**
> Visit mometrix.com/academy and enter code: 437248

### FORESHADOWING

Foreshadowing uses hints in a narrative to let the audience **anticipate** future events in the plot. Foreshadowing can be indicated by a number of literary devices and figures of speech, as well as through dialogue between characters.

## DRAWING CONCLUSIONS

In addition to inference and prediction, readers must often **draw conclusions** about the information they have read. When asked for a *conclusion* that may be drawn, look for critical "hedge" phrases, such as *likely, may, can, will often,* among many others. When you are being tested on this knowledge, remember the question that writers insert into these hedge phrases to cover every possibility. Often an answer will be wrong simply because there is no room for exception. Extreme positive or negative answers (such as always or never) are usually not correct. The reader should not use any outside knowledge that is not gathered from the passage to answer the related questions. Correct answers can be derived *straight from the passage.*

## THEMES IN PRINT AND OTHER SOURCES

Themes are seldom expressed directly in a text and can be difficult to identify. A **theme** is *an issue, an idea, or a question raised by the text.* For instance, a theme of *Cinderella* (the Charles Perrault version) is perseverance as the title character serves her step-sisters and step-mother, and the prince seeks to find the girl with the missing slipper. A passage may have many themes, and you, as a dedicated reader, must take care to identify only themes that you are asked to find. One common characteristic of themes is that they raise more questions than they answer. In a good piece of fiction, authors are trying to elevate the reader's perspective and encourage him or her to consider the themes in a deeper way. In the process of reading, one can identify themes by constantly *asking about the general issues that the text is addressing.* A good way to evaluate an author's approach to a theme is to begin reading with a question in mind (e.g., How does this text approach the theme of love?) and to look for evidence in the text that addresses that question.

> **Review Video: Theme**
> Visit mometrix.com/academy and enter code: 732074

## SIMILAR THEMES ACROSS CULTURES

A brief study of world literature suggests that writers from vastly different cultures address **similar themes**. For instance, works like the *Odyssey* and *Hamlet* both consider the individual's battle for self-control and independence. In most cultures, authors address themes of *personal growth and the struggle for maturity.* Another universal theme is the *conflict between the individual and society.* Works that are as culturally disparate as *Native Son*, the *Aeneid*, and *1984* dramatize how people struggle to maintain their personalities and dignity in large (sometimes) oppressive groups. Finally, many cultures have versions of the *hero's or heroine's journey* in which an adventurous person must overcome many obstacles in order to gain greater knowledge, power, and perspective. Some famous works that treat this theme are the *Epic of Gilgamesh*, Dante's *Divine Comedy*, and Cervantes' *Don Quixote.*

## DIFFERENCES IN ADDRESSING THEMES IN VARIOUS CULTURES AND GENRES

Authors from different **genres** and **cultures** may address similar themes, but they do so in different ways. For instance, poets are likely to address subject matter indirectly through the use of *images and allusions.* In a play, the author is more likely to dramatize themes by using characters to express opposing viewpoints; this disparity is known as a *dialectical approach.* In a passage, the author does not need to express themes directly; indeed, they can be expressed through *events and actions.* In some regional literatures, such as Greece or England, authors tend to use more irony. In the 1950s, Latin American authors popularized the use of unusual and surreal events to show themes about real life in the genre of magical realism. Japanese authors use the well-established poetic form of the haiku to organize their treatment of common themes.

## EVALUATING AN ARGUMENT

Argumentative and persuasive passages take a **stand** on a debatable issue, seek to explore all sides of the issue, and find the best possible solution. Argumentative and persuasive passages should not be combative or abusive. The word *argument* may remind you of two or more people shouting at each other and walking away in anger. However, an argumentative or persuasive passage should be a *calm and reasonable presentation of an author's ideas* for others to consider. When an author writes reasonable arguments, his or her goal is not to win or have the last word. Instead, authors want to reveal current understanding of the question at hand and suggest a **solution** to a problem. The purpose of argument and persuasion in a free society is to reach the best solution.

### EVIDENCE

The term **text evidence** refers to information that supports a **main point** or **minor points** and can help lead the reader to a conclusion. Information used as text evidence is precise, descriptive, and factual. A main point is often followed by **supporting details** that provide evidence to back up a claim. For example, a passage may include the claim that winter occurs during opposite months in the Northern and Southern hemispheres. Text evidence based on this claim may include countries where winter occurs in opposite months along with reasons that winter occurs at different times of the year in separate hemispheres (due to the tilt of the Earth as it rotates around the sun).

> **Review Video: Text Evidence**
> Visit mometrix.com/academy and enter code: 486236

Evidence needs to be provided that supports the thesis and additional arguments. Most arguments must be supported by facts or statistics. A **fact** is something that is *known with certainty* and has been verified by several independent individuals. **Examples** and **illustrations** add an emotional component to arguments. With this component, you persuade readers in ways that facts and statistics cannot. The emotional component is effective when used with objective information that can be confirmed.

### CREDIBILITY

The text used to support an argument can be the argument's downfall if the text is not credible. A text is **credible**, or believable, when the author is knowledgeable and objective, or unbiased. The author's **motivations** for writing the text play a critical role in determining the credibility of the text and must be evaluated when assessing that credibility. Reports written about the ozone layer by an environmental scientist and a hairdresser will have different levels of credibility.

### APPEAL TO EMOTION

Sometimes, authors will **appeal to the reader's emotion** in an attempt to *persuade or to distract the reader from the weakness of the argument*. For instance, the author may try to inspire the **pity** of the reader by delivering a heart-rending story. An author also might use the **bandwagon** approach, in which he suggests that his opinion is correct because it is held by the majority. Some authors resort to **name-calling**, in which insults and harsh words are delivered to the opponent in an attempt to distract. In advertising, a common appeal is the **celebrity testimonial**, in which a famous person endorses a product. Of course, the fact that a famous person likes something should not really mean anything to the reader. These and other emotional appeals are usually evidence of poor reasoning and a weak argument.

## COUNTERARGUMENTS

When authors give both sides to the argument, they build trust with their readers. As a reader, you should start with an undecided or neutral position. If an author presents only his or her side to the argument, then you will need to be concerned at best.

Building common ground with neutral or opposed readers can be appealing to skeptical readers. Sharing values with undecided readers can allow people to switch positions without giving up what they feel is important. For people who may oppose a position, they need to feel that they can change their minds without betraying who they are as a person. This *appeal to having an open mind* can be a powerful tool in arguing a position without antagonizing other views. Objections can be countered on a point-by-point basis or in a summary paragraph. Be mindful of how an author points out flaws in **counterarguments**. If they are unfair to the other side of the argument, then you should lose trust with the author.

## DATA FROM DIFFERENT SOURCES AND IN DIFFERENT FORMATS

### JOURNAL ARTICLES

Although published journal articles listed in library databases have been reviewed and edited to be acceptable for publication, you should still evaluate them by six criteria.

1. **Source**: Articles by experts in their subjects, published in scholarly journals, are more *reliable*. They also contain *references* to more publications on the same topic. Try to start your search with a database that includes searching by article type (e.g., reviews, clinical trials, editorials, and research articles).
2. **Length**: The citation states an article's number of pages, an indication of its research utility.
3. **Authority**: Research sources should be authoritative, written by *experts* affiliated with academic institutions.
4. **Date**: Many research fields are constantly changing, so research must be as *current* as possible. In areas with new research breakthroughs, some articles are not up-to-date.
5. **Audience**: If an author wrote an article for professional colleagues, it will include subject-specific language and terminology.
6. **Usefulness**: Evaluate whether an article is *relevant* to one's own research topic.

> **Review Video: Media**
> Visit mometrix.com/academy and enter code: 785859

### LINE GRAPH

A line graph is a type of graph that is typically used for measuring trends over time. The graph is set up along a vertical and a horizontal **axis**. The variables being measured are listed along the left side and the bottom side of the axes. Points are then plotted along the graph as they correspond with their values for each variable. For instance, imagine a line graph measuring a person's income for each month of the year. If the person earned $1500 in January, there should be a point directly above January (perpendicular to the horizontal axis) and directly to the right of $1500 (perpendicular to the vertical axis). Once all of the lines are plotted, they are connected with a line from left to right. This line provides a nice visual illustration of the general **trends**. For instance, using the earlier example, if the line sloped up, then one would see that the person's income had increased over the course of the year.

### BAR GRAPH

The bar graph is one of the most common visual representations of information. **Bar graphs** are used to illustrate sets of numerical **data**. The graph has a vertical axis (along which numbers are listed) and a horizontal axis (along which categories, words, or some other indicators are placed).

One example of a bar graph is a depiction of the respective heights of famous basketball players: the vertical axis would contain numbers ranging from five to eight feet, and the horizontal axis would contain the names of the players. The length of the bar above the player's name would illustrate his height, and the top of the bar would stop perpendicular to the height listed along the left side. In this representation, one would see that Yao Ming is taller than Michael Jordan because Yao's bar would be higher.

## PIE CHART

A pie chart, also known as a circle graph, is useful for depicting how a single unit or category is divided. The standard pie chart is a circle with designated wedges. Each wedge is **proportional** in size to a part of the whole. For instance, consider a pie chart representing a student's budget. If the student spends half of his or her money on rent, then the pie chart will represent that amount with a line through the center of the pie. If she spends a quarter of her money on food, there will be a line extending from the edge of the circle to the center at a right angle to the line depicting rent. This illustration would make it clear that the student spends twice the amount of money on rent as she does on food.

A pie chart is effective at showing how a single entity is divided into parts. They are not effective at demonstrating the relationships between parts of different wholes. For example, an unhelpful use of a pie chart would be to compare the respective amounts of state and federal spending devoted to infrastructure since these values are only meaningful in the context of the entire budget.

## RESEARCH ASSISTANCE

Today's **library media specialists** are important figures in contemporary learning communities, which now consist of administrators, teachers, and parents; and international, national, state, regional, and local communities. Such communities transcend the borders of disciplinary field, occupation, age, time, and place. They are connected by shared needs, interests, and rapidly increasing technologies in telecommunications. Library media specialists and student-centered library media programs aim to aid students in attaining and improving their **information literacy**. As such, library media specialists and library media programs have the objective of helping every student to creatively and actively find, evaluate, and use information toward the ends of fulfilling their own curiosities and imaginations by pursuing reading and research activities and of exercising and developing their own critical thinking abilities.

## INFORMATION SPECIALIST

In fulfilling the function of an **information specialist**, library media specialists bring their skills for finding and evaluating information in a variety of formats as resources for learners and educators. They bring an awareness of various issues related to information to the attention of students, teachers, administrators, and other involved parties. Library media specialists also serve to model for students the **strategies** they can learn to find, access, and evaluate information inside and outside of the library media centers. The environment of the library media center has experienced a critical impact from the development of technology. Accordingly, the library media specialist not only attains mastery over current advanced electronic resources, but she or he must also continually sustain attention focused on how information—both in more traditional forms and in the newest technological forms—is used ethically, as well as its quality and its character.

## ORGANIZING AND SYNTHESIZING DATA

### ORGANIZING INFORMATION

Organizing information effectively is an important part of research. The data must be organized in a useful manner so that it can be effectively used. Three basic ways to organize information are:

1. **Spatial Organization** – This is useful as it lets the user "see" the information, to fix it in *space*. This has benefits for those individuals who are visually adept at processing information.
2. **Chronological Organization** – This is the most common presentation of information. This method places information in the *sequence* with which it occurs. Chronological organization is very useful in explaining a process that occurs in a step-by-step pattern.
3. **Logical Organization** – This includes presenting material in a logical *pattern* that makes intuitive sense. Some patterns that are frequently used are illustrated, definition, compare/contrast, cause/effect, problem/solution, and division/classification.

### LOGICAL ORGANIZATION

There are six major types of logical organization that are frequently used:

1. **Illustrations** may be used to support the thesis. Examples are the most common form of this organization.
2. **Definitions** say what something is or is not. A helpful question for this type of organization is, "What are the characteristics of the topic?"
3. **Dividing** or **classifying** information into separate items according to their similarities is a common and effective organizing method.
4. **Comparing** (focusing on the similarities of things) and **contrasting** (highlighting the differences between things) are excellent tools to use with certain kinds of information.
5. **Cause and effect** is a simple tool to logically understand relationships between things. A phenomenon may be traced to its causes for organizing a subject logically.
6. **Problem and solution** is a simple and effective manner of logically organizing material. It is very commonly used and lucidly presents information.

### SYNTHESIS OF RESEARCH

When you must generate questions about what the data that you have collected, you realize whether you understand it and whether you can answer your own questions. You can learn to ask yourself questions which require that you **synthesize** content from different portions of the data, such as asking questions about the data's important information.

Understanding how to **summarize** what you have collected allows you to discern what is important in the data, and to be able to express the important content in your own words. When you learn to summarize your data, you are better able to identify the main ideas of the research, and to connect these main ideas. Then, you will be better able to generate central ideas from your research. Also, you will be able to avoid irrelevant information and to remember what you have researched.

# Mathematics

## Numbers

**Numbers** are the basic building blocks of mathematics. Specific features of numbers are identified by the following terms:

**Integer** – any positive or negative whole number, including zero. Integers do not include fractions $\left(\frac{1}{3}\right)$, decimals (0.56), or mixed numbers $\left(7\frac{3}{4}\right)$.

**Prime number** – any whole number greater than 1 that has only two factors, itself and 1; that is, a number that can be divided evenly only by 1 and itself.

**Composite number** – any whole number greater than 1 that has more than two different factors; in other words, any whole number that is not a prime number. For example: The composite number 8 has the factors of 1, 2, 4, and 8.

**Even number** – any integer that can be divided by 2 without leaving a remainder. For example: 2, 4, 6, 8, and so on.

**Odd number** – any integer that cannot be divided evenly by 2. For example: 3, 5, 7, 9, and so on.

**Decimal number** – any number that uses a decimal point to show the part of the number that is less than one. Example: 1.234.

**Decimal point** – a symbol used to separate the ones place from the tenths place in decimals or dollars from cents in currency.

**Decimal place** – the position of a number to the right of the decimal point. In the decimal 0.123, the 1 is in the first place to the right of the decimal point, indicating tenths; the 2 is in the second place, indicating hundredths; and the 3 is in the third place, indicating thousandths.

The **decimal**, or base 10, system is a number system that uses ten different digits (0, 1, 2, 3, 4, 5, 6, 7, 8, 9). An example of a number system that uses something other than ten digits is the **binary**, or base 2, number system, used by computers, which uses only the numbers 0 and 1. It is thought that the decimal system originated because people had only their 10 fingers for counting.

**Rational numbers** include all integers, decimals, and fractions. Any terminating or repeating decimal number is a rational number.

**Irrational numbers** cannot be written as fractions or decimals because the number of decimal places is infinite and there is no recurring pattern of digits within the number. For example, pi ($\pi$) begins with 3.141592 and continues without terminating or repeating, so $\pi$ is an irrational number.

**Real numbers** are the set of all rational and irrational numbers.

> **Review Video: <u>Numbers and Their Classifications</u>**
> Visit mometrix.com/academy and enter code: 461071
>
> **Review Video: <u>Rational and Irrational Numbers</u>**
> Visit mometrix.com/academy and enter code: 280645

## THE NUMBER LINE

A number line is a graph to see the distance between numbers. Basically, this graph shows the relationship between numbers. So, a number line may have a point for zero and may show negative numbers on the left side of the line. Also, any positive numbers are placed on the right side of the line. For example, consider the points labeled on the following number line:

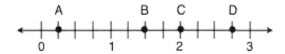

We can use the dashed lines on the number line to identify each point. Each dashed line between two whole numbers is $\frac{1}{4}$. The line halfway between two numbers is $\frac{1}{2}$.

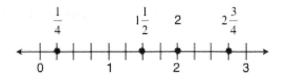

| **Review Video: Negative and Positive Number Line** |
| :---: |
| Visit mometrix.com/academy and enter code: 816439 |

## NUMBERS IN WORD FORM AND PLACE VALUE

When writing numbers out in word form or translating word form to numbers, it is essential to understand how a place value system works. In the decimal or base-10 system, each digit of a number represents how many of the corresponding place value—a specific factor of 10—are contained in the number being represented. To make reading numbers easier, every three digits to the left of the decimal place is preceded by a comma. The following table demonstrates some of the place values:

| **Power of 10** | $10^3$ | $10^2$ | $10^1$ | $10^0$ | $10^{-1}$ | $10^{-2}$ | $10^{-3}$ |
| :---: | :---: | :---: | :---: | :---: | :---: | :---: | :---: |
| **Value** | 1,000 | 100 | 10 | 1 | 0.1 | 0.01 | 0.001 |
| **Place** | thousands | hundreds | tens | ones | tenths | hundredths | thousandths |

For example, consider the number 4,546.09, which can be separated into each place value like this:

4: thousands
5: hundreds
4: tens
6: ones
0: tenths
9: hundredths

This number in word form would be *four thousand five hundred forty-six and nine hundredths*.

| **Review Video: Number Place Value** |
| :---: |
| Visit mometrix.com/academy and enter code: 205433 |

## MULTIPLES AND LEAST COMMON MULTIPLE

Often listed out in multiplication tables, **multiples** are integer increments of a given factor. In other words, dividing a multiple by the factor number will result in an integer. For example, the multiples of 7 include: $1 \times 7 = 7$, $2 \times 7 = 14$, $3 \times 7 = 21$, $4 \times 7 = 28$, $5 \times 7 = 35$. Dividing 7, 14, 21, 28, or 35 by 7 will result in the integers 1, 2, 3, 4, and 5, respectively.

The least common multiple (**LCM**) is the smallest number that is a multiple of two or more numbers. For example, the multiples of 3 include 3, 6, 9, 12, 15, etc.; the multiples of 5 include 5, 10, 15, 20, etc. Therefore, the least common multiple of 3 and 5 is 15.

> **Review Video: Multiples**
> Visit mometrix.com/academy and enter code: 626738

## FACTORS AND GREATEST COMMON FACTOR

Factors are numbers that are multiplied together to obtain a **product**. For example, in the equation $2 \times 3 = 6$, the numbers 2 and 3 are factors. A **prime number** has only two factors (1 and itself), but other numbers can have many factors.

A **common factor** is a number that divides exactly into two or more other numbers. For example, the factors of 12 are 1, 2, 3, 4, 6, and 12, while the factors of 15 are 1, 3, 5, and 15. The common factors of 12 and 15 are 1 and 3.

A **prime factor** is also a prime number. Therefore, the prime factors of 12 are 2 and 3. For 15, the prime factors are 3 and 5.

The **greatest common factor** (**GCF**) is the largest number that is a factor of two or more numbers. For example, the factors of 15 are 1, 3, 5, and 15; the factors of 35 are 1, 5, 7, and 35. Therefore, the greatest common factor of 15 and 35 is 5.

> **Review Video: Factors**
> Visit mometrix.com/academy and enter code: 920086
>
> **Review Video: GCF and LCM**
> Visit mometrix.com/academy and enter code: 838699

## PRACTICE

**P1**. Write the place value of each digit in 14,059.826

**P2**. Write out each of the following in words:

   **(a)** 29
   **(b)** 478
   **(c)** 98,542
   **(d)** 0.06
   **(e)** 13.113

**P3.** Write each of the following in numbers:

    **(a)** nine thousand four hundred thirty-five
    **(b)** three hundred two thousand eight hundred seventy-six
    **(c)** nine hundred one thousandths
    **(d)** nineteen thousandths
    **(e)** seven thousand one hundred forty-two and eighty-five hundredths

## PRACTICE SOLUTIONS

**P1.** The place value for each digit would be as follows:

| Digit | Place Value |
|-------|-------------|
| 1 | ten-thousands |
| 4 | thousands |
| 0 | hundreds |
| 5 | tens |
| 9 | ones |
| 8 | tenths |
| 2 | hundredths |
| 6 | thousandths |

**P2.** Each written out in words would be:

    **(a)** twenty-nine
    **(b)** four hundred seventy-eight
    **(c)** ninety-eight thousand five hundred forty-two
    **(d)** six hundredths
    **(e)** thirteen and one hundred thirteen thousandths

**P3.** Each in numeric form would be:

    **(a)** 9,435
    **(b)** 302,876
    **(c)** 0.901
    **(d)** 0.019
    **(e)** 7,142.85

# Operations

## OPERATIONS

An **operation** is simply a mathematical process that takes some value(s) as input(s) and produces an output. Elementary operations are often written in the following form: *value operation value*. For instance, in the expression $1 + 2$ the values are 1 and 2 and the operation is addition. Performing the operation gives the output of 3. In this way we can say that $1 + 2$ and 3 are equal, or $1 + 2 = 3$.

## ADDITION

**Addition** increases the value of one quantity by the value of another quantity (both called **addends**). For example, $2 + 4 = 6$; $8 + 9 = 17$. The result is called the **sum**. With addition, the order does not matter, $4 + 2 = 2 + 4$.

When adding signed numbers, if the signs are the same simply add the absolute values of the addends and apply the original sign to the sum. For example, $(+4) + (+8) = +12$ and $(-4) + (-8) = -12$. When the original signs are different, take the absolute values of the addends and subtract the smaller value from the larger value, then apply the original sign of the larger value to the difference. For instance, $(+4) + (-8) = -4$ and $(-4) + (+8) = +4$.

## SUBTRACTION

**Subtraction** is the opposite operation to addition; it decreases the value of one quantity (the **minuend**) by the value of another quantity (the **subtrahend**). For example, $6 - 4 = 2$; $17 - 8 = 9$. The result is called the **difference**. Note that with subtraction, the order does matter, $6 - 4 \neq 4 - 6$.

For subtracting signed numbers, change the sign of the subtrahend and then follow the same rules used for addition. For example, $(+4) - (+8) = (+4) + (-8) = -4$.

## MULTIPLICATION

**Multiplication** can be thought of as repeated addition. One number (the **multiplier**) indicates how many times to add the other number (the **multiplicand**) to itself. For example, $3 \times 2$ (three times two) $= 2 + 2 + 2 = 6$. With multiplication, the order does not matter: $2 \times 3 = 3 \times 2$ or $3 + 3 = 2 + 2 + 2$, either way the result (the **product**) is the same.

If the signs are the same, the product is positive when multiplying signed numbers. For example, $(+4) \times (+8) = +32$ and $(-4) \times (-8) = +32$. If the signs are opposite, the product is negative. For example, $(+4) \times (-8) = -32$ and $(-4) \times (+8) = -32$. When more than two factors are multiplied together, the sign of the product is determined by how many negative factors are present. If there are an odd number of negative factors then the product is negative, whereas an even number of negative factors indicates a positive product. For instance, $(+4) \times (-8) \times (-2) = +64$ and $(-4) \times (-8) \times (-2) = -64$.

## DIVISION

**Division** is the opposite operation to multiplication; one number (the **divisor**) tells us how many parts to divide the other number (the **dividend**) into. The result of division is called the **quotient**. For example, $20 \div 4 = 5$; if 20 is split into 4 equal parts, each part is 5. With division, the order of the numbers does matter, $20 \div 4 \neq 4 \div 20$.

The rules for dividing signed numbers are similar to multiplying signed numbers. If the dividend and divisor have the same sign, the quotient is positive. If the dividend and divisor have opposite signs, the quotient is negative. For example, $(-4) \div (+8) = -0.5$.

> **Review Video: Addition, Subtraction, Multiplication, and Division**
> Visit mometrix.com/academy and enter code: 208095

## PARENTHESES

**Parentheses** are used to designate which operations should be done first when there are multiple operations. Example: $4 - (2 + 1) = 1$; the parentheses tell us that we must add 2 and 1, and then subtract the sum from 4, rather than subtracting 2 from 4 and then adding 1 (this would give us an answer of 3).

> **Review Video: Mathematical Parentheses**
> Visit mometrix.com/academy and enter code: 978600

## ORDER OF OPERATIONS

**Order of operations** is a set of rules that dictates the order in which we must perform each operation in an expression so that we will evaluate it accurately. If we have an expression that includes multiple different operations, order of operations tells us which operations to do first. The most common mnemonic for order of operations is **PEMDAS**, or "Please Excuse My Dear Aunt Sally." PEMDAS stands for parentheses, exponents, multiplication, division, addition, and subtraction. It is important to understand that multiplication and division have equal precedence, as do addition and subtraction, so those pairs of operations are simply worked from left to right in order.

For example, evaluating the expression $5 + 20 \div 4 \times (2 + 3) - 6$ using the correct order of operations would be done like this:

- **P:** Perform the operations inside the parentheses: $(2 + 3) = 5$
- **E:** Simplify the exponents. (Not required on the ATI TEAS)
  - The equation now looks like this: $5 + 20 \div 4 \times 5 - 6$
- **MD:** Perform multiplication and division from left to right: $20 \div 4 = 5$; then $5 \times 5 = 25$
  - The equation now looks like this: $5 + 25 - 6$
- **AS:** Perform addition and subtraction from left to right: $5 + 25 = 30$; then $30 - 6 = 24$

> **Review Video: Order of Operations**
> Visit mometrix.com/academy and enter code: 259675

## SUBTRACTION WITH REGROUPING

A great way to make use of some of the features built into the decimal system would be regrouping when attempting longform subtraction operations. When subtracting within a place value, sometimes the minuend is smaller than the subtrahend, **regrouping** enables you to 'borrow' a unit from a place value to the left in order to get a positive difference. For example, consider subtracting 189 from 525 with regrouping.

> **Review Video: Subtracting Large Numbers**
> Visit mometrix.com/academy and enter code: 603350

First, set up the subtraction problem in vertical form:

$$
\begin{array}{r}
525 \\
-\ 189 \\
\hline
\end{array}
$$

Notice that the numbers in the ones and tens columns of 525 are smaller than the numbers in the ones and tens columns of 189. This means you will need to use regrouping to perform subtraction:

| | 5 | 2 | 5 |
|---|---|---|---|
| − | 1 | 8 | 9 |

To subtract 9 from 5 in the ones column you will need to borrow from the 2 in the ten's columns:

| | 5 | 1 | 15 |
|---|---|---|---|
| − | 1 | 8 | 9 |
| | | | 6 |

Next, to subtract 8 from 1 in the tens column you will need to borrow from the 5 in the hundred's column:

| | 4 | 11 | 15 |
|---|---|---|---|
| − | 1 | 8 | 9 |
| | | 3 | 6 |

Last, subtract the 1 from the 4 in the hundred's column:

| | 4 | 11 | 15 |
|---|---|---|---|
| − | 1 | 8 | 9 |
| | 3 | 3 | 6 |

# Rational Numbers

## FRACTIONS

A **fraction** is a number that is expressed as one integer written above another integer, with a dividing line between them $\left(\frac{x}{y}\right)$. It represents the **quotient** of the two numbers "x divided by y." It can also be thought of as x out of y equal parts.

The top number of a fraction is called the **numerator**, and it represents the number of parts under consideration. The 1 in $\frac{1}{4}$ means that 1 part out of the whole is being considered in the calculation. The bottom number of a fraction is called the **denominator**, and it represents the total number of equal parts. The 4 in $\frac{1}{4}$ means that the whole consists of 4 equal parts. A fraction cannot have a denominator of zero; this is referred to as "*undefined*."

Fractions can be manipulated, without changing the value of the fraction, by multiplying or dividing (but not adding or subtracting) both the numerator and denominator by the same number. If you divide both numbers by a common factor, you are **reducing** or simplifying the fraction. Two fractions that have the same value but are expressed differently are known as **equivalent fractions**. For example, $\frac{2}{10}, \frac{3}{15}, \frac{4}{20}$, and $\frac{5}{25}$ are all equivalent fractions. They can also all be reduced or simplified to $\frac{1}{5}$.

When two fractions are manipulated so that they have the same denominator, this is known as finding a **common denominator**. The number chosen to be that common denominator should be the least common multiple of the two original denominators. Example: $\frac{3}{4}$ and $\frac{5}{6}$; the least common multiple of 4 and 6 is 12. Manipulating to achieve the common denominator: $\frac{3}{4} = \frac{9}{12}$; $\frac{5}{6} = \frac{10}{12}$.

## PROPER FRACTIONS AND MIXED NUMBERS

A fraction whose denominator is greater than its numerator is known as a **proper fraction**, while a fraction whose numerator is greater than its denominator is known as an **improper fraction**. Proper fractions have values *less than one* and improper fractions have values *greater than one*.

A **mixed number** is a number that contains both an integer and a fraction. Any improper fraction can be rewritten as a mixed number. Example: $\frac{8}{3} = \frac{6}{3} + \frac{2}{3} = 2 + \frac{2}{3} = 2\frac{2}{3}$. Similarly, any mixed number can be rewritten as an improper fraction. Example: $1\frac{3}{5} = 1 + \frac{3}{5} = \frac{5}{5} + \frac{3}{5} = \frac{8}{5}$.

> **Review Video: <u>Proper and Improper Fractions and Mixed Numbers</u>**
> Visit mometrix.com/academy and enter code: 211077
>
> **Review Video: <u>Fractions</u>**
> Visit mometrix.com/academy and enter code: 262335

## ADDING AND SUBTRACTING FRACTIONS

If two fractions have a common denominator, they can be added or subtracted simply by adding or subtracting the two numerators and retaining the same denominator. If the two fractions do not already have the same denominator, one or both of them must be manipulated to achieve a common denominator before they can be added or subtracted. Example: $\frac{1}{2} + \frac{1}{4} = \frac{2}{4} + \frac{1}{4} = \frac{3}{4}$.

> **Review Video: <u>Adding and Subtracting Fractions</u>**
> Visit mometrix.com/academy and enter code: 378080

## MULTIPLYING FRACTIONS

Two fractions can be multiplied by multiplying the two numerators to find the new numerator and the two denominators to find the new denominator. Example: $\frac{1}{3} \times \frac{2}{3} = \frac{1 \times 2}{3 \times 3} = \frac{2}{9}$.

## DIVIDING FRACTIONS

Two fractions can be divided by flipping the numerator and denominator of the second fraction and then proceeding as though it were a multiplication. Example: $\frac{2}{3} \div \frac{3}{4} = \frac{2}{3} \times \frac{4}{3} = \frac{8}{9}$.

> **Review Video: <u>Multiplying and Dividing Fractions</u>**
> Visit mometrix.com/academy and enter code: 473632

## MULTIPLYING A MIXED NUMBER BY A WHOLE NUMBER OR A DECIMAL

When multiplying a mixed number by something, it is usually best to convert it to an improper fraction first. Additionally, if the multiplicand is a decimal, it is most often simplest to convert it to a fraction. For instance, to multiply $4\frac{3}{8}$ by 3.5, begin by rewriting each quantity as a whole number plus a proper fraction. Remember, a mixed number is a fraction added to a whole number and a decimal is a representation of the sum of fractions, specifically tenths, hundredths, thousandths, and so on:

$$4\frac{3}{8} \times 3.5 = \left(4 + \frac{3}{8}\right) \times \left(3 + \frac{1}{2}\right)$$

Next, the quantities being added need to be expressed with the same denominator. This is achieved by multiplying and dividing the whole number by the denominator of the fraction. Recall that a whole number is equivalent to that number divided by 1:

$$= \left(\frac{4}{1} \times \frac{8}{8} + \frac{3}{8}\right) \times \left(\frac{3}{1} \times \frac{2}{2} + \frac{1}{2}\right)$$

When multiplying fractions, remember to multiply the numerators and denominators separately:

$$= \left(\frac{4 \times 8}{1 \times 8} + \frac{3}{8}\right) \times \left(\frac{3 \times 2}{1 \times 2} + \frac{1}{2}\right)$$
$$= \left(\frac{32}{8} + \frac{3}{8}\right) \times \left(\frac{6}{2} + \frac{1}{2}\right)$$

Now that the fractions have the same denominators, they can be added:

$$= \frac{35}{8} \times \frac{7}{2}$$

Finally, perform the last multiplication and then simplify:

$$= \frac{35 \times 7}{8 \times 2} = \frac{245}{16} = \frac{240}{16} + \frac{5}{16} = 15\frac{5}{16}$$

## DECIMALS

Decimals are one way to represent parts of a whole. Using the place value system, each digit to the right of a decimal point denotes the number of units of a corresponding *negative* power of ten. For example, consider the decimal 0.24. We can use a model to represent the decimal. Since a dime is worth one-tenth of a dollar and a penny is worth one-hundredth of a dollar, one possible model to represent this fraction is to have 2 dimes representing the 2 in the tenths place and 4 pennies representing the 4 in the hundredths place:

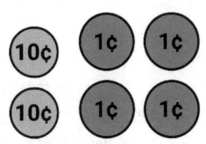

To write the decimal as a fraction, put the decimal in the numerator with 1 in the denominator. Multiply the numerator and denominator by tens until there are no more decimal places. Then simplify the fraction to lowest terms. For example, converting 0.24 to a fraction:

$$0.24 = \frac{0.24}{1} = \frac{0.24 \times 100}{1 \times 100} = \frac{24}{100} = \frac{6}{25}$$

> **Review Video: Decimals**
> Visit mometrix.com/academy and enter code: 837268

## OPERATIONS WITH DECIMALS
### ADDING AND SUBTRACTING DECIMALS

When adding and subtracting decimals, the decimal points must always be aligned. Adding decimals is just like adding regular whole numbers. Example: $4.5 + 2.0 = 6.5$.

If the problem-solver does not properly align the decimal points, an incorrect answer of 4.7 may result. An easy way to add decimals is to align all of the decimal points in a vertical column visually. This will allow one to see exactly where the decimal should be placed in the final answer. Begin adding from right to left. Add each column in turn, making sure to carry the number to the left if a column adds up to more than 9. The same rules apply to the subtraction of decimals.

> **Review Video: Adding and Subtracting Decimals**
> Visit mometrix.com/academy and enter code: 381101

### MULTIPLYING DECIMALS

A simple multiplication problem has two components: a **multiplicand** and a **multiplier**. When multiplying decimals, work as though the numbers were whole rather than decimals. Once the final product is calculated, count the number of places to the right of the decimal in both the multiplicand and the multiplier. Then, count that number of places from the right of the product and place the decimal in that position.

For example, $12.3 \times 2.56$ has a total of three places to the right of the respective decimals. Multiply $123 \times 256$ to get 31,488. Now, beginning on the right, count three places to the left and insert the decimal. The final product will be 31.488.

> **Review Video: Multiplying Decimals**
> Visit mometrix.com/academy and enter code: 731574

### DIVIDING DECIMALS

Every division problem has a **divisor** and a **dividend**. The dividend is the number that is being divided. In the problem $14 \div 7$, 14 is the dividend and 7 is the divisor. In a division problem with decimals, the divisor must be converted into a whole number. Begin by moving the decimal in the divisor to the right until a whole number is created. Next, move the decimal in the dividend the same number of spaces to the right. For example, 4.9 into 24.5 would become 49 into 245. The decimal was moved one space to the right to create a whole number in the divisor, and then the same was done for the dividend. Once the whole numbers are created, the problem is carried out normally: $245 \div 49 = 5$.

> **Review Video: Dividing Decimals**
> Visit mometrix.com/academy and enter code: 560690

## PERCENTAGES

**Percentages** can be thought of as fractions that are based on a whole of 100; that is, one whole is equal to 100%. The word **percent** means "per hundred." Percentage problems are often presented in three main ways:

- Find what percentage of some number another number is.
  - Example: What percentage of 40 is 8?
- Find what number is some percentage of a given number.
  - Example: What number is 20% of 40?
- Find what number another number is a given percentage of.
  - Example: What number is 8 20% of?

There are three components in each of these cases: a **whole** ($W$), a **part** ($P$), and a **percentage** (%). These are related by the equation: $P = W \times \%$. This can easily be rearranged into other forms that may suit different questions better: $\% = \frac{P}{W}$ and $W = \frac{P}{\%}$. Percentage problems are often also word problems. As such, a large part of solving them is figuring out which quantities are what. For example, consider the following word problem:

*In a school cafeteria, 7 students choose pizza, 9 choose hamburgers, and 4 choose tacos. What percentage of student choose tacos?*

To find the whole, you must first add all of the parts: $7 + 9 + 4 = 20$. The percentage can then be found by dividing the part by the whole ($\% = \frac{P}{W}$): $\frac{4}{20} = \frac{20}{100} = 20\%$.

> **Review Video: Calculation of a Percentage**
> Visit mometrix.com/academy and enter code: 456247

## CONVERTING BETWEEN PERCENTAGES, FRACTIONS, AND DECIMALS

Converting decimals to percentages and percentages to decimals is as simple as moving the decimal point. To *convert from a decimal to a percentage*, move the decimal point **two places to the right**. To *convert from a percentage to a decimal*, move it **two places to the left**. It may be helpful to remember that the percentage number will always be larger than the equivalent decimal number. For example:

$$0.23 = 23\% \quad 5.34 = 534\% \quad 0.007 = 0.7\%$$
$$700\% = 7.00 \quad 86\% = 0.86 \quad 0.15\% = 0.0015$$

To convert a fraction to a decimal, simply divide the numerator by the denominator in the fraction. To convert a decimal to a fraction, put the decimal in the numerator with 1 in the denominator. Multiply the numerator and denominator by tens until there are no more decimal places. Then simplify the fraction to lowest terms. For example, converting 0.24 to a fraction:

$$0.24 = \frac{0.24}{1} = \frac{0.24 \times 100}{1 \times 100} = \frac{24}{100} = \frac{6}{25}$$

Fractions can be converted to a percentage by finding equivalent fractions with a denominator of 100. For example,

$$\frac{7}{10} = \frac{70}{100} = 70\% \quad \frac{1}{4} = \frac{25}{100} = 25\%$$

To convert a percentage to a fraction, divide the percentage number by 100 and reduce the fraction to its simplest possible terms. For example,

$$60\% = \frac{60}{100} = \frac{3}{5} \quad 96\% = \frac{96}{100} = \frac{24}{25}$$

> **Review Video: <u>Converting Fractions to Percentages and Decimals</u>**
> Visit mometrix.com/academy and enter code: 306233
>
> **Review Video: <u>Converting Percentages to Decimals and Fractions</u>**
> Visit mometrix.com/academy and enter code: 287297

## RATIONAL NUMBERS

The term **rational** means that the number can be expressed as a ratio or fraction. That is, a number, $r$, is rational if and only if it can be represented by a fraction $\frac{a}{b}$ where $a$ and $b$ are integers and $b$ does not equal 0. The set of rational numbers includes integers and decimals. If there is no finite way to represent a value with a fraction of integers, then the number is **irrational**. Common examples of irrational numbers include: $\sqrt{5}, \left(1 + \sqrt{2}\right)$, and $\pi$.

> **Review Video: <u>Rational and Irrational Numbers</u>**
> Visit mometrix.com/academy and enter code: 280645

## PRACTICE

**P1.** What is 30% of 120?

**P2.** What is 150% of 20?

**P3.** What is 14.5% of 96?

**P4.** Simplify the following expressions:

**(a)** $\left(\frac{2}{5}\right)/\left(\frac{4}{7}\right)$
**(b)** $\frac{7}{8} - \frac{8}{16}$
**(c)** $\frac{1}{2} + \left(3\left(\frac{3}{4}\right) - 2\right) + 4$
**(d)** $0.22 + 0.5 - (5.5 + 3.3 \div 3)$
**(e)** $\frac{3}{2} + (4(0.5) - 0.75) + 2$

**P5.** Convert the following to a fraction and to a decimal: **(a)** 15%; **(b)** 24.36%

**P6.** Convert the following to a decimal and to a percentage. **(a)** 4/5; **(b)** $3\frac{2}{5}$

**P7.** A woman's age is thirteen more than half of 60. How old is the woman?

**P8.** A patient was given pain medicine at a dosage of 0.22 grams. The patient's dosage was then increased to 0.80 grams. By how much was the patient's dosage increased?

**P9.** At a hotel, $\frac{3}{4}$ of the 100 rooms are occupied today. Yesterday, $\frac{4}{5}$ of the 100 rooms were occupied. On which day were more of the rooms occupied and by how much more?

**P10.** At a school, 40% of the teachers teach English. If 20 teachers teach English, how many teachers work at the school?

**P11.** A patient was given blood pressure medicine at a dosage of 2 grams. The patient's dosage was then decreased to 0.45 grams. By how much was the patient's dosage decreased?

**P12.** Two weeks ago, $\frac{2}{3}$ of the 60 customers at a skate shop were male. Last week, $\frac{3}{6}$ of the 80 customers were male. During which week were there more male customers?

**P13.** Jane ate lunch at a local restaurant. She ordered a $4.99 appetizer, a $12.50 entrée, and a $1.25 soda. If she wants to tip her server 20%, how much money will she spend in all?

**P14.** According to a survey, about 82% of engineers were highly satisfied with their job. If 145 engineers were surveyed, how many reported that they were highly satisfied?

**P15.** A patient was given 40 mg of a certain medicine. Later, the patient's dosage was increased to 45 mg. What was the percent increase in his medication?

## PRACTICE SOLUTIONS

**P1.** The word *of* indicates multiplication, so 30% of 120 is found by multiplying 120 by 30%. Change 30% to a decimal, then multiply: $120 \times 0.3 = 36$

**P2.** The word *of* indicates multiplication, so 150% of 20 is found by multiplying 20 by 150%. Change 150% to a decimal, then multiply: $20 \times 1.5 = 30$

**P3.** Change 14.5% to a decimal before multiplying. $0.145 \times 96 = 13.92$.

**P4.** Follow the order of operations and utilize properties of fractions to solve each:

(a) Rewrite the problem as a multiplication problem: $\frac{2}{5} \times \frac{7}{4} = \frac{2 \times 7}{5 \times 4} = \frac{14}{20}$. Make sure the fraction is reduced to lowest terms. Both 14 and 20 can be divided by 2.

$$\frac{14}{20} = \frac{14 \div 2}{20 \div 2} = \frac{7}{10}$$

(b) The denominators of $\frac{7}{8}$ and $\frac{8}{16}$ are 8 and 16, respectively. The lowest common denominator of 8 and 16 is 16 because 16 is the least common multiple of 8 and 16. Convert the first fraction to its equivalent with the newly found common denominator of 16: $\frac{7 \times 2}{8 \times 2} = \frac{14}{16}$. Now that the fractions have the same denominator, you can subtract them.

$$\frac{14}{16} - \frac{8}{16} = \frac{6}{16} = \frac{3}{8}$$

**(c)** When simplifying expressions, first perform operations within groups. Within the set of parentheses are multiplication and subtraction operations. Perform the multiplication first to get $\frac{1}{2} + \left(\frac{9}{4} - 2\right) + 4$. Then, subtract two to obtain $\frac{1}{2} + \frac{1}{4} + 4$. Finally, perform addition from left to right:

$$\frac{1}{2} + \frac{1}{4} + 4 = \frac{2}{4} + \frac{1}{4} + \frac{16}{4} = \frac{19}{4} = 4\frac{3}{4}$$

**(d)** First, evaluate the terms in the parentheses $(5.5 + 3.3 \div 3)$ using order of operations. $3.3 \div 3 = 1.1$, and $5.5 + 1.1 = 6.6$. Next, rewrite the problem: $0.22 + 0.5 - 6.6$. Finally, add and subtract from left to right: $0.22 + 0.5 = 0.72$; $0.72 - 6.6 = -5.88$. The answer is $-5.88$.

**(e)** First, simplify within the parentheses, then change the fraction to a decimal and perform addition from left to right:

$$\frac{3}{2} + (2 - 0.75) + 2 =$$
$$\frac{3}{2} + 1.25 + 2 =$$
$$1.5 + 1.25 + 2 = 4.75$$

**P5. (a)** 15% can be written as $\frac{15}{100}$. Both 15 and 100 can be divided by 5: $\frac{15 \div 5}{100 \div 5} = \frac{3}{20}$

When converting from a percentage to a decimal, drop the percent sign and move the decimal point two places to the left: $15\% = 0.15$

**(b)** 24.36% written as a fraction is $\frac{24.36}{100}$, or $\frac{2436}{10,000}$, which reduces to $\frac{609}{2500}$. 24.36% written as a decimal is 0.2436. Recall that dividing by 100 moves the decimal two places to the left.

**P6. (a)** Recall that in the decimal system the first decimal place is one tenth: $\frac{4 \times 2}{5 \times 2} = \frac{8}{10} = 0.8$

Percent means "per hundred." $\frac{4 \times 20}{5 \times 20} = \frac{80}{100} = 80\%$

**(b)** The mixed number $3\frac{2}{5}$ has a whole number and a fractional part. The fractional part $\frac{2}{5}$ can be written as a decimal by dividing 5 into 2, which gives 0.4. Adding the whole to the part gives 3.4.

To find the equivalent percentage, multiply the decimal by 100. $3.4(100) = 340\%$. Notice that this percentage is greater than 100%. This makes sense because the original mixed number $3\frac{2}{5}$ is greater than 1.

**P7.** "More than" indicates addition, and "of" indicates multiplication. The expression can be written as $\frac{1}{2}(60) + 13$. So, the woman's age is equal to $\frac{1}{2}(60) + 13 = 30 + 13 = 43$. The woman is 43 years old.

**P8.** The first step is to determine what operation (addition, subtraction, multiplication, or division) the problem requires. Notice the keywords and phrases "by how much" and "increased." "Increased" means that you go from a smaller amount to a larger amount. This change can be found by subtracting the smaller amount from the larger amount: 0.80 grams– 0.22 grams = 0.58 grams.

Remember to line up the decimal when subtracting:

$$\begin{array}{r} 0.80 \\ -\ \ 0.22 \\ \hline 0.58 \end{array}$$

**P9.** First, find the number of rooms occupied each day. To do so, multiply the fraction of rooms occupied by the number of rooms available:

$$\text{Number occupied} = \text{Fraction occupied} \times \text{Total number}$$
$$\text{Number of rooms occupied today} = \frac{3}{4} \times 100 = 75$$
$$\text{Number of rooms occupied} = \frac{4}{5} \times 100 = 80$$

The difference in the number of rooms occupied is: $80 - 75 = 5$ rooms

**P10.** To answer this problem, first think about the number of teachers that work at the school. Will it be more or less than the number of teachers who work in a specific department such as English? More teachers work at the school, so the number you find to answer this question will be greater than 20.

40% of the teachers are English teachers. "Of" indicates multiplication, and words like "is" and "are" indicate equivalence. Translating the problem into a mathematical sentence gives $40\% \times t = 20$, where $t$ represents the total number of teachers. Solving for $t$ gives $t = \frac{20}{40\%} = \frac{20}{0.40} = 50$. Fifty teachers work at the school.

**P11.** The decrease is represented by the difference between the two amounts:

$$2 \text{ grams} - 0.45 \text{ grams} = 1.55 \text{ grams}.$$

Remember to line up the decimal point before subtracting.

$$\begin{array}{r} 2.00 \\ -\ \ 0.45 \\ \hline 1.55 \end{array}$$

**P12.** First, you need to find the number of male customers that were in the skate shop each week. You are given this amount in terms of fractions. To find the actual number of male customers, multiply the fraction of male customers by the number of customers in the store.

$$\text{Actual number of male customers} = \text{fraction of male customers} \times \text{total customers}$$
$$\text{Number of male customers two weeks ago} = \frac{2}{3} \times 60 = \frac{120}{3} = 40$$
$$\text{Number of male customers last week} = \frac{3}{6} \times 80 = \frac{1}{2} \times 80 = \frac{80}{2} = 40$$

The number of male customers was the same both weeks.

**P13.** To find total amount, first find the sum of the items she ordered from the menu and then add 20% of this sum to the total.

$$\$4.99 + \$12.50 + \$1.25 = \$18.74$$

$$\$18.74 \times 20\% = (0.20)(\$18.74) = \$3.748 \approx \$3.75$$

$$\text{Total} = \$18.74 + \$3.75 = \$22.49$$

**P14.** 82% of 145 is 0.82 × 145 = 118.9. Because you can't have 0.9 of a person, we must round up to say that 119 engineers reported that they were highly satisfied with their jobs.

**P15.** To find the percent increase, first compare the original and increased amounts. The original amount was 40 mg, and the increased amount is 45 mg, so the dosage of medication was increased by 5 mg (45– 40 = 5). Note, however, that the question asks not by how much the dosage increased but by what percentage it increased.

$$\text{Percent increase} = \frac{\text{new amount} - \text{original amount}}{\text{original amount}} \times 100\%$$
$$= \frac{45 \text{ mg} - 40 \text{ mg}}{40 \text{ mg}} \times 100\% = \frac{5}{40} \times 100\% = 0.125 \times 100\% = 12.5\%$$

# Proportions and Ratios

## PROPORTIONS

A proportion is a relationship between two quantities that dictates how one changes when the other changes. A **direct proportion** describes a relationship in which a quantity increases by a set amount for every increase in the other quantity, or decreases by that same amount for every decrease in the other quantity. Example: Assuming a constant driving speed, the time required for a car trip increases as the distance of the trip increases. The distance to be traveled and the time required to travel are directly proportional.

**Inverse proportion** is a relationship in which an increase in one quantity is accompanied by a decrease in the other, or vice versa. Example: the time required for a car trip decreases as the speed increases, and increases as the speed decreases, so the time required is inversely proportional to the speed of the car.

| **Review Video: Proportions** |
| :---: |
| Visit mometrix.com/academy and enter code: 505355 |

## RATIOS

A **ratio** is a comparison of two quantities in a particular order. Example: If there are 14 computers in a lab, and the class has 20 students, there is a student to computer ratio of 20 to 14, commonly written as 20:14. Ratios are normally reduced to their smallest whole number representation, so 20:14 would be reduced to 10:7 by dividing both sides by 2.

| **Review Video: Ratios** |
| :---: |
| Visit mometrix.com/academy and enter code: 996914 |

## CONSTANT OF PROPORTIONALITY

When two quantities have a proportional relationship, there exists a **constant of proportionality** between the quantities; the product of this constant and one of the quantities is equal to the other quantity. For example, if one lemon costs $0.25, two lemons cost $0.50, and three lemons cost $0.75, there is a proportional relationship between the total cost of lemons and the number of lemons purchased. The constant of proportionality is the **unit price**, namely $0.25/lemon. Notice that the total price of lemons, $t$, can be found by multiplying the unit price of lemons, $p$, and the number of lemons, $n$: $t = pn$.

## WORK/UNIT RATE

**Unit rate** expresses a quantity of one thing in terms of one unit of another. For example, if you travel 30 miles every two hours, a unit rate expresses this comparison in terms of one hour: in one hour you travel 15 miles, so your unit rate is 15 miles per hour. Other examples are how much one ounce of food costs (price per ounce) or figuring out how much one egg costs out of the dozen (price per 1 egg, instead of price per 12 eggs). The denominator of a unit rate is always 1. Unit rates are used to compare different situations to solve problems. For example, to make sure you get the best deal when deciding which kind of soda to buy, you can find the unit rate of each. If soda #1 costs $1.50 for a 1-liter bottle, and soda #2 costs $2.75 for a 2-liter bottle, it would be a better deal to buy soda #2, because its unit rate is only $1.375 per 1-liter, which is cheaper than soda #1. Unit rates can also help determine the length of time a given event will take. For example, if you can paint 2 rooms in 4.5 hours, you can determine how long it will take you to paint 5 rooms by solving for the unit rate per room and then multiplying that by 5.

> **Review Video: Rates and Unit Rates**
> Visit mometrix.com/academy and enter code: 185363

## SLOPE

On a graph with two points, $(x_1, y_1)$ and $(x_2, y_2)$, the **slope** is found with the formula $m = \frac{y_2 - y_1}{x_2 - x_1}$, where $x_1 \neq x_2$ and m stands for slope. If the value of the slope is **positive**, the line has an *upward direction* from left to right. If the value of the slope is **negative**, the line has a *downward direction* from left to right. Consider the following example:

A new book goes on sale in bookstores and online stores. In the first month, 5,000 copies of the book are sold. Over time, the book continues to grow in popularity. The data for the number of copies sold is in the table below.

| # of Months on Sale | 1 | 2 | 3 | 4 | 5 |
|---|---|---|---|---|---|
| # of Copies Sold (In Thousands) | 5 | 10 | 15 | 20 | 25 |

So, the number of copies that are sold and the time that the book is on sale is a proportional relationship. In this example, an equation can be used to show the data: $y = 5x$, where $x$ is the number of months that the book is on sale. Also, y is the number of copies sold. So, the slope of the corresponding line is $\frac{\text{rise}}{\text{run}} = \frac{5}{1} = 5$.

> **Review Video: Finding the Slope of a Line**
> Visit mometrix.com/academy and enter code: 766664

### FINDING AN UNKNOWN IN EQUIVALENT EXPRESSIONS

It is often necessary to apply information given about a rate or proportion to a new scenario. For example, if you know that Jedha can run a marathon (26 miles) in 3 hours, how long would it take her to run 10 miles at the same pace? Start by setting up equivalent expressions:

$$\frac{26 \text{ mi}}{3 \text{ hr}} = \frac{10 \text{ mi}}{x \text{ hr}}$$

Now, cross multiply and solve for $x$:

$$26x = 30$$
$$x = \frac{30}{26} = \frac{15}{13}$$
$$x \cong 1.15 \text{ hrs } or \text{ 1 hr 9 min}$$

So, at this pace, Jedha could run 10 miles in about 1.15 hours or about 1 hour and 9 minutes.

> **Review Video: Cross Multiplying Fractions**
> Visit mometrix.com/academy and enter code: 893904

### PRACTICE

**P1.** Solve the following for $x$.

(a) $\frac{45}{12} = \frac{15}{x}$

(b) $\frac{0.50}{2} = \frac{1.50}{x}$

(c) $\frac{40}{8} = \frac{x}{24}$

**P2.** At a school, for every 20 female students there are 15 male students. This same student ratio happens to exist at another school. If there are 100 female students at the second school, how many male students are there?

**P3.** In a hospital emergency room, there are 4 nurses for every 12 patients. What is the ratio of nurses to patients? If the nurse-to-patient ratio remains constant, how many nurses must be present to care for 24 patients?

**P4.** In a bank, the banker-to-customer ratio is 1:2. If seven bankers are on duty, how many customers are currently in the bank?

**P5.** Janice made $40 during the first 5 hours she spent babysitting. She will continue to earn money at this rate until she finishes babysitting in 3 more hours. Find how much money Janice earns per hour and the total she earned babysitting.

**P6.** The McDonalds are taking a family road trip, driving 300 miles to their cabin. It took them 2 hours to drive the first 120 miles. They will drive at the same speed all the way to their cabin. Find the speed at which the McDonalds are driving and how much longer it will take them to get to their cabin.

**P7.** It takes Andy 10 minutes to read 6 pages of his book. He has already read 150 pages in his book that is 210 pages long. Find how long it takes Andy to read 1 page and also find how long it will take him to finish his book if he continues to read at the same speed.

## PRACTICE SOLUTIONS

**P1.** Cross multiply, then solve for $x$:

**(a)** $45x = 12 \times 15$
$$45x = 180$$
$$x = \frac{180}{45} = 4$$

**(b)** $0.5x = 1.5 \times 2$
$$0.5x = 3$$
$$x = \frac{3}{0.5} = 6$$

**(c)** $8x = 40 \times 24$
$$8x = 960$$
$$x = \frac{960}{8} = 120$$

**P2.** One way to find the number of male students is to set up and solve a proportion.

$$\frac{\text{number of female students}}{\text{number of male students}} = \frac{20}{15} = \frac{100}{\text{number of male students}}$$

Represent the unknown number of male students as the variable x: $\frac{20}{15} = \frac{100}{x}$

Cross multiply and then solve for $x$:

$$20x = 15 \times 100$$
$$x = \frac{1500}{20}$$
$$x = 75$$

**P3.** The ratio of nurses to patients can be written as 4 to 12, 4:12, or $\frac{4}{12}$. Because four and twelve have a common factor of four, the ratio should be reduced to 1:3, which means that there is one nurse present for every three patients. If this ratio remains constant, there must be eight nurses present to care for 24 patients.

**P4.** Use proportional reasoning or set up a proportion to solve. Because there are twice as many customers as bankers, there must be fourteen customers when seven bankers are on duty. Setting up and solving a proportion gives the same result:

$$\frac{\text{number of bankers}}{\text{number of customers}} = \frac{1}{2} = \frac{7}{\text{number of customers}}$$

Represent the unknown number of patients as the variable $x$: $\frac{1}{2} = \frac{7}{x}$.

To solve for $x$, cross multiply: $1 \times x = 7 \times 2$, so $x = 14$.

**P5.** Janice earns \$8 per hour. This can be found by taking her initial amount earned, \$40, and dividing it by the number of hours worked, 5. Since $\frac{40}{5} = 8$, Janice makes \$8 in one hour. This can also be found by finding the unit rate, money earned per hour: $\frac{40}{5} = \frac{x}{1}$. Since cross multiplying yields $5x = 40$, and division by 5 shows that $x = 8$, Janice earns \$8 per hour.

Janice will earn \$64 babysitting in her 8 total hours (adding the first 5 hours to the remaining 3 gives the 8-hour total). Since Janice earns \$8 per hour and she worked 8 hours, $\frac{\$8}{\text{hr}} \times 8 \text{ hrs} = \$64$. This can also be found by setting up a proportion comparing money earned to babysitting hours. Since she earns \$40 for 5 hours and since the rate is constant, she will earn a proportional amount in 8 hours: $\frac{40}{5} = \frac{x}{8}$. Cross multiplying will yield $5x = 320$, and division by 5 shows that $x = 64$.

**P6.** The McDonalds are driving 60 miles per hour. This can be found by setting up a proportion to find the unit rate, the number of miles they drive per one hour: $\frac{120}{2} = \frac{x}{1}$. Cross multiplying yields $2x = 120$ and division by 2 shows that $x = 60$.

Since the McDonalds will drive this same speed, it will take them another 3 hours to get to their cabin. This can be found by first finding how many miles the McDonalds have left to drive, which is $300 - 120 = 180$. The McDonalds are driving at 60 miles per hour, so a proportion can be set up to determine how many hours it will take them to drive 180 miles: $\frac{180}{x} = \frac{60}{1}$. Cross multiplying yields $60x = 180$, and division by 60 shows that $x = 3$. This can also be found by using the formula $D = r \times t$ (or distance = rate × time), where $180 = 60 \times t$, and division by 60 shows that $t = 3$.

**P7.** It takes Andy 10 minutes to read 6 pages, $\frac{10}{6} = 1\frac{2}{3}$ minutes, which is 1 minute and 40 seconds.

Next, determine how many pages Andy has left to read, $210 - 150 = 60$. Since it is now known that it takes him $1\frac{2}{3}$ minutes to read each page, that rate must be multiplied by however many pages he has left to read (60) to find the time he'll need: $60 \times 1\frac{2}{3} = 100$, so it will take him 100 minutes, or 1 hour and 40 minutes, to read the rest of his book.

---

**Review Video: Word Problems with Ratios**
Visit mometrix.com/academy and enter code: 104804

---

# Expressions, Equations, and Inequalities

## TERMS, COEFFICIENTS, AND EXPRESSIONS

**Mathematical expressions** consist of a combination of one or more values arranged in terms that are added together. As such, an expression could be just a single number, including zero. A **variable term** is the product of a real number, also called a **coefficient**, and one or more variables. Expressions may also include numbers without a variable, called **constants** or **constant terms**.

A **single variable linear expression** is the sum of a single variable term and a constant, which may be zero. For instance, the expression $2w + 7$ has $2w$ as the variable term and 7 as the constant term. It is important to realize that terms are separated by addition or subtraction. Since an expression is a sum of terms, expressions such as $5x - 3$ can be written as $5x + (-3)$ to emphasize that the constant term is negative. A real-world example of a single variable linear expression is the perimeter of a square, four times the side length, often expressed as $4s$.

## LINEAR EQUATIONS

Equations that can be written as $ax + b = 0$, where $a \neq 0$, are referred to as **one variable linear equations**. A solution to such an equation is called a **root**. In the case where we have the equation $5x + 10 = 0$, if we solve for $x$, we get a solution of $x = -2$. In other words, the root of the equation is -2. This is found by first subtracting 10 from both sides, which gives $5x = -10$. Next, simply divide both sides by the coefficient of the variable, in this case 5, to get $x = -2$. This can be checked by plugging -2 back into the original equation $(5)(-2) + 10 = -10 + 10 = 0$.

The **solution set** is the set of all solutions of an equation. In our example, the solution set would simply be -2. If there were more solutions (there usually are in multivariable equations), then they would also be included in the solution set. When an equation has no true solutions, this is referred to as an **empty set**. Equations with identical solution sets are **equivalent equations**. An **identity** is a term whose value or determinant is equal to 1.

Linear equations can be written many ways. Below is a list of some forms linear equations can take:

- **Standard Form**: $Ax + By = C$; the slope is $\frac{-A}{B}$ and the y-intercept is $\frac{C}{B}$
- **Slope Intercept Form**: $y = mx + b$, where $m$ is the slope and $b$ is the $y$-intercept
- **Point-Slope Form**: $y - y_1 = m(x - x_1)$, where m is the slope and $(x_1, y_1)$ is a point on the line
- **Two-Point Form**: $\frac{y - y_1}{x - x_1} = \frac{y_2 - y_1}{x_2 - x_1}$, where $(x_1, y_1)$ and $(x_2, y_2)$ are two points on the given line
- **Intercept Form**: $\frac{x}{x_1} + \frac{y}{y_1} = 1$, where $(x_1, 0)$ is the point at which a line intersects the x-axis, and $(0, y_1)$ is the point at which the same line intersects the y-axis

> **Review Video: Slope-Intercept and Point-Slope Forms**
> Visit mometrix.com/academy and enter code: 113216

## SOLVING ONE-VARIABLE LINEAR EQUATIONS

Multiply all terms by the lowest common denominator to eliminate any fractions. Look for addition or subtraction to undo so you can isolate the variable on one side of the equal sign. Divide both sides by the coefficient of the variable. When you have a value for the variable, substitute this value into the original equation to make sure you have a true equation. Consider the following example:

Kim's savings are represented by the table below. Represent her savings, using an equation.

| X (Months) | Y (Total Savings) |
|------------|-------------------|
| 2          | $1300             |
| 5          | $2050             |
| 9          | $3050             |
| 11         | $3550             |
| 16         | $4800             |

The table shows a function with a constant rate of change, or slope, of 250. Given the points on the table, the slopes can be calculated as $\frac{2050-1300}{5-2}$, $\frac{3050-2050}{9-5}$, $\frac{3550-3050}{11-9}$, and $\frac{4800-3550}{16-11}$, each of which equals 250. Thus, the table shows a constant rate of change, indicating a linear function. The slope-intercept form of a linear equation is written as $y = mx + b$, where m represents the slope and b represents the y-intercept. Substituting the slope into this form gives $y = 250x + b$. Substituting corresponding x- and y-values from any point into this equation will give the y-intercept, or b. Using the point, (2,1300), gives $1300 = 250(2) + b$, which simplifies as $b = 800$. Thus, her savings may be represented by the equation, $y = 250x + 800$.

## RULES FOR MANIPULATING EQUATIONS

### CARRYING OUT THE SAME OPERATION ON BOTH SIDES OF AN EQUATION

When solving an equation, the general procedure is to carry out a series of operations on both sides of an equation, choosing operations that will tend to simplify the equation when doing so. The reason why the same operation must be carried out on both sides of the equation is because that leaves the meaning of the equation unchanged, and yields a result that is equivalent to the original equation. This would not be the case if we carried out an operation on one side of an equation and not the other. Consider what an equation means: it is a statement that two values or expressions are equal. If we carry out the same operation on both sides of the equation—add 3 to both sides, for example—then the two sides of the equation are changed in the same way, and so remain equal. If we do that to only one side of the equation—add 3 to one side but not the other—then that wouldn't be true; if we change one side of the equation but not the other then the two sides are no longer equal.

### ADVANTAGE OF COMBINING LIKE TERMS

**Combining like terms** refers to adding or subtracting like terms—terms with the same variable—and therefore reducing sets of like terms to a single term. The main advantage of doing this is that it simplifies the equation. Often, combining like terms can be done as the first step in solving an equation, though it can also be done later, such as after distributing terms in a product.

For example, consider the equation $2(x + 3) + 3(2 + x + 3) = -4$. The 2 and the 3 in the second set of parentheses are like terms, and we can combine them, yielding $2(x + 3) + 3(x + 5) = -4$. Now we can carry out the multiplications implied by the parentheses, distributing the outer 2 and 3 accordingly: $2x + 6 + 3x + 15 = -4$. The $2x$ and the $3x$ are like terms, and we can add them together: $5x + 6 + 15 = -4$. Now, the constants 6, 15, and –4 are also like terms, and we can combine them as well: subtracting 6 and 15 from both sides of the equation, we get $5x = -4 - 6 - 15$, or $5x = -25$, which simplifies further to $x = -5$.

### CANCELING TERMS ON OPPOSITE SIDES OF AN EQUATION

Two terms on opposite sides of an equation can be canceled if and only if they *exactly* match each other. They must have the same variable raised to the same power and the same coefficient. For example, in the equation $3x + 2x^2 + 6 = 2x^2 - 6$, $2x^2$ appears on both sides of the equation and can be canceled, leaving $3x + 6 = -6$. The 6 on each side of the equation *cannot* be canceled, because it is added on one side of the equation and subtracted on the other. While they cannot be canceled, however, the 6 and –6 are like terms and can be combined, yielding $3x = -12$, which simplifies further to $x = -4$.

It's also important to note that the terms to be canceled must be independent terms and cannot be part of a larger term. For example, consider the equation $2(x + 6) = 3(x + 4) + 1$. We cannot cancel the $x$'s, because even though they match each other they are part of the larger terms $2(x + 6)$ and $3(x + 4)$. We must first distribute the 2 and 3, yielding $2x + 12 = 3x + 12 + 1$. Now we see that the terms with the $x$'s do not match, but the 12s do, and can be canceled, leaving $2x = 3x + 1$, which simplifies to $x = -1$.

> **Review Video: <u>Rules for Manipulating Equations</u>**
> Visit mometrix.com/academy and enter code: 838871

## PROCESS FOR MANIPULATING EQUATIONS

### ISOLATING VARIABLES

To **isolate a variable** means to manipulate the equation so that the variable appears by itself on one side of the equation and does not appear at all on the other side. Generally, an equation or inequality is considered to be solved once the variable is isolated and the other side of the equation or inequality is simplified as much as possible. In the case of a two-variable equation or inequality, only one variable needs to be isolated; it will not usually be possible to simultaneously isolate both variables.

For a linear equation—an equation in which the variable only appears raised to the first power—isolating a variable can be done by first moving all the terms with the variable to one side of the equation and all other terms to the other side. (*Moving* a term really means adding the inverse of the term to both sides; when a term is *moved* to the other side of the equation, its sign is flipped.) Then combine like terms on each side. Finally, divide both sides by the coefficient of the variable, if applicable. The steps need not necessarily be done in this order, but this order will always work.

## WORKING WITH INEQUALITIES

Commonly in algebra and other upper-level fields of math you find yourself working with mathematical expressions that do not equal each other. The statement comparing such expressions with symbols such as < (less than) or > (greater than) is called an *inequality*. An example of an inequality is $7x > 5$. To solve for $x$, simply divide both sides by 7 and the solution is shown to be $x > \frac{5}{7}$. Graphs of the solution set of inequalities are represented on a number line. Open circles are used to show that an expression approaches a number but is never quite equal to that number.

> **Review Video: <u>Inequalities</u>**
> Visit mometrix.com/academy and enter code: 347842

**Conditional inequalities** are those with certain values for the variable that will make the condition true and other values for the variable where the condition will be false. **Absolute inequalities** can have any real number as the value for the variable to make the condition true, while there is no real number value for the variable that will make the condition false. Solving inequalities is done by following the same rules for solving equations with the exception that when multiplying or dividing by a negative number the direction of the inequality sign must be flipped or reversed. **Double inequalities** are situations where two inequality statements apply to the same variable expression. An example of this is $-c < ax + b < c$.

> **Review Video: <u>Conditional and Absolute Inequalities</u>**
> Visit mometrix.com/academy and enter code: 980164

## DETERMINING SOLUTIONS TO INEQUALITIES

To determine whether a coordinate is a solution of an inequality, you can substitute the values of the coordinate into the inequality, simplify, and check whether the resulting statement holds true. For instance, to determine whether $(-2,4)$ is a solution of the inequality $y \geq -2x + 3$, substitute the values into the inequality, $4 \geq -2(-2) + 3$. Simplify the right side of the inequality and the result is $4 \geq 7$, which is a false statement. Therefore, the coordinate is not a solution of the inequality. You can also use this method to determine which part of the graph of an inequality is shaded. The graph of $y \geq -2x + 3$ includes the solid line $y = -2x + 3$ and, since it excludes the point $(-2,4)$ to the left of the line, it is shaded to the right of the line.

## FLIPPING INEQUALITY SIGNS

When given an inequality, we can always turn the entire inequality around, swapping the two sides of the inequality and changing the inequality sign. For instance, $x + 2 > 2x - 3$ is equivalent to $2x - 3 < x + 2$. Aside from that, normally the inequality does not change if we carry out the same operation on both sides of the inequality. There is, however, one principal exception: if we *multiply* or *divide* both sides of the inequality by a *negative number*, the inequality is flipped. For example, if we take the inequality $-2x < 6$ and divide both sides by $-2$, the inequality flips and we are left with $x > -3$. This *only* applies to multiplication and division, and only with negative numbers. Multiplying or dividing both sides by a positive number, or adding or subtracting any number regardless of sign, does not flip the inequality.

## GRAPHICAL SOLUTIONS TO EQUATIONS AND INEQUALITIES

When equations are shown graphically, they are usually shown on a **Cartesian coordinate plane**. The Cartesian coordinate plane consists of two number lines placed perpendicular to each other and intersecting at the zero point, also known as the origin. The horizontal number line is known as the $x$-axis, with positive values to the right of the origin, and negative values to the left of the origin. The vertical number line is known as the $y$-axis, with positive values above the origin, and negative values below the origin. Any point on the plane can be identified by an ordered pair in the form $(x, y)$, called coordinates. The $x$-value of the coordinate is called the abscissa, and the $y$-value of the coordinate is called the ordinate. The two number lines divide the plane into **four quadrants**: I, II, III, and IV.

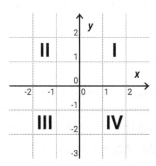

Note that in quadrant I $x > 0$ and $y > 0$, in quadrant II $x < 0$ and $y > 0$, in quadrant III $x < 0$ and $y < 0$, and in quadrant IV $x > 0$ and $y < 0$.

Recall that if the value of the slope of a line is positive, the line slopes upward from left to right. If the value of the slope is negative, the line slopes downward from left to right. If the $y$-coordinates are the same for two points on a line, the slope is 0 and the line is a **horizontal line**. If the $x$-coordinates are the same for two points on a line, there is no slope and the line is a **vertical line**.

Two or more lines that have equivalent slopes are **parallel lines**. **Perpendicular lines** have slopes that are negative reciprocals of each other, such as $\frac{a}{b}$ and $\frac{-b}{a}$.

### GRAPHING SIMPLE INEQUALITIES

To graph a simple inequality, we first mark on the number line the value that signifies the end point of the inequality. If the inequality is strict (involves a less than or greater than), we use a hollow circle; if it is not strict (less than or equal to or greater than or equal to), we use a solid circle. We then fill in the part of the number line that satisfies the inequality: to the left of the marked point for less than (or less than or equal to), to the right for greater than (or greater than or equal to).

For example, we would graph the inequality $x < 5$ by putting a hollow circle at 5 and filling in the part of the line to the left:

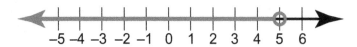

### PRACTICE

**P1.** Seeing the equation $2x + 4 = 4x + 7$, a student divides the first terms on each side by 2, yielding $x + 4 = 2x + 7$, and then combines like terms to get $x = -3$. However, this is incorrect, as can be seen by substituting –3 into the original equation. Explain what is wrong with the student's reasoning.

**P2.** Describe the steps necessary to solve the equation $2x + 1 - x = 4 + 3x + 7$.

**P3.** Describe the steps necessary to solve the equation $2(x + 5) = 7(4 - x)$.

**P4.** Ray earns \$10 an hour at his job. Write an equation for his earnings as a function of time spent working. Determine how long Ray has to work in order to earn \$360.

### PRACTICE SOLUTIONS

**P1.** As stated, it's easy to verify that the student's solution is incorrect: $2(-3) + 4 = -2$ and $4(-3) + 7 = -5$; clearly $-2 \neq -5$. The mistake was in the first step, which illustrates a common type of error in solving equations. The student tried to simplify the two variable terms by dividing them by 2. However, it's not valid to multiply or divide only one term on each side of an equation by a number; when multiplying or dividing, the operation must be applied to *every* term in the equation. So, dividing by 2 would yield not $x + 4 = 2x + 7$, but $x + 2 = 2x + \frac{7}{2}$. While this is now valid, that fraction is inconvenient to work with, so this may not be the best first step in solving the equation. Rather, it may have been better to first combine like terms. Subtracting $4x$ from both sides yields $-2x + 4 = 7$; subtracting 4 from both sides yields $-2x = 3$; *now* we can divide both sides by –2 to get $x = -\frac{3}{2}$.

**P2.** Our ultimate goal is to isolate the variable, $x$. To that end we first move all the terms containing $x$ to the left side of the equation, and all the constant terms to the right side. Note that when we move a term to the other side of the equation its sign changes. We are therefore now left with $2x - x - 3x = 4 + 7 - 1$.

Next, we combine the like terms on each side of the equation, adding and subtracting the terms as appropriate. This leaves us with $-2x = 10$.

At this point, we're almost done; all that remains is to divide both sides by $-2$ to leave the $x$ by itself. We now have our solution, $x = -5$. We can verify that this is a correct solution by substituting it back into the original equation.

**P3.** Generally, in equations that have a sum or difference of terms multiplied by another value or expression, the first step is to multiply those terms, distributing as necessary: $2(x + 5) = 2(x) + 2(5) = 2x + 10$, and $7(4 - x) = 7(4) - 7(x) = 28 - 7x$. So, the equation becomes $2x + 10 = 28 - 7x$. We can now add $7x$ to both sides to eliminate the variable from the right-hand side: $9x + 10 = 28$. Similarly, we can subtract 10 from both sides to move all the constants to the right: $9x = 18$. Finally, we can divide both sides by 9, yielding the final answer, $x = 2$.

**P4.** The number of dollars that Ray earns is dependent on the number of hours he works, so earnings will be represented by the dependent variable $y$ and hours worked will be represented by the independent variable $x$. He earns 10 dollars per hour worked, so his earnings can be calculated as $y = 10x$. To calculate the number of hours Ray must work in order to earn \$360, plug in 360 for $y$ and solve for $x$:

$$360 = 10x$$
$$x = \frac{360}{10} = 36$$

# Measurement Principles

### PRECISION, ACCURACY, AND ERROR

**Precision**: How reliable and repeatable a measurement is. The more consistent the data is with repeated testing, the more precise it is. For example, hitting a target consistently in the same spot, which may or may not be the center of the target, is precision.

**Accuracy**: How close the data is to the correct data. For example, hitting a target consistently in the center area of the target, whether or not the hits are all in the same spot, is accuracy.

Note: it is possible for data to be precise without being accurate. If a scale is off balance, the data will be precise, but will not be accurate. For data to have precision and accuracy, it must be repeatable and correct.

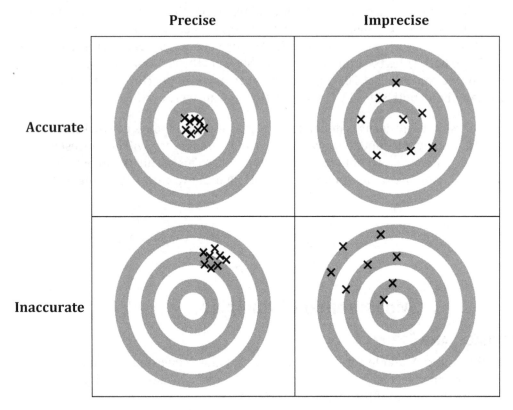

**Approximate error**: The amount of error in a physical measurement. Approximate error is often reported as the measurement, followed by the ± symbol and the amount of the approximate error.

**Maximum possible error**: Half the magnitude of the smallest unit used in the measurement. For example, if the unit of measurement is 1 centimeter, the maximum possible error is $\frac{1}{2}$ cm, written as $\pm 0.5$ cm following the measurement. It is important to apply significant figures in reporting maximum possible error. Do not make the answer appear more accurate than the least accurate of your measurements.

## ROUNDING AND ESTIMATION

**Rounding** is reducing the digits in a number while still trying to keep the value similar. The result will be less accurate, but it will be in a simpler form and will be easier to use. Whole numbers can be rounded to the nearest ten, hundred or thousand.

When you are asked to estimate the solution to a problem, you will need to provide only an approximate figure or **estimation** for your answer. In this situation, you will need to round each number in the calculation to the level indicated (nearest hundred, nearest thousand, etc.) or to a level that makes sense for the numbers involved. When estimating a sum **all numbers must be** rounded to the same level. You cannot round one number to the nearest thousand while rounding another to the nearest hundred.

**Review Video: Rounding and Estimation**
Visit mometrix.com/academy and enter code: 126243

# Units of Measurement

## METRIC MEASUREMENT PREFIXES

Giga-: one billion (1 *giga*watt is one billion watts)
Mega-: one million (1 *mega*hertz is one million hertz)
Kilo-: one thousand (1 *kilo*gram is one thousand grams)
Deci-: one-tenth (1 *deci*meter is one-tenth of a meter)
Centi-: one-hundredth (1 *centi*meter is one-hundredth of a meter)
Milli-: one-thousandth (1 *milli*liter is one-thousandth of a liter)
Micro-: one-millionth (1 *micro*gram is one-millionth of a gram)

## MEASUREMENT CONVERSION

When converting between units, the goal is to maintain the same meaning but change the way it is displayed. In order to go from a larger unit to a smaller unit, multiply the number of the known amount by the equivalent amount. When going from a smaller unit to a larger unit, divide the number of the known amount by the equivalent amount.

For complicated conversions, it may be helpful to set up conversion fractions. In these fractions, one fraction is the **conversion factor**. The other fraction has the unknown amount in the numerator. So, the known value is placed in the denominator. Sometimes, the second fraction has the known value from the problem in the numerator and the unknown in the denominator. Multiply the two fractions to get the converted measurement. Note that since the numerator and the denominator of the factor are equivalent, the value of the fraction is 1. That is why we can say that the result in the new units is equal to the result in the old units even though they have different numbers.

It can often be necessary to chain known conversion factors together. As an example, consider converting 512 square inches to square meters. We know that there are 2.54 centimeters in an inch and 100 centimeters in a meter and that we will need to square each of these factors to achieve the conversion we are looking for.

$$\frac{512 \text{ in}^2}{1} \times \left(\frac{2.54 \text{ cm}}{1 \text{ in}}\right)^2 \times \left(\frac{1 \text{ m}}{100 \text{ cm}}\right)^2 = \frac{512 \text{ in}^2}{1} \times \left(\frac{6.4516 \text{ cm}^2}{1 \text{ in}^2}\right) \times \left(\frac{1 \text{ m}^2}{10000 \text{ cm}^2}\right) = 0.330 \text{ m}^2$$

**Review Video: Measurement Conversion**
Visit mometrix.com/academy and enter code: 316703

## COMMON UNITS AND EQUIVALENTS

### METRIC EQUIVALENTS

| | |
|---|---|
| 1000 µg (microgram) | 1 mg |
| 1000 mg (milligram) | 1 g |
| 1000 g (gram) | 1 kg |
| 1000 kg (kilogram) | 1 metric ton |
| 1000 mL (milliliter) | 1 L |
| 1000 µm (micrometer) | 1 mm |
| 1000 mm (millimeter) | 1 m |
| 100 cm (centimeter) | 1 m |
| 1000 m (meter) | 1 km |

### DISTANCE AND AREA MEASUREMENT

| Unit | Abbreviation | US equivalent | Metric equivalent |
|---|---|---|---|
| Inch | in | 1 inch | 2.54 centimeters |
| Foot | ft | 12 inches | 0.305 meters |
| Yard | yd | 3 feet | 0.914 meters |
| Mile | mi | 5280 feet | 1.609 kilometers |
| Acre | ac | 4840 square yards | 0.405 hectares |
| Square Mile | sq. mi. or mi.$^2$ | 640 acres | 2.590 square kilometers |

### CAPACITY MEASUREMENTS

| Unit | Abbreviation | US equivalent | Metric equivalent |
|---|---|---|---|
| Fluid Ounce | fl oz | 8 fluid drams | 29.573 milliliters |
| Cup | c | 8 fluid ounces | 0.237 liter |
| Pint | pt. | 16 fluid ounces | 0.473 liter |
| Quart | qt. | 2 pints | 0.946 liter |
| Gallon | gal. | 4 quarts | 3.785 liters |
| Teaspoon | t or tsp. | 1 fluid dram | 5 milliliters |
| Tablespoon | T or tbsp. | 4 fluid drams | 15 or 16 milliliters |
| Cubic Centimeter | cc or cm.$^3$ | 0.271 drams | 1 milliliter |

### WEIGHT MEASUREMENTS

| Unit | Abbreviation | US equivalent | Metric equivalent |
|---|---|---|---|
| Ounce | oz | 16 drams | 28.35 grams |
| Pound | lb | 16 ounces | 453.6 grams |
| Ton | tn. | 2,000 pounds | 907.2 kilograms |

## PRACTICE

**P1.** Perform the following conversions:

    **(a)** 1.4 meters to centimeters

    **(b)** 218 centimeters to meters

    **(c)** 42 inches to feet

    **(d)** 15 kilograms to pounds

    **(e)** 80 ounces to pounds

    **(f)** 2 miles to kilometers

    **(g)** 5 feet to centimeters

    **(h)** 15.14 liters to gallons

    **(i)** 8 quarts to liters

    **(j)** 13.2 pounds to grams

## PRACTICE SOLUTIONS

**P1. (a)** $\frac{100 \text{ cm}}{1 \text{ m}} = \frac{x \text{ cm}}{1.4 \text{ m}}$ Cross multiply to get $x = 140$

    **(b)** $\frac{100 \text{ cm}}{1 \text{ m}} = \frac{218 \text{ cm}}{x \text{ m}}$ Cross multiply to get $100x = 218$, or $x = 2.18$

    **(c)** $\frac{12 \text{ in}}{1 \text{ ft}} = \frac{42 \text{ in}}{x \text{ ft}}$ Cross multiply to get $12x = 42$, or $x = 3.5$

    **(d)** 15 kilograms $\times \frac{2.2 \text{ pounds}}{1 \text{ kilogram}} = 33$ pounds

    **(e)** 80 ounces $\times \frac{1 \text{ pound}}{16 \text{ ounces}} = 5$ pounds

    **(f)** 2 miles $\times \frac{1.609 \text{ kilometers}}{1 \text{ mile}} = 3.218$ kilometers

    **(g)** 5 feet $\times \frac{12 \text{ inches}}{1 \text{ foot}} \times \frac{2.54 \text{ centimeters}}{1 \text{ inch}} = 152.4$ centimeters

    **(h)** 15.14 liters $\times \frac{1 \text{ gallon}}{3.785 \text{ liters}} = 4$ gallons

    **(i)** 8 quarts $\times \frac{1 \text{ gallon}}{4 \text{ quarts}} \times \frac{3.785 \text{ liters}}{1 \text{ gallon}} = 7.57$ liters

    **(j)** 13.2 pounds $\times \frac{1 \text{ kilogram}}{2.2 \text{ pounds}} \times \frac{1000 \text{ grams}}{1 \text{ kilogram}} = 6000$ grams

# Two-Dimensional Shapes

## POLYGONS

A **polygon** is a closed, two-dimensional figure with three or more straight line segments called **sides**. The point at which two sides of a polygon intersect is called the **vertex**. In a polygon, the number of sides is always equal to the number of vertices. A polygon with all sides congruent and all angles equal is called a **regular polygon**. Common polygons are:

Triangle = 3 sides
Quadrilateral = 4 sides
Pentagon = 5 sides
Hexagon = 6 sides
Heptagon = 7 sides
Octagon = 8 sides
Nonagon = 9 sides
Decagon = 10 sides
Dodecagon = 12 sides

More generally, an *n*-gon is a polygon that has *n* angles and *n* sides.

The sum of the interior angles of an *n*-sided polygon is $(n - 2) \times 180°$. For example, in a triangle $n = 3$. So the sum of the interior angles is $(3 - 2) \times 180° = 180°$. In a quadrilateral, $n = 4$, and the sum of the angles is $(4 - 2) \times 180° = 360°$.

> **Review Video: Polygons**
> Visit mometrix.com/academy and enter code: 271869

## TRIANGLES

A triangle is a three-sided figure with the sum of its interior angles being 180°. The **perimeter of any triangle** is found by summing the three side lengths; $P = a + b + c$. For an equilateral triangle, this is the same as $P = 3a$, where $a$ is any side length, since all three sides are the same length.

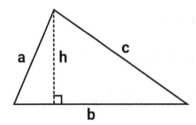

The **area of any triangle** can be found by taking half the product of one side length referred to as the base, often given the variable $b$ and the perpendicular distance from that side to the opposite vertex called the altitude or height and given the variable $h$. In equation form that is $A = \frac{1}{2}bh$.

> **Review Video: Area and Perimeter of a Triangle**
> Visit mometrix.com/academy and enter code: 853779

## QUADRILATERALS

A **quadrilateral** is a closed two-dimensional geometric figure that has four straight sides. The sum of the interior angles of any quadrilateral is 360°.

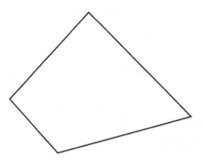

## KITE

A **kite** is a quadrilateral with two pairs of adjacent sides that are congruent. A result of this is perpendicular diagonals. A kite can be concave or convex and has one line of symmetry.

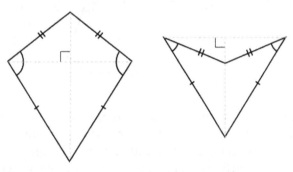

## TRAPEZOID

**Trapezoid**: A trapezoid is defined as a quadrilateral that has at least one pair of parallel sides. There are no rules for the second pair of sides. So there are no rules for the diagonals and no lines of symmetry for a trapezoid.

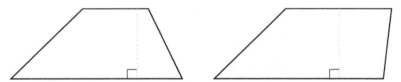

The **area of a trapezoid** is found by the formula $A = \frac{1}{2}h(b_1 + b_2)$, where $h$ is the height (segment joining and perpendicular to the parallel bases), and $b_1$ and $b_2$ are the two parallel sides (bases). Do not use one of the other two sides as the height unless that side is also perpendicular to the parallel bases.

The **perimeter of a trapezoid** is found by the formula $P = a + b_1 + c + b_2$, where $a$, $b_1$, $c$, and $b_2$ are the four sides of the trapezoid.

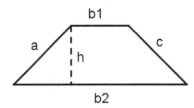

**Isosceles trapezoid**: A trapezoid with equal base angles. This gives rise to other properties including: the two nonparallel sides have the same length, the two non-base angles are also equal, and there is one line of symmetry through the midpoints of the parallel sides.

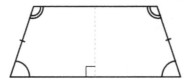

*PARALLELOGRAM*

A **parallelogram** is a quadrilateral that has two pairs of opposite parallel sides. As such it is a special type of trapezoid. The sides that are parallel are also congruent. The opposite interior angles are always congruent, and the consecutive interior angles are supplementary. The diagonals of a parallelogram divide each other. Each diagonal divides the parallelogram into two congruent triangles. A parallelogram has no line of symmetry, but does have 180-degree rotational symmetry about the midpoint.

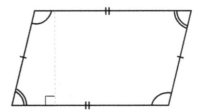

The **area of a parallelogram** is found by the formula $A = bh$, where $b$ is the length of the base, and $h$ is the height. Note that the base and height correspond to the length and width in a rectangle, so this formula would apply to rectangles as well. Do not confuse the height of a parallelogram with the length of the second side. The two are only the same measure in the case of a rectangle.

The **perimeter of a parallelogram** is found by the formula $P = 2a + 2b$ or $P = 2(a + b)$, where $a$ and $b$ are the lengths of the two sides.

## RECTANGLE

A **rectangle** is a quadrilateral with four right angles. All rectangles are parallelograms and trapezoids, but not all parallelograms or trapezoids are rectangles. The diagonals of a rectangle are congruent. Rectangles have two lines of symmetry (through each pair of opposing midpoints) and 180-degree rotational symmetry about the midpoint.

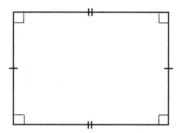

The **area of a rectangle** is found by the formula $A = lw$, where $A$ is the area of the rectangle, $l$ is the length (usually considered to be the longer side) and $w$ is the width (usually considered to be the shorter side). The numbers for $l$ and $w$ are interchangeable.

The **perimeter of a rectangle** is found by the formula $P = 2l + 2w$ or $P = 2(l + w)$, where $l$ is the length, and $w$ is the width. It may be easier to add the length and width first and then double the result, as in the second formula.

## RHOMBUS

A **rhombus** is a quadrilateral with four congruent sides. All rhombuses are parallelograms and kites; thus, they inherit all the properties of both types of quadrilaterals. The diagonals of a rhombus are perpendicular to each other. Rhombi have two lines of symmetry (along each of the diagonals) and 180° rotational symmetry. The **area of a rhombus** is half the product of the diagonals: $A = \frac{d_1 d_2}{2}$ and the perimeter of a rhombus is: $P = 2\sqrt{(d_1)^2 + (d_2)^2}$

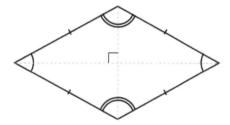

## SQUARE

A **square** is a quadrilateral with four right angles and four congruent sides. Squares satisfy the criteria of all other types of quadrilaterals. The diagonals of a square are congruent and perpendicular to each other. Squares have four lines of symmetry (through each pair of opposing midpoints and along each of the diagonals) as well as 90° rotational symmetry about the midpoint.

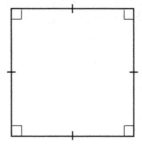

The **area of a square** is found by using the formula $A = s^2$, where $s$ is the length of one side. The **perimeter of a square** is found by using the formula $P = 4s$, where $s$ is the length of one side. Because all four sides are equal in a square, it is faster to multiply the length of one side by 4 than to add the same number four times. You could use the formulas for rectangles and get the same answer.

**Review Video: <u>How to Find the Area and Perimeter</u>**
Visit mometrix.com/academy and enter code: 471797

### HIERARCHY OF QUADRILATERALS

The hierarchy of quadrilaterals can be shown as follows:

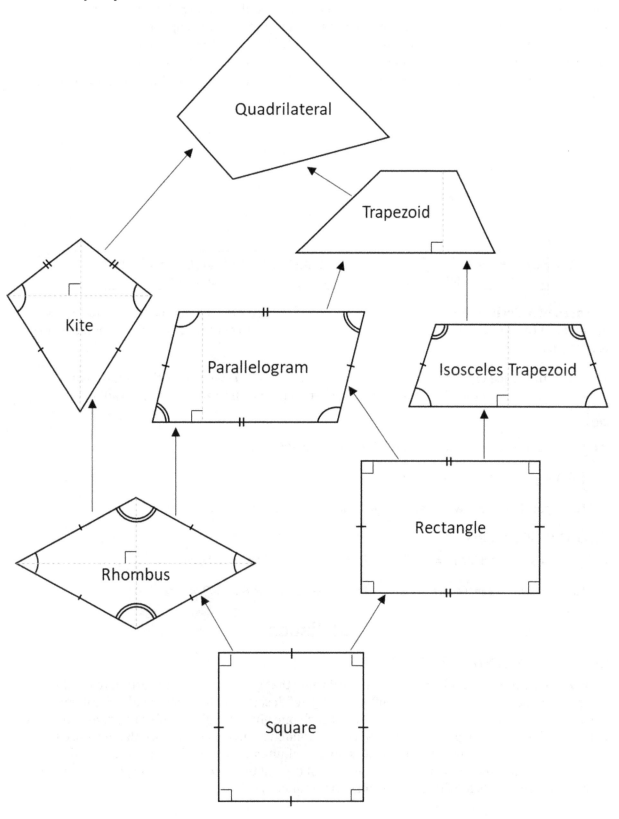

### CIRCLES

The **center** of a circle is the single point from which every point on the circle is **equidistant**. The **radius** is a line segment that joins the center of the circle and any one point on the circle. All radii of a circle are equal. Circles that have the same center but not the same length of radii are **concentric**. The **diameter** is a line segment that passes through the center of the circle and has both endpoints on the circle. The length of the diameter is exactly twice the length of the radius. Point $O$ in the diagram below is the center of the circle, segments $\overline{OX}$, $\overline{OY}$, and $\overline{OZ}$ are radii; and segment $\overline{XZ}$ is a diameter.

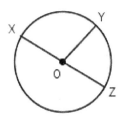

> **Review Video: The Diameter, Radius, and Circumference of Circles**
> Visit mometrix.com/academy and enter code: 448988

The **area of a circle** is found by the formula $A = \pi r^2$, where $r$ is the length of the radius. If the diameter of the circle is given, remember to divide it in half to get the length of the radius before proceeding.

The **circumference** of a circle is found by the formula $C = 2\pi r$, where $r$ is the radius. Again, remember to convert the diameter if you are given that measure rather than the radius.

### PRACTICE

**P1.** Find the area and perimeter of the following quadrilaterals:

**(a)** A square with side length 2.5 cm.

**(b)** A parallelogram with height 3 m, base 4 m, and other side 6 m.

### PRACTICE SOLUTIONS

**P1. (a)** $A = s^2 = (2.5 \text{ cm})^2 = 6.25 \text{ cm}^2$; $P = 4s = 4 \times 2.5 \text{ cm} = 10 \text{ cm}$

**(b)** $A = bh = (3 \text{ m})(4 \text{ m}) = 12 \text{ m}^2$; $P = 2a + 2b = 2 \times 6 \text{ m} + 2 \times 4 \text{ m} = 20 \text{ m}$

# Statistics

### MEASURES OF CENTRAL TENDENCY

A **measure of central tendency** is a statistical value that gives a reasonable estimate for the center of a group of data. There are several different ways of describing the measure of central tendency. Each one has a unique way it is calculated, and each one gives a slightly different perspective on the data set. Whenever you give a measure of central tendency, always make sure the units are the same. If the data has different units, such as hours, minutes, and seconds, convert all the data to the same unit, and use the same unit in the measure of central tendency. If no units are given in the data, do not give units for the measure of central tendency.

## MEAN

The **statistical mean** of a group of data is the same as the arithmetic average of that group. To find the mean of a set of data, first convert each value to the same units, if necessary. Then find the sum of all the values, and count the total number of data values, making sure you take into consideration each individual value. If a value appears more than once, count it more than once. Divide the sum of the values by the total number of values and apply the units, if any. Note that the mean does not have to be one of the data values in the set, and may not divide evenly.

$$\text{mean} = \frac{\text{sum of the data values}}{\text{quantity of data values}}$$

For instance, the mean of the data set {88, 72, 61, 90, 97, 68, 88, 79, 86, 93, 97, 71, 80, 84, 89} would be the sum of the fifteen numbers divided by 15:

$$\frac{88 + 72 + 61 + 90 + 97 + 68 + 88 + 79 + 86 + 93 + 97 + 71 + 80 + 84 + 88}{15} = \frac{1242}{15}$$
$$= 82.8$$

While the mean is relatively easy to calculate and averages are understood by most people, the mean can be very misleading if used as the sole measure of central tendency. If the data set has outliers (data values that are unusually high or unusually low compared to the rest of the data values), the mean can be very distorted, especially if the data set has a small number of values. If unusually high values are countered with unusually low values, the mean is not affected as much. For example, if five of twenty students in a class get a 100 on a test, but the other 15 students have an average of 60 on the same test, the class average would appear as 70. Whenever the mean is skewed by outliers, it is always a good idea to include the median as an alternate measure of central tendency.

A **weighted mean**, or weighted average, is a mean that uses "weighted" values. The formula is weighted mean $= \frac{w_1 x_1 + w_2 x_2 + w_3 x_3 \ldots + w_n x_n}{w_1 + w_2 + w_3 + \cdots + w_n}$. Weighted values, such as $w_1, w_2, w_3, \ldots w_n$ are assigned to each member of the set $x_1, x_2, x_3, \ldots x_n$. If calculating weighted mean, make sure a weight value for each member of the set is used.

## MEDIAN

The **statistical median** is the value in the middle of the set of data. To find the median, list all data values in order from smallest to largest or from largest to smallest. Any value that is repeated in the set must be listed the number of times it appears. If there are an odd number of data values, the median is the value in the middle of the list. If there is an even number of data values, the median is the arithmetic mean of the two middle values.

For example, the median of the data set {88, 72, 61, 90, 97, 68, 88, 79, 86, 93, 97, 71, 80, 84, 88} is 86 since the ordered set is {61, 68, 71, 72, 79, 80, 84, **86**, 88, 88, 88, 90, 93, 97, 97}.

The big disadvantage of using the median as a measure of central tendency is that is relies solely on a value's relative size as compared to the other values in the set. When the individual values in a set of data are evenly dispersed, the median can be an accurate tool. However, if there is a group of rather large values or a group of rather small values that are not offset by a different group of values, the information that can be inferred from the median may not be accurate because the distribution of values is skewed.

## MODE

The **statistical mode** is the data value that occurs the greatest number of times in the data set. It is possible to have exactly one mode, more than one mode, or no mode. To find the mode of a set of data, arrange the data like you do to find the median (all values in order, listing all multiples of data values). Count the number of times each value appears in the data set. If all values appear an equal number of times, there is no mode. If one value appears more than any other value, that value is the mode. If two or more values appear the same number of times, but there are other values that appear fewer times and no values that appear more times, all of those values are the modes.

For example, the mode of the data set {**88**, 72, 61, 90, 97, 68, **88**, 79, 86, 93, 97, 71, 80, 84, **88**} is 88.

The main disadvantage of the mode is that the values of the other data in the set have no bearing on the mode. The mode may be the largest value, the smallest value, or a value anywhere in between in the set. The mode only tells which value or values, if any, occurred the greatest number of times. It does not give any suggestions about the remaining values in the set.

> **Review Video: Mean, Median, and Mode**
> Visit mometrix.com/academy and enter code: 286207

## DISPERSION

A **measure of dispersion** is a single value that helps to "interpret" the measure of central tendency by providing more information about how the data values in the set are distributed about the measure of central tendency. The measure of dispersion helps to eliminate or reduce the disadvantages of using the mean, median, or mode as a single measure of central tendency, and give a more accurate picture of the dataset as a whole. To have a measure of dispersion, you must know or calculate the range, standard deviation, or variance of the data set.

## RANGE

The **range** of a set of data is the difference between the greatest and lowest values of the data in the set. To calculate the range, you must first make sure the units for all data values are the same, and then identify the greatest and lowest values. If there are multiple data values that are equal for the highest or lowest, just use one of the values in the formula. Write the answer with the same units as the data values you used to do the calculations.

## SKEWNESS

**Skewness** is a way to describe the symmetry or asymmetry of the distribution of values in a dataset. If the distribution of values is symmetrical, there is no skew. In general the closer the mean of a data set is to the median of the data set, the less skew there is. Generally, if the mean is to the right of the median, the data set is *positively skewed*, or right-skewed, and if the mean is to the left of the median, the data set is *negatively skewed*, or left-skewed. However, this rule of thumb is not infallible. When the data values are graphed on a curve, a set with no skew will be a perfect bell curve.

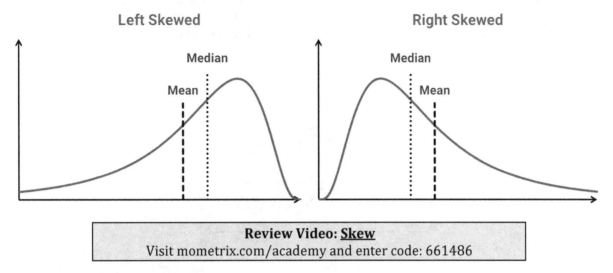

**Review Video: Skew**
Visit mometrix.com/academy and enter code: 661486

### UNIMODAL VS. BIMODAL

If a distribution has a single peak, it would be considered **unimodal**. If it has two discernible peaks it would be considered **bimodal**. Bimodal distributions may be an indication that the set of data being considered is actually the combination of two sets of data with significant differences. A **uniform distribution** is a distribution in which there is *no distinct peak or variation* in the data. No values or ranges are particularly more common than any other values or ranges.

# Displaying Information

### FREQUENCY TABLES

**Frequency tables** show how frequently each unique value appears in the set. A **relative frequency table** is one that shows the proportions of each unique value compared to the entire set. Relative frequencies are given as percentages; however, the total percent for a relative frequency table will not necessarily equal 100 percent due to rounding. An example of a frequency table with relative frequencies is below.

| Favorite Color | Frequency | Relative Frequency |
|---|---|---|
| Blue | 4 | 13% |
| Red | 7 | 22% |
| Green | 3 | 9% |
| Purple | 6 | 19% |
| Cyan | 12 | 38% |

**Review Video: Data Interpretation of Graphs**
Visit mometrix.com/academy and enter code: 200439

### LINE GRAPHS

**Line graphs** have one or more lines of varying styles (solid or broken) to show the different values for a set of data. The individual data are represented as ordered pairs, much like on a Cartesian plane. In this case, the *x*- and *y*-axes are defined in terms of their units, such as dollars or time. The individual plotted points are joined by line segments to show whether the value of the data is increasing (line sloping upward), decreasing (line sloping downward), or staying the same (horizontal line). Multiple sets of data can be graphed on the same line graph to give an easy visual comparison. An example of this would be graphing achievement test scores for different groups of students over the same time period to see which group had the greatest increase or decrease in performance from year to year (as shown below).

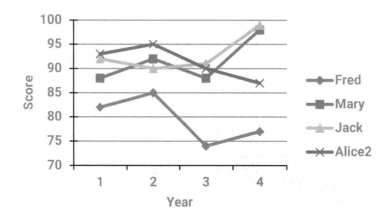

**Review Video: <u>Line Graphs</u>**
Visit mometrix.com/academy and enter code: 480147

## LINE PLOTS

A **line plot**, also known as a *dot plot*, has plotted points that are not connected by line segments. In this graph, the horizontal axis lists the different possible values for the data, and the vertical axis lists the number of times the individual value occurs. A single dot is graphed for each value to show the number of times it occurs. This graph is more closely related to a bar graph than a line graph. Do not connect the dots in a line plot or it will misrepresent the data.

**Review Video: <u>Line Plot</u>**
Visit mometrix.com/academy and enter code: 754610

## BAR GRAPHS

A **bar graph** is one of the few graphs that can be drawn correctly in two different configurations – both horizontally and vertically. A bar graph is similar to a line plot in the way the data is organized on the graph. Both axes must have their categories defined for the graph to be useful. Rather than placing a single dot to mark the point of the data's value, a bar, or thick line, is drawn from zero to the exact value of the data, whether it is a number, percentage, or other numerical value. Longer bar lengths correspond to greater data values. To read a bar graph, read the labels for the axes to find the units being reported. Then, look where the bars end in relation to the scale given on the corresponding axis and determine the associated value.

The bar chart below represents the responses from our favorite-color survey.

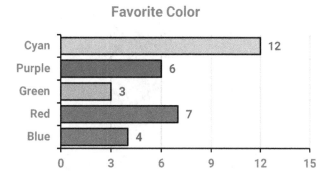

## HISTOGRAMS

At first glance, a **histogram** looks like a vertical bar graph. The difference is that a bar graph has a separate bar for each piece of data and a histogram has one continuous bar for each *range* of data. For example, a histogram may have one bar for the range 0–9, one bar for 10–19, etc. While a bar graph has numerical values on one axis, a histogram has numerical values on both axes. Each range is of equal size, and they are ordered left to right from lowest to highest. The height of each column on a histogram represents the number of data values within that range. Like a stem and leaf plot, a histogram makes it easy to glance at the graph and quickly determine which range has the greatest quantity of values. A simple example of a histogram is below.

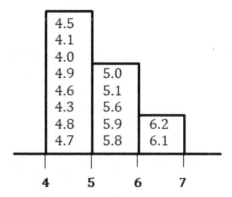

## BIVARIATE DATA

**Bivariate data** is simply data from two different variables. (The prefix *bi-* means *two.*) In a *scatter plot*, each value in the set of data is plotted on a grid similar to a Cartesian plane, where each axis represents one of the two variables. By looking at the pattern formed by the points on the grid, you can often determine whether or not there is a relationship between the two variables, and what that relationship is, if it exists. The variables may be directly proportionate, inversely proportionate, or show no proportion at all. It may also be possible to determine if the data is linear, and if so, to find an equation to relate the two variables. The following scatter plot shows the relationship between preference for brand "A" and the age of the consumers surveyed.

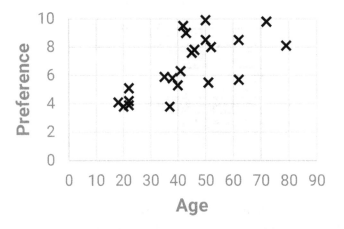

## SCATTER PLOTS

**Scatter plots** are also useful in determining the type of function represented by the data and finding the simple regression. Linear scatter plots may be positive or negative. Nonlinear scatter plots are generally exponential or quadratic. Below are some common types of scatter plots:

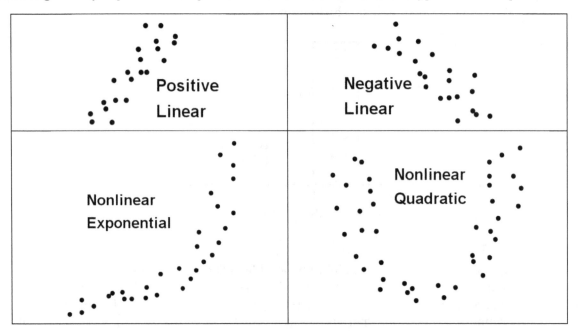

**Review Video: Scatter Plot**
Visit mometrix.com/academy and enter code: 596526

# Science

## Human Anatomy and Physiology

Note: If you already have a solid foundation in Anatomy and Physiology, reviewing this section of the study guide should be sufficient to get you up to speed for the exam. However, if A&P is not a strength for you, and you know you're not close to where you need to be for the TEAS, check out our Anatomy and Physiology Addendum, available on our Additional Bonus Material link: mometrix.com/bonus948/teas6. It approaches the subject more like a textbook would, going into greater depth on each of the A&P topics covered on the TEAS. Good luck!

### GENERAL ANATOMY AND PHYSIOLOGY

#### CELL

The cell is the basic *organizational unit* of all living things. Each piece within a cell has a function that helps organisms grow and survive. There are many different types of cells, but cells are unique to each type of organism. The one thing that all cells have in common is a **membrane**, which is comparable to a semi-permeable plastic bag. The membrane is composed of **phospholipids**. There are also some **transport holes**, which are proteins that help certain molecules and ions move in and out of the cell. The cell is filled with a fluid called **cytoplasm** or cytosol.

Within the cell are a variety of **organelles**, groups of complex molecules that help a cell survive, each with its own unique membrane that has a different chemical makeup from the cell membrane. The larger the cell, the more organelles it will need to live.

> **Review Video: Plant and Animal Cells**
> Visit mometrix.com/academy and enter code: 115568

All organisms, whether plants, animals, fungi, protists, or bacteria, exhibit structural organization on the cellular and organism level. All cells contain **DNA** and **RNA** and can synthesize proteins. Cells are the basic structural units of all organisms. All organisms have a highly organized cellular structure. Each cell consists of **nucleic acids**, **cytoplasm**, and a **cell membrane**. Specialized organelles such as **mitochondria** and **chloroplasts** have specific functions within the cell. In single-celled organisms, that single cell contains all of the components necessary for life. In multicellular organisms, cells can become specialized. Different types of cells can have different functions. Life begins as a single cell whether by **asexual** or **sexual reproduction**. Cells are grouped together in **tissues**. Tissues are grouped together in **organs**. Organs are grouped together in **systems**. An **organism** is a complete individual.

### CELL STRUCTURE

**Ribosomes**: Ribosomes are involved in *synthesizing proteins from amino acids*. They are numerous, making up about one quarter of the cell. Some cells contain thousands of ribosomes. Some are mobile and some are embedded in the rough **endoplasmic reticulum**.

**Golgi complex** (Golgi apparatus): This is involved in *synthesizing materials* such as proteins that are transported out of the cell. It is located near the nucleus and consists of layers of **membranes**.

**Vacuoles**: These are sacs used for *storage, digestion, and waste removal*. There is one large vacuole in plant cells. Animal cells have small, sometimes numerous vacuoles.

**Vesicle**: This is a small organelle within a cell. It has a membrane and performs varying functions, including *moving materials within a cell.*

**Cytoskeleton**: This consists of **microtubules** that help *shape and support the cell.*

**Microtubules**: These are part of the **cytoskeleton** and help *support the cell.* They are made of protein.

**Cytosol**: This is the *liquid material in the cell.* It is mostly water, but also contains some floating molecules.

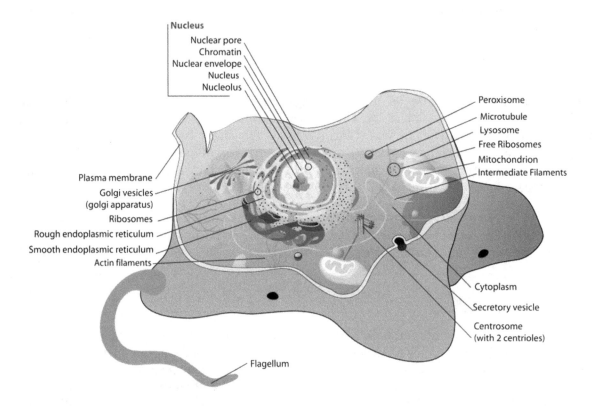

**Cytoplasm**: This is a general term that refers to cytosol and the substructures (organelles) found *within the plasma membrane*, but not within the nucleus.

**Cell membrane** (plasma membrane): This defines the cell by acting as a *barrier*. It helps keeps cytoplasm in and substances located outside the cell out. It also determines what is allowed to enter and exit the cell.

**Endoplasmic reticulum**: The two types of endoplasmic reticulum are **rough** (has ribosomes on the surface) and **smooth** (does not have ribosomes on the surface). It is a tubular network that comprises the *transport system of a cell.* It is fused to the nuclear membrane and extends through the cytoplasm to the cell membrane.

**Mitochondrion** (pl. mitochondria): These cell structures vary in terms of size and quantity. Some cells may have one mitochondrion, while others have thousands. This structure performs various functions such as *generating ATP*, and is also involved in *cell growth and death.* Mitochondria contain their own DNA that is separate from that contained in the nucleus.

MITOCHONDRIA FUNCTIONS

Four functions of mitochondria are: the production of **cell energy**, **cell signaling** (how communications are carried out within a cell, **cellular differentiation** (the process whereby a non-differentiated cell becomes transformed into a cell with a more specialized purpose), and **cell cycle and growth regulation** (the process whereby the cell gets ready to reproduce and reproduces). Mitochondria are numerous in eukaryotic cells. There may be hundreds or even thousands of mitochondria in a single cell. Mitochondria can be involved in many functions, their main one being *supplying the cell with energy*. Mitochondria consist of an inner and outer membrane. The inner membrane encloses the **matrix**, which contains the **mitochondrial DNA** (mtDNA) and ribosomes. Between the inner and outer membranes are **folds** (cristae). Chemical reactions occur here that release energy, control water levels in cells, and recycle and create proteins and fats. **Aerobic respiration** also occurs in the mitochondria.

ANIMAL CELL STRUCTURE

**Centrosome**: This is comprised of the pair of **centrioles** located at right angles to each other and surrounded by protein. The centrosome is involved in *mitosis and the cell cycle*.

**Centrioles**: These are cylinder-shaped structures near the nucleus that are involved in *cellular division*. Each cylinder consists of nine groups of three **microtubules**. Centrioles occur in pairs.

**Lysosome**: This *digests proteins, lipids, and carbohydrates*, and also *transports undigested substances* to the cell membrane so they can be removed. The shape of a lysosome depends on the material being transported.

**Cilia** (singular: cilium): These are appendages extending from the surface of the cell, the movement of which *causes the cell to move*. They can also result in fluid being moved by the cell.

**Flagella**: These are tail-like structures on cells that use whip-like movements to *help the cell move*. They are similar to cilia, but are usually longer and not as numerous. A cell usually only has one or a few flagella.

*NUCLEAR PARTS OF A CELL*

- **Nucleus** (pl. nuclei): This is a small structure that contains the **chromosomes** and regulates the **DNA** of a cell. The nucleus is the defining structure of **eukaryotic cells**, and all eukaryotic cells have a nucleus. The nucleus is responsible for the passing on of genetic traits between generations. The nucleus contains a *nuclear envelope, nucleoplasm, a nucleolus, nuclear pores, chromatin, and ribosomes*.
- **Chromosomes**: These are highly condensed, threadlike rods of **DNA**. Short for **deoxyribonucleic acid**, DNA is the genetic material that *stores information about the plant or animal*.
- **Chromatin**: This consists of the DNA and protein that make up **chromosomes**.
- **Nucleolus**: This structure contained within the nucleus consists of protein. It is small, round, does not have a membrane, is involved in **protein synthesis**, and synthesizes and stores **RNA** (**ribonucleic acid**).
- **Nuclear envelope**: This encloses the structures of the nucleus. It consists of inner and outer membranes made of **lipids**.
- **Nuclear pores**: These are involved in the exchange of material between the nucleus and the **cytoplasm**.
- **Nucleoplasm**: This is the liquid within the nucleus, and is similar to cytoplasm.

┌─────────────────────────────────────────────────┐
│ **Review Video: Chromosomes**                   │
│ Visit mometrix.com/academy and enter code: 132083 │
└─────────────────────────────────────────────────┘

## CELL MEMBRANES

The cell membrane, also referred to as the **plasma membrane**, is a thin semipermeable membrane of lipids and proteins. The cell membrane isolates the cell from its external environment while still enabling the cell to communicate with that outside environment. It consists of a **phospholipid bilayer**, or double layer, with the **hydrophilic ends** of the outer layer facing the external environment, the inner layer facing the inside of the cell, and the **hydrophobic ends** facing each other. **Cholesterol** in the cell membrane adds stiffness and flexibility. **Glycolipids** help the cell to recognize other cells of the organisms. The **proteins** in the cell membrane help give the cells shape. Special proteins help the cell communicate with its external environment. Other proteins transport molecules across the cell membrane.

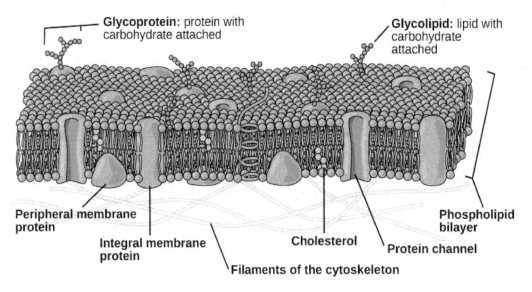

### SELECTIVE PERMEABILITY

The cell membrane, or plasma membrane, has **selective permeability** with regard to size, charge, and solubility. With regard to molecule size, the cell membrane allows only small molecules to diffuse through it. **Oxygen** and **water** molecules are small and typically can pass through the cell membrane. The charge of the **ions** on the cell's surface also either attracts or repels ions. Ions with like charges are repelled, and ions with opposite charges are attracted to the cell's surface. Molecules that are soluble in **phospholipids** can usually pass through the cell membrane. Many molecules are not able to diffuse the cell membrane, and, if needed, those molecules must be moved through by active transport and **vesicles**.

## CELL CYCLE

The term cell cycle refers to the process by which a cell **reproduces**, which involves *cell growth, the duplication of genetic material, and cell division*. Complex organisms with many cells use the cell cycle to replace cells as they lose their functionality and wear out. The entire cell cycle in animal cells can take 24 hours. The time required varies among different cell types. Human skin cells, for example, are constantly reproducing. Some other cells only divide infrequently. Once neurons are mature, they do not grow or divide. The two ways that cells can reproduce are through meiosis and mitosis. When cells replicate through **mitosis**, the "daughter cell" is an *exact replica* of the parent cell. When cells divide through **meiosis**, the daughter cells have *different genetic coding* than the parent cell. Meiosis only happens in specialized reproductive cells called **gametes**.

## CELL DIFFERENTIATION

The human body is filled with many different types of cells. The process that helps to determine the cell type for each cell is known as **differentiation**. Another way to say this is when *a less-specialized cell becomes a more-specialized cell*. This process is controlled by the genes of each cell among a group of cells known as a **zygote**. Following the directions of the genes, a cell builds certain proteins and other pieces that set it apart as a specific type of cell.

An example occurs with **gastrulation**—an early phase in the embryonic development of most animals. During gastrulation, the cells are organized into three primary germ layers: **ectoderm**, **mesoderm**, and **endoderm**. Then, the cells in these layers differentiate into special tissues and organs. For example, the *nervous system* develops from the ectoderm. The *muscular system* develops from the mesoderm. Much of the *digestive system* develops from the endoderm.

## MITOSIS

The primary events that occur during mitosis are:

- **Interphase**: The cell prepares for division by replicating its genetic and cytoplasmic material. Interphase can be further divided into $G_1$, S, and $G_2$.
- **Prophase**: The **chromatin** thickens into chromosomes and the **nuclear membrane** begins to disintegrate. Pairs of **centrioles** move to opposite sides of the cell and spindle fibers begin to form. The **mitotic spindle**, formed from cytoskeleton parts, moves chromosomes around within the cell.
- **Metaphase**: The spindle moves to the center of the cell and chromosome pairs align along the center of the spindle structure.
- **Anaphase**: The pairs of chromosomes, called sisters, begin to pull apart, and may bend. When they are separated, they are called **daughter chromosomes**. Grooves appear in the cell membrane.
- **Telophase**: The spindle disintegrates, the nuclear membranes reform, and the chromosomes revert to chromatin. In animal cells, the membrane is pinched. In plant cells, a new cell wall begins to form.
- **Cytokinesis**: This is the physical splitting of the cell (including the cytoplasm) into two cells. Some believe this occurs following telophase. Others say it occurs from anaphase, as the cell begins to furrow, through telophase, when the cell actually splits into two.

> **Review Video: Cellular Division: Mitosis and Meiosis**
> Visit mometrix.com/academy and enter code: 109813

## MEIOSIS

Meiosis has the same phases as mitosis, but they happen twice. In addition, different events occur during some phases of meiosis than mitosis. The events that occur during the first phase of meiosis are interphase (I), prophase (I), metaphase (I), anaphase (I), telophase (I), and cytokinesis (I). During this first phase of meiosis, *chromosomes cross over, genetic material is exchanged, and tetrads of four chromatids are formed*. The nuclear membrane dissolves. Homologous pairs of chromatids are separated and travel to different poles. At this point, there has been one cell division resulting in two cells. Each cell goes through a second cell division, which consists of prophase (II), metaphase (II), anaphase (II), telophase (II), and cytokinesis (II). The result is *four daughter cells* with different sets of chromosomes. The daughter cells are **haploid**, which means they contain half the genetic material of the parent cell. The second phase of meiosis is similar to the process of mitosis. Meiosis encourages genetic diversity.

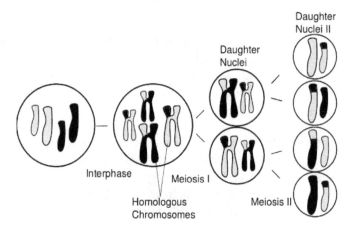

### TISSUES

Tissues are groups of cells that work together to perform a specific function. Tissues are divided into broad categories based on their function. Animal tissues may be divided into seven categories:

- **Epithelial** – Tissue in which cells are joined together tightly. *Skin* tissue is an example.
- **Connective** – Connective tissue may be dense, loose, or fatty. It protects and binds body parts. Connective tissues include *bone tissue, cartilage, tendons, ligaments, fat, blood, and lymph.*
- **Cartilage** – Cushions and provides structural support for body parts. It has a jelly-like base and is fibrous.
- **Blood** – Blood transports oxygen to cells and removes wastes. It also carries hormones and defends against disease.
- **Bone** – Bone is a hard tissue that supports and protects softer tissues and organs. Its marrow produces red blood cells.
- **Muscle** – Muscle tissue helps support and move the body. The three types of muscle tissue are *smooth, cardiac, and skeletal.*
- **Nervous** – Nerve tissue is located in the *brain, spinal cord, and nerves.* Cells called neurons form a network through the body that control responses to changes in the external and internal environment. Some send signals to muscles and glands to trigger responses.

### ORGANS

Organs are groups of tissues that work together to perform specific functions. Complex animals have several organs that are grouped together in multiple **systems**. For example, the **heart** is specifically designed to pump blood throughout an organism's body. The heart is composed mostly of muscle tissue in the myocardium, but it also contains connective tissue in the blood and membranes, nervous tissue that controls the heart rate, and epithelial tissue in the membranes. Gills in fish and lungs in reptiles, birds, and mammals are specifically designed to exchange gases. In birds, crops are designed to store food and gizzards are designed to grind food.

Organ systems are groups of organs that work together to perform specific functions. In mammals, there are 11 major organ systems: **integumentary system**, **respiratory system**, **cardiovascular system**, **endocrine system**, **nervous system**, **immune system**, **digestive system**, **excretory system**, **muscular system**, **skeletal system**, and **reproductive system**.

## TERMS OF DIRECTION

**Medial** means *nearer to the midline* of the body. In anatomical position, the little finger is medial to the thumb.

**Lateral** is the opposite of medial. It refers to structures *further away from the body's midline*, at the sides. In anatomical position, the thumb is lateral to the little finger.

**Proximal** refers to structures *closer to the center* of the body. The hip is proximal to the knee.

**Distal** refers to structures *further away from the center* of the body. The knee is distal to the hip.

**Anterior** refers to structures in *front*.

**Posterior** refers to structures *behind*.

**Cephalad** and **cephalic** are adverbs meaning towards the *head*. **Cranial** is the adjective, meaning of the *skull*.

**Caudad** is an adverb meaning towards the *tail* or posterior. **Caudal** is the adjective, meaning of the *hindquarters*.

**Superior** means *above*, or closer to the head.

**Inferior** means *below*, or closer to the feet.

## THE THREE PRIMARY BODY PLANES

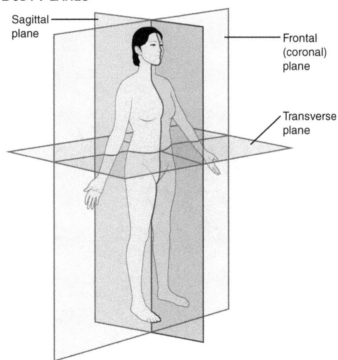

The **transverse (or horizontal) plane** divides the patient's body into imaginary upper (*superior*) and lower (*inferior or caudal*) halves.

The **sagittal plane** divides the body, or any body part, vertically into right and left sections. The sagittal plane runs parallel to the midline of the body.

The **coronal (or frontal) plane** divides the body, or any body structure, vertically into front and back (*anterior* and *posterior*) sections. The coronal plane runs vertically through the body at right angles to the midline.

## RESPIRATORY SYSTEM
### STRUCTURE OF THE RESPIRATORY SYSTEM

The respiratory system can be divided into the upper and lower respiratory system. The **upper respiratory system** includes the nose, nasal cavity, mouth, pharynx, and larynx. The **lower respiratory system** includes the trachea, lungs, and bronchial tree. Alternatively, the components of the respiratory system can be categorized as part of the airway, the lungs, or the respiratory muscles. The **airway** includes the nose, nasal cavity, mouth, pharynx, (throat), larynx (voice box), trachea (windpipe), bronchi, and bronchial network. The airway is lined with **cilia** that trap microbes and debris and sweep them back toward the mouth. The **lungs** are structures that house the **bronchi** and bronchial network, which extend into the lungs and terminate in millions of **alveoli** (air sacs). The walls of the alveoli are only one cell thick, allowing for the exchange of gases with the blood capillaries that surround them. The right lung has three lobes. The left lung only has two lobes, leaving room for the heart on the left side of the body. The lungs are surrounded by a **pleural membrane**, which reduces friction between surfaces when breathing. The respiratory muscles include the **diaphragm** and the **intercostal muscles**. The diaphragm is a dome-shaped muscle that separates the thoracic and abdominal cavities. The intercostal muscles are located between the ribs.

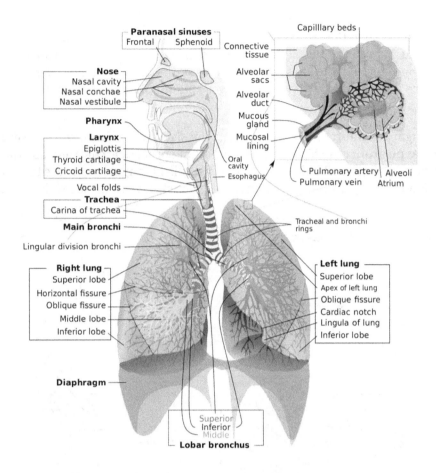

**Review Video: Respiratory System**
Visit mometrix.com/academy and enter code: 783075

## FUNCTIONS OF THE RESPIRATORY SYSTEM

The main function of the respiratory system is to supply the body with **oxygen** and rid the body of **carbon dioxide**. This exchange of gases occurs in millions of tiny **alveoli**, which are surrounded by blood capillaries.

The respiratory system also filters air. Air is warmed, moistened, and filtered as it passes through the nasal passages before it reaches the lungs.

The respiratory system is responsible for speech. As air passes through the throat, it moves through the **larynx** (voice box), which vibrates and produces sound, before it enters the **trachea** (windpipe). The respiratory system is vital in cough production. Foreign particles entering the nasal passages or airways are expelled from the body by the respiratory system.

The respiratory system functions in the sense of smell. **Chemoreceptors** that are located in the nasal cavity respond to airborne chemicals. The respiratory system also helps the body maintain acid-base **homeostasis**. Hyperventilation can increase blood pH during **acidosis** (low pH). Slowing breathing during **alkalosis** (high pH) helps to lower blood pH.

### BREATHING PROCESS

During the breathing process, the **diaphragm** and the **intercostal muscles** contract to expand the lungs.

During **inspiration** or inhalation, the diaphragm contracts and moves down, increasing the size of the chest cavity. The intercostal muscles contract and the ribs expand, increasing the size of the **chest cavity**. As the volume of the chest cavity increases, the pressure inside the chest cavity decreases. Because the outside air is under a greater amount of pressure than the air inside the lungs, air rushes into the lungs.

When the diaphragm and intercostal muscles relax, the size of the chest cavity decreases, forcing air out of the lungs (**expiration** or exhalation). The breathing process is controlled by the portion of the brain stem called the **medulla oblongata**. The medulla oblongata monitors the level of carbon dioxide in the blood and signals the breathing rate to increase when these levels are too high.

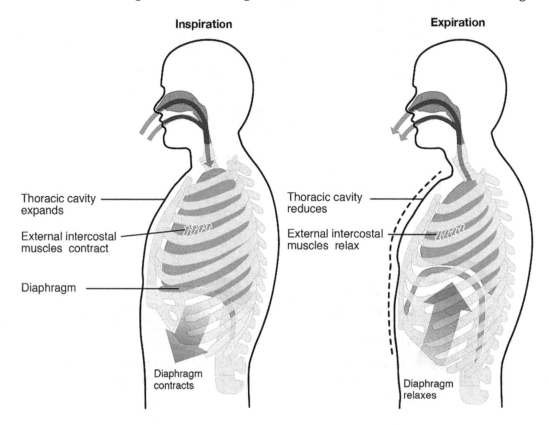

## CARDIOVASCULAR SYSTEM

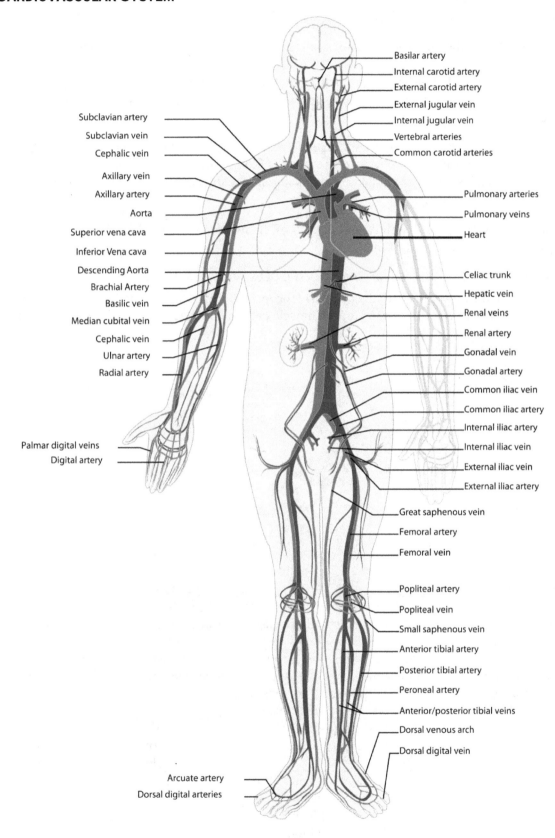

The **circulatory system** is responsible for the internal transport of substances to and from the cells. The circulatory system usually consists of the following three parts:

- **Blood** – Blood is composed of water, solutes, and other elements in a fluid connective tissue.
- **Blood Vessels** – Tubules of different sizes that transport blood.
- **Heart** – The heart is a muscular pump providing the pressure necessary to keep blood flowing.

Circulatory systems can be either **open** or **closed**. Most animals have closed systems, where the *heart and blood vessels are continually connected*. As the blood moves through the system from larger tubules through smaller ones, the rate slows down. The flow of blood in the **capillary beds**, the smallest tubules, is quite slow.

A supplementary system, the **lymph vascular system**, cleans up excess fluids and proteins and returns them to the circulatory system.

### ARTERIAL AND VENOUS SYSTEMS (ARTERIES, ARTERIOLES, VENULES, VEINS)

The walls of all blood vessels (except the capillaries) consist of three layers: the innermost **tunica intima**, the **tunica media** consisting of smooth muscle cells and elastic fibers, and the outer **tunica adventitia**.

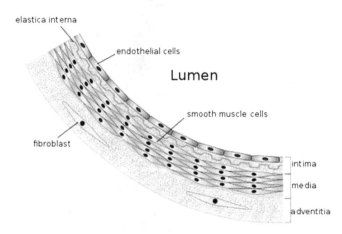

| Vessel | Structure | Function |
|---|---|---|
| Elastic arteries | Includes the aorta and major branches Tunica media has more elastin than any other vessels Largest vessels in the arterial system | Stretch when blood is forced out of the heart, and recoil under low pressure |
| Muscular arteries | Includes the arteries that branch off of the elastic arteries Tunica media has a higher proportion of smooth muscle cells, and fewer elastic fibers as compared to elastic arteries | Regulate blood flow by vasoconstriction / vasodilation |
| Arterioles | Tiny vessels that lead to the capillary beds Tunica media is thin, but composed almost entirely smooth muscle cells | Primary vessels involved in vasoconstriction / vasodilation Control blood flow to capillaries |
| Venules | Tiny vessels that exit the capillary beds Thin, porous walls; few muscle cells and elastic fibers | Empty blood into larger veins |
| Veins | Thin tunica media and tunica intima Wide lumen Valves prevent backflow of blood | Carry blood back to the heart |

## Blood

Blood helps maintain a healthy internal environment in animals by *carrying raw materials to cells* and *removing waste products*. It helps stabilize internal pH and hosts various kinds of infection fighters.

An adult human has about five quarts of blood. Blood is composed of **red and white blood cells**, **platelets**, and **plasma**. Plasma constitutes over half of the blood volume. It is mostly water and serves as a solvent. Plasma contains plasma proteins, ions, glucose, amino acids, hormones, and dissolved gases.

Red blood cells transport **oxygen** to cells. Red blood cells form in the bone marrow and can live for about four months. These cells are constantly being replaced by fresh ones, keeping the total number relatively stable.

White blood cells defend the body against **infection** and remove various wastes. The types of white blood cells include lymphocytes, neutrophils, monocytes, eosinophils, and basophils. **Platelets** are fragments of stem cells and serve an important function in *blood clotting*.

## Heart

The heart is a muscular pump made of **cardiac muscle tissue**. It has four chambers; each half contains both an **atrium** and a **ventricle**, and the halves are separated by a valve, known as the AV valve. It is located between the ventricle and the artery leading away from the heart. Valves keep blood moving in a single direction and prevent any backwash into the chambers.

The heart has its own circulatory system with its own **coronary arteries**.

The heart functions by contracting and relaxing. **Atrial contraction** fills the ventricles and **ventricular contraction** empties them, forcing circulation. This sequence is called the **cardiac cycle**.

Cardiac muscles are attached to each other and signals for contractions spread rapidly. A complex electrical system controls the heartbeat as cardiac muscle cells produce and conduct electric signals. These muscles are said to be **self-exciting**, needing no external stimuli.

## Cardiac Cycle

The cardiac cycle consists of **diastole** and **systole** phases, which can be further divided into the first and second phases to describe the events of the right and left sides of the heart. However, these events are simultaneously occurring. During the first diastole phase, blood flows through the **superior** and **inferior venae cavae**. Because the heart is relaxed, blood flows passively from the atrium through the open **atrioventricular valve** (tricuspid valve) to the right ventricle. The **sinoatrial (SA) node**, the cardiac pacemaker located in the wall of the right atrium, generates electrical signals, which are carried by the **Purkinje fibers** to the rest of the atrium, stimulating it to contract and fill the right ventricle with blood. The impulse from the SA node is transmitted to the ventricle through the atrioventricular (AV) node, signaling the right ventricle to contract and initiating the first systole phase. The tricuspid valve closes, and the **pulmonary semilunar valve** opens. Blood is pumped out the **pulmonary arteries** to the lungs. Blood returning from the lungs fills the left atrium as part of the second diastole phase. The SA node triggers the **mitral valve** to open, and blood fills the left ventricle. During the second systole phase, the mitral valve closes and the **aortic semilunar valve** opens. The left ventricle contracts, and blood is pumped out of the aorta to the rest of the body. The path of blood through the heart is traced in the diagram below:

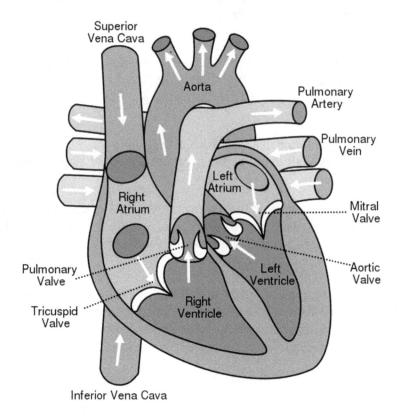

## TYPES OF CIRCULATION

The **circulatory system** includes coronary circulation, pulmonary circulation, and systemic circulation. **Coronary circulation** is the flow of blood to the heart tissue. Blood enters the **coronary arteries**, which branch off the aorta, supplying major arteries, which enter the heart with oxygenated blood. The deoxygenated blood returns to the right atrium through the **cardiac veins**, which empty into the **coronary sinus**. **Pulmonary circulation** is the flow of blood between the heart and the lungs. Deoxygenated blood flows from the right ventricle to the lungs through **pulmonary arteries**. Oxygenated blood flows back to the left atrium through the **pulmonary veins**. **Systemic circulation** is the flow of blood to the entire body with the exception of coronary circulation and pulmonary circulation. Blood exits the left ventricle through the aorta, which branches into the *carotid arteries, subclavian arteries, common iliac arteries, and the renal artery*. Blood returns to the heart through the *jugular veins, subclavian veins, common iliac veins, and renal veins*, which empty into the **superior** and **inferior venae cavae**. Included in systemic circulation is **portal circulation**, which is the flow of blood from the digestive system to the liver and then to the heart, and **renal circulation**, which is the flow of blood between the heart and the kidneys.

## BLOOD PRESSURE

Blood pressure is the fluid pressure generated by the cardiac cycle.

**Arterial blood pressure** functions by transporting oxygen-poor blood into the lungs and oxygen-rich blood to the body tissues. **Arteries** branch into smaller arterioles which contract and expand based on signals from the body. **Arterioles** are where adjustments are made in blood delivery to specific areas based on complex communication from body systems.

**Capillary beds** are diffusion sites for exchanges between blood and interstitial fluid. A capillary has the thinnest wall of any blood vessel, consisting of a single layer of **endothelial cells**.

Capillaries merge into venules, which in turn merge with larger diameter tubules called **veins**. Veins transport blood from body tissues *back to the heart*. Valves inside the veins facilitate this transport. The walls of veins are thin and contain smooth muscle and also function as blood volume reserves.

## LYMPHATIC SYSTEM

The main function of the **lymphatic system** is to *return excess tissue fluid to the bloodstream*. This system consists of transport vessels and lymphoid organs. The lymph vascular system consists of **lymph capillaries**, **lymph vessels**, and **lymph ducts**. The major functions of the lymph vascular system are:

- The return of excess fluid to the blood.
- The return of protein from the capillaries.
- The transport of fats from the digestive tract.
- The disposal of debris and cellular waste.

**Lymphoid organs** include the lymph nodes, spleen, appendix, adenoids, thymus, tonsils, and small patches of tissue in the small intestine. **Lymph nodes** are located at intervals throughout the lymph vessel system. Each node contains **lymphocytes** and **plasma cells**. The **spleen** filters blood stores of red blood cells and macrophages. The **thymus** secretes hormones and is the major site of lymphocyte production.

## SPLEEN

The spleen is in the upper left of the abdomen. It is located behind the stomach and immediately below the diaphragm. It is about the size of a thick paperback book and weighs just over half a pound. It is made up of **lymphoid tissue**. The blood vessels are connected to the spleen by **splenic sinuses** (modified capillaries). The following **peritoneal ligaments** support the spleen:

- The **gastrolienal ligament** connects the stomach to the spleen.
- The **lienorenal ligament** connects the kidney to the spleen.
- The middle section of the **phrenicocolic ligament** (connects the left colic flexure to the thoracic diaphragm).

The main functions of the spleen are to *filter unwanted materials* from the blood (including old red blood cells) and to help *fight infections*. Up to ten percent of the population has one or more accessory spleens that tend to form at the **hilum** of the original spleen.

## GASTROINTESTINAL SYSTEM

Most digestive systems function by the following means:

- **Movement** – Movement mixes and passes nutrients through the system and eliminates waste.
- **Secretion** – Enzymes, hormones, and other substances necessary for digestion are secreted into the digestive tract.

- **Digestion** – Includes the chemical breakdown of nutrients into smaller units that enter the internal environment.
- **Absorption** – The passage of nutrients through plasma membranes into the blood or lymph and then to the body.

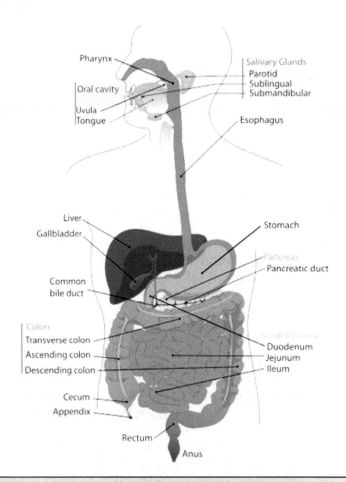

| Review Video: **Gastrointestinal System** |
| :---: |
| Visit mometrix.com/academy and enter code: 378740 |

### MOUTH AND STOMACH

Digestion begins in the mouth with the chewing and mixing of nutrients with **saliva**. Only humans and other mammals actually chew their food. **Salivary glands** are stimulated and secrete saliva. Saliva contains **enzymes** that initiate the breakdown of starch in digestion. Once swallowed, the food moves down the **pharynx** into the **esophagus** en route to the stomach.

The **stomach** is a flexible, muscular sac. It has three main functions:

- Mixing and storing food
- Dissolving and degrading food via secretions
- Controlling passage of food into the small intestine

Protein digestion begins in the stomach. Stomach acidity helps break down the food and make nutrients available for absorption. Smooth muscle moves the food by **peristalsis**, contracting and relaxing to move nutrients along. Smooth muscle contractions move nutrients into the small intestine where the **absorption** process begins.

## LIVER

The liver is the largest solid organ of the body. It is also the largest gland. It weighs about three pounds and is located below the diaphragm on the right side of the chest. The liver is made up of four **lobes**. They are called the *right, left, quadrate, and caudate lobes*. The liver is secured to the diaphragm and abdominal walls by five **ligaments**. They are called the *falciform* (that forms a membrane-like barrier between the right and left lobes), *coronary, right triangular, left triangular, and round ligaments*.

The liver processes all of the blood that passes through the digestive system. Nutrient-rich blood is supplied to the liver via the **hepatic portal vein**. The **hepatic artery** supplies oxygen-rich blood. Blood leaves the liver through the **hepatic veins**. The liver's functional units are called **lobules** (made up of layers of liver cells). Blood enters the lobules through branches of the portal vein and hepatic artery. The blood then flows through small channels called **sinusoids**.

The liver is responsible for performing many vital functions in the body including:

- Production of **bile**
- Production of certain **blood plasma proteins**
- Production of **cholesterol** (and certain proteins needed to carry fats)
- Storage of excess glucose in the form of **glycogen** (that can be converted back to glucose when needed)
- Regulation of **amino acids**
- Processing of **hemoglobin** (to store iron)
- Conversion of ammonia (that is poisonous to the body) to **urea** (a waste product excreted in urine)
- **Purification** of the blood (clears out drugs and other toxins)
- Regulation of **blood clotting**
- Controlling infections by boosting **immune factors** and removing bacteria.

The nutrients (and drugs) that pass through the liver are converted into forms that are appropriate for the body to use.

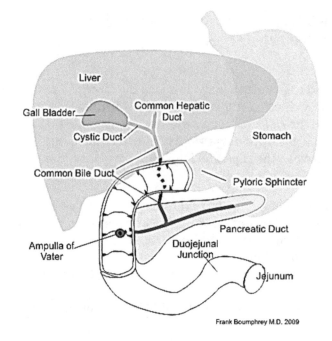

Frank Boumphrey M.D. 2009

## PANCREAS

The pancreas is six to ten inches long and located at the back of the abdomen behind the stomach. It is a long, tapered organ. The wider (right) side is called the **head** and the narrower (left) side is called the **tail**. The head lies near the **duodenum** (the first part of the small intestine) and the tail ends near the **spleen**. The body of the pancreas lies between the head and the tail. The pancreas is made up of exocrine and endocrine tissues. The **exocrine tissue** secretes digestive enzymes from a series of ducts that collectively form the main pancreatic duct (that runs the length of the pancreas). The **main pancreatic duct** connects to the common bile duct near the duodenum. The **endocrine tissue** secretes hormones (such as insulin) into the bloodstream. Blood is supplied to the pancreas from the *splenic artery, gastroduodenal artery, and the superior mesenteric artery.*

### DIGESTIVE ROLE OF PANCREAS

The pancreas assists in the digestion of foods by secreting **enzymes** (to the small intestine) that help to break down many foods, especially fats and proteins.

The precursors to these enzymes (called **zymogens**) are produced by groups of exocrine cells (called **acini**). They are converted, through a chemical reaction in the gut, to the active enzymes (such as **pancreatic lipase** and **amylase**) once they enter the small intestine. The pancreas also secretes large amounts of **sodium bicarbonate** to neutralize the stomach acid that reaches the small intestine.

The **exocrine** functions of the pancreas are controlled by hormones released by the stomach and small intestine (duodenum) when food is present. The exocrine secretions of the pancreas flow into the main pancreatic duct (**Wirsung's duct**) and are delivered to the duodenum through the pancreatic duct.

## SMALL INTESTINE

In the digestive process, most nutrients are absorbed in the **small intestine**. Enzymes from the pancreas, liver, and stomach are transported to the small intestine to aid digestion. These enzymes act on *fats, carbohydrates, nucleic acids, and proteins*. **Bile** is a secretion of the liver and is particularly useful in breaking down fats. It is stored in the **gall bladder** between meals.

By the time food reaches the lining of the small intestine, it has been reduced to small molecules. The lining of the small intestine is covered with **villi**, tiny absorptive structures that greatly increase the surface area for interaction with chyme (the semi-liquid mass of partially digested food). Epithelial cells at the surface of the villi, called **microvilli**, further increase the ability of the small intestine to serve as the *main absorption organ* of the digestive tract.

### LARGE INTESTINE

Also called the **colon**, the large intestine concentrates, mixes, and stores waste material. A little over a meter in length, the colon ascends on the right side of the abdominal cavity, cuts across transversely to the left side, then descends and attaches to the **rectum**, a short tube for waste disposal.

When the rectal wall is distended by waste material, the nervous system triggers an impulse in the body to expel the waste from the rectum. A muscle **sphincter** at the end of the **anus** is stimulated to facilitate the expelling of waste matter.

The speed at which waste moves through the colon is influenced by the volume of fiber and other undigested material present. Without adequate bulk in the diet, it takes longer to move waste along, sometimes with negative effects. Lack of bulk in the diet has been linked to a number of disorders.

## NERVOUS SYSTEM

The human nervous system senses, interprets, and issues commands as a response to conditions in the body's environment. This process is made possible by a very complex communication system organized as a grid of **neurons**.

Messages are sent across the plasma membrane of neurons through a process called **action potential**. These messages occur when a neuron is stimulated past a necessary threshold. These stimulations occur in a sequence from the stimulation point of one neuron to its contact with another neuron. At the point of contact, called a **chemical synapse**, a substance is released that stimulates or inhibits the action of the adjoining cell. This network fans out across the body and forms the framework for the nervous system. The direction the information flows depends on the specific organizations of nerve circuits and pathways.

### FUNCTIONAL TYPES OF NEURONS

The three general functional types of neurons are the sensory neurons, motor neurons, and interneurons. **Sensory neurons** transmit signals to the **central nervous system** (CNS) from the sensory receptors associated with touch, pain, temperature, hearing, sight, smell, and taste. **Motor neurons** transmit signals from the CNS to the rest of the body such as by signaling muscles or glands to respond. **Interneurons** transmit signals between neurons; for example, interneurons receive transmitted signals between sensory neurons and motor neurons. In general, a neuron consists of three basic parts: the cell body, the axon, and many dendrites. The **dendrites** receive **impulses** from sensory receptors or interneurons and transmit them toward the cell body. The **cell body** (soma) contains the nucleus of the neuron. The **axon** transmits the impulses away from the cell body. The axon is insulated by **oligodendrocytes** and the **myelin sheath** with gaps known as the **nodes of Ranvier**. The axon terminates at the synapse.

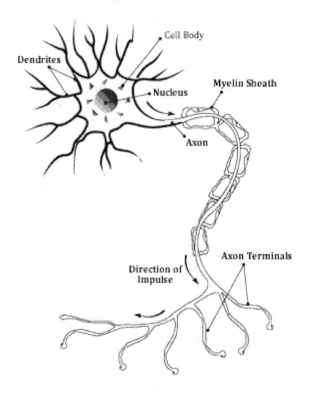

## ORGANIZATION OF VERTEBRATE NERVOUS SYSTEM

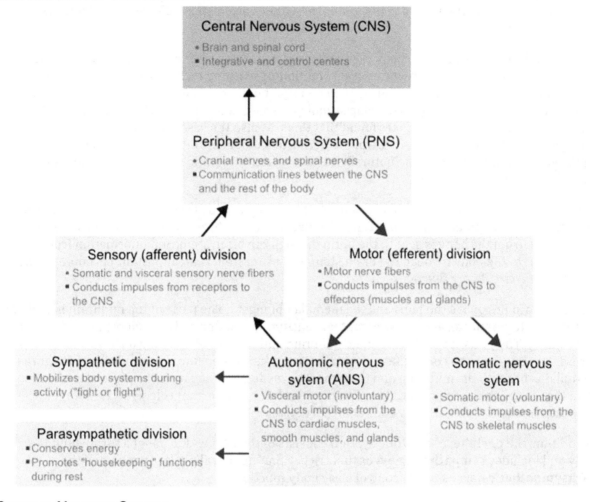

## CENTRAL NERVOUS SYSTEM

There are two primary components of the central nervous system:

### SPINAL CORD

The spinal cord is encased in the bony structure of the **vertebrae**, which protects and supports it. Its nervous tissue functions mainly with respect to limb movement and internal organ activity. Major nerve tracts ascend and descend from the spinal cord to the brain.

### BRAIN

The brain consists of the hindbrain, midbrain, and forebrain. The **hindbrain** includes the **medulla oblongata**, **cerebellum**, and **pons**. The **midbrain** integrates sensory signals and orchestrates responses to these signals. The **forebrain** includes the **cerebrum**, **thalamus**, and **hypothalamus**. The **cerebral cortex** is a thin layer of gray matter covering the cerebrum. The brain is divided into two hemispheres, with each responsible for multiple functions. The brain is divided into four main **lobes**, the frontal lobe, the parietal lobe, the occipital lobe, and the temporal lobes. The **frontal lobe** located in the front of the brain is responsible for a short term and working *memory and information processing* as well as *decision-making, planning, and judgment*. The **parietal lobe** is located slightly toward the back of the brain and the top of the head and is responsible for *sensory input* as well as *spatial positioning of the body*. The **occipital lobe** is located at the back of the head just above the brain stem. This lobe is responsible for *visual input, processing, and output*;

specifically nerves from the eyes enter directly into this lobe. Finally, the **temporal lobes** are located at the left and right sides of the brain. These lobes are responsible for all *auditory input, processing, and output.*

The **cerebellum** plays a role in the processing and storing of *implicit memories.* Specifically, for those memories developed during classical conditioning learning techniques. The role of the cerebellum was discovered by exploring the memory of individuals with damaged cerebellums. These individuals were unable to develop stimulus responses when presented via a classical conditioning technique. Researchers found that this was also the case for automatic responses. For example, when these individuals were presented with a puff of air into their eyes, they did not blink, which would have been the naturally occurring and automatic response in an individual with no brain damage.

The **posterior** area of the brain that is connected to the spinal cord is known as the **brain stem**. The **midbrain**, the **pons**, and the **medulla oblongata** are the three parts of the brain stem. Information from the body is sent to the brain through the brain stem, and information from the brain is sent to the body through the brain stem. The brain stem is an important part of *respiratory, digestive, and circulatory functions.*

The **midbrain** lies above the pons and the medulla oblongata. The parts of the midbrain include the **tectum**, the **tegmentum**, and the **ventral tegmentum**. The midbrain is an important part of *vision and hearing.* The **pons** comes between the midbrain and the medulla oblongata. Information is sent across the pons from the cerebrum to the medulla and the cerebellum. The **medulla oblongata** (or medulla) is beneath the midbrain and the pons. The medulla oblongata is the piece of the brain stem that connects the spinal cord to the brain. So, it has an important role with the autonomic nervous system in the *circulatory and respiratory system.*

In addition, the **peripheral nervous system** consists of the nerves and ganglia throughout the body and includes **sympathetic nerves** that trigger the "fight or flight" response, and the **parasympathetic nerves** which control basic body function.

### AUTONOMIC NERVOUS SYSTEM

The autonomic nervous system (**ANS**) maintains **homeostasis** within the body. In general, the ANS controls the functions of the *internal organs, blood vessels, smooth muscle tissues, and glands.* This is accomplished through the direction of the **hypothalamus**, which is located above the midbrain. The hypothalamus controls the ANS through the brain stem. With this direction from the hypothalamus, the ANS helps maintain a stable body environment (homeostasis) by regulating numerous factors including heart rate, breathing rate, body temperature, and blood pH.

The ANS consists of two divisions: the sympathetic nervous system and the parasympathetic nervous system. The **sympathetic nervous system** controls the body's reaction to extreme, stressful, and emergency situations. For example, the sympathetic nervous system increases the heart rate, signals the adrenal glands to secrete adrenaline, triggers the dilation of the pupils, and slows digestion. The **parasympathetic nervous system** counteracts the effects of the sympathetic nervous system. For example, the parasympathetic nervous system decreases heart rate, signals the adrenal glands to stop secreting adrenaline, constricts the pupils, and returns the digestion process to normal.

> **Review Video: The Nervous System**
> Visit mometrix.com/academy and enter code: 708428

## THE SOMATIC NERVOUS SYSTEM AND THE REFLEX ARC

The somatic nervous system (**SNS**) controls the five senses and the voluntary movement of skeletal muscle. So, this system has all of the neurons that are connected to sense organs. Efferent (motor) and afferent (sensory) nerves help the somatic nervous system operate the senses and the movement of skeletal muscle. **Efferent nerves** bring signals from the central nervous system to the sensory organs and the muscles. **Afferent nerves** bring signals from the sensory organs and the muscles to the central nervous system. The somatic nervous system also performs involuntary movements which are known as reflex arcs.

A **reflex**, the simplest act of the nervous system, is an automatic response without any conscious thought to a stimulus via the reflex arc. The **reflex arc** is the simplest nerve pathway, which bypasses the brain and is controlled by the spinal cord. For example, in the classic knee-jerk response (patellar tendon reflex), the stimulus is the reflex hammer hitting the tendon, and the response is the muscle contracting, which jerks the foot upward. The stimulus is detected by sensory receptors, and a message is sent along a **sensory** (afferent) neuron to one or more **interneurons** in the spinal cord. The interneuron(s) transmit this message to a **motor** (efferent) neuron, which carries the message to the correct **effector** (muscle).

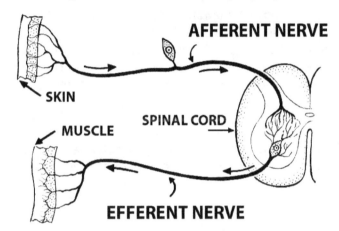

## MUSCULAR SYSTEM

There are three types of muscle tissue: **skeletal**, **cardiac**, and **smooth**. There are over 600 muscles in the human body. All muscles have these three properties in common:

- **Excitability** – All muscle tissues have an *electric gradient* which can reverse when stimulated.
- **Contraction** – All muscle tissues have the ability to contract, or *shorten*.
- **Elongate** – All muscle tissues share the capacity to elongate, or *relax*.

> **Review Video: Muscular System**
> Visit mometrix.com/academy and enter code: 967216

## TYPES OF MUSCULAR TISSUE

The three types of muscular tissue are skeletal muscle, smooth muscle, and cardiac muscle.

**Skeletal muscles** are *voluntary* muscles that work in pairs to move various parts of the skeleton. Skeletal muscles are composed of **muscle fibers** (cells) that are bound together in parallel **bundles**. Skeletal muscles are also known as **striated muscle** due to their striped appearance under a microscope.

**Smooth muscle tissues** are *involuntary* muscles that are found in the walls of internal organs such as the stomach, intestines, and blood vessels. Smooth muscle tissues or **visceral tissue** is nonstriated. Smooth muscle cells are shorter and wider than skeletal muscle fibers. Smooth muscle tissue is also found in sphincters or valves that control various openings throughout the body.

**Cardiac muscle** tissue is *involuntary* muscle that is found only in the heart. Like skeletal muscle cells, cardiac muscle cells are also striated.

Only skeletal muscle interacts with the skeleton to move the body. When they contract, the muscles transmit **force** to the attached bones. Working together, the muscles and bones act as a system of levers which move around the joints. A small contraction of a muscle can produce a large movement. A limb can be extended and rotated around a joint due to the way the muscles are arranged.

### SKELETAL MUSCLE CONTRACTION

Skeletal muscles consist of numerous muscle fibers. Each muscle fiber contains a bundle of **myofibrils**, which are composed of multiple repeating contractile units called **sarcomeres**.

Myofibrils contain two protein **microfilaments**: a thick filament and a thin filament. The thick filament is composed of the protein **myosin**. The thin filament is composed of the protein **actin**. The dark bands (**striations**) in skeletal muscles are formed when thick and thin filaments overlap. Light bands occur where the thin filament is overlapped. Skeletal muscle attraction occurs when the thin filaments slide over the thick filaments, shortening the sarcomere.

When an **action potential** (electrical signal) reaches a muscle fiber, **calcium ions** are released. According to the sliding filament model of muscle contraction, these calcium ions bind to the myosin and actin, which assists in the binding of the **myosin heads** of the thick filaments to the **actin molecules** of the thin filaments. **Adenosine triphosphate** released from glucose provides the energy necessary for the contraction.

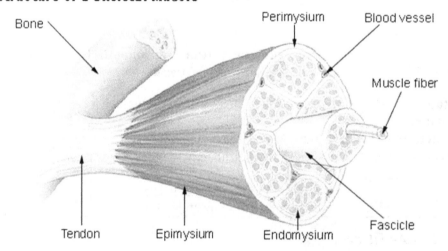

**Structure of a Skeletal Muscle**

## MAJOR MUSCLES OF THE BODY

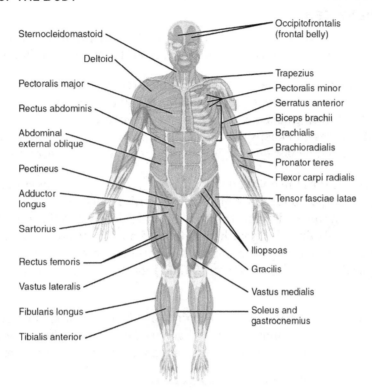

Sternocleidomastoid

Deltoid

Pectoralis major

Rectus abdominis

Abdominal external oblique

Pectineus

Adductor longus

Sartorius

Rectus femoris

Vastus lateralis

Fibularis longus

Tibialis anterior

Occipitofrontalis (frontal belly)

Trapezius

Pectoralis minor

Serratus anterior

Biceps brachii

Brachialis

Brachioradialis

Pronator teres

Flexor carpi radialis

Tensor fasciae latae

Iliopsoas

Gracilis

Vastus medialis

Soleus and gastrocnemius

Major muscles of the body.
Right side: superficial; left side:
deep (anterior view)

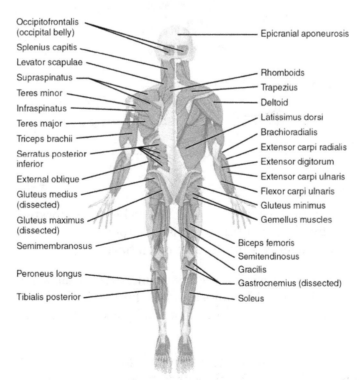

Occipitofrontalis (occipital belly)

Splenius capitis

Levator scapulae

Supraspinatus

Teres minor

Infraspinatus

Teres major

Triceps brachii

Serratus posterior inferior

External oblique

Gluteus medius (dissected)

Gluteus maximus (dissected)

Semimembranosus

Peroneus longus

Tibialis posterior

Epicranial aponeurosis

Rhomboids

Trapezius

Deltoid

Latissimus dorsi

Brachioradialis

Extensor carpi radialis

Extensor digitorum

Extensor carpi ulnaris

Flexor carpi ulnaris

Gluteus minimus

Gemellus muscles

Biceps femoris

Semitendinosus

Gracilis

Gastrocnemius (dissected)

Soleus

Major muscles of the body.
Right side: superficial; left side:
deep (posterior view)

## REPRODUCTIVE SYSTEM
### *MALE REPRODUCTIVE SYSTEM*

The functions of the male reproductive system are to produce, maintain, and transfer **sperm** and **semen** into the female reproductive tract and to produce and secrete **male hormones**.

The external structure includes the penis, scrotum, and testes. The **penis**, which contains the **urethra**, can fill with blood and become erect, enabling the deposition of semen and sperm into the female reproductive tract during sexual intercourse. The **scrotum** is a sac of skin and smooth muscle that houses the testes and keeps the testes at the proper temperature for **spermatogenesis**. The **testes**, or testicles, are the male gonads, which produce sperm and testosterone.

The internal structure includes the epididymis, vas deferens, ejaculatory ducts, urethra, seminal vesicles, prostate gland, and bulbourethral glands. The **epididymis** stores the sperm as it matures. Mature sperm moves from the epididymis through the **vas deferens** to the **ejaculatory duct**. The **seminal vesicles** secrete alkaline fluids with proteins and mucus into the ejaculatory duct, also. The **prostate gland** secretes a milky white fluid with proteins and enzymes as part of the semen. The **bulbourethral**, or Cowper's, glands secrete a fluid into the urethra to neutralize the acidity in the urethra.

Additionally, the hormones associated with the male reproductive system include **follicle-stimulating hormone**, which stimulates spermatogenesis; **luteinizing hormone**, which stimulates testosterone production; and **testosterone**, which is responsible for the male sex characteristics.

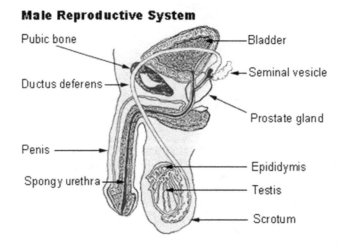

### *FEMALE REPRODUCTIVE SYSTEM*

The functions of the female reproductive system are to produce **ova** (oocytes, or egg cells), transfer the ova to the **fallopian tubes** for fertilization, receive the sperm from the male, and to provide a protective, nourishing environment for the developing **embryo**.

The external portion of the female reproductive system includes the labia majora, labia minora, Bartholin's glands and clitoris. The **labia majora** and the **labia minora** enclose and protect the vagina. The **Bartholin's glands** secrete a lubricating fluid. The **clitoris** contains erectile tissue and nerve endings for sensual pleasure.

The internal portion of the female reproductive system includes the ovaries, fallopian tubes, uterus, and vagina. The **ovaries**, which are the female gonads, produce the ova and secrete **estrogen** and **progesterone**. The **fallopian tubes** carry the mature egg toward the uterus. Fertilization typically occurs in the fallopian tubes. If fertilized, the egg travels to the **uterus**, where it implants in the uterine wall. The uterus protects and nourishes the developing embryo until birth. The **vagina** is a muscular tube that extends from the **cervix** of the uterus to the outside of the body. The vagina receives the semen and sperm during sexual intercourse and provides a birth canal when needed.

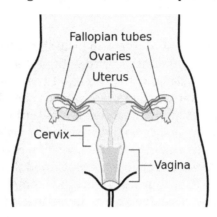

### FEMALE REPRODUCTIVE CYCLE

The female reproductive cycle is characterized by changes in both the ovaries and the uterine lining (endometrium).

The ovarian cycle has three phases: the follicular phase, ovulation, and the luteal phase. During the **follicular phase**, FSH stimulates the maturation of the follicle, which then secretes estrogen. Estrogen helps to regenerate the uterine lining that was shed during menstruation. **Ovulation**, the release of a secondary oocyte from the ovary, is induced by a surge in LH. The **luteal phase** begins with the formation of the corpus luteum from the remnants of the follicle. The corpus luteum secretes progesterone and estrogen, which inhibit FSH and LH. Progesterone also maintains the thickness of the endometrium. Without the implantation of a fertilized egg, the corpus luteum begins to regress, and the levels of estrogen and progesterone drop. FSH and LH are no longer inhibited, and the cycle renews.

The uterine cycle also consists of three phases: the proliferative phase, secretory phase, and menstrual phase. The **proliferative phase** is characterized by the regeneration of the uterine lining. During the **secretory phase**, the endometrium becomes increasingly vascular, and nutrients are secreted to prepare for implantation. Without implantation, the endometrium is shed during **menstruation**.

### PREGNANCY, PARTURITION, LACTATION

*Pregnancy*: When a blastocyst implants in the uterine lining, it releases hCG. This hormone prevents the corpus luteum from degrading, and it continues to produce estrogen and progesterone. These hormones are necessary to maintain the uterine lining. By the second trimester, the placenta secretes enough of its own estrogen and progesterone to sustain pregnancy and the levels continue to increase throughout pregnancy, while hCG hormone levels decrease.

*Parturition*: The precise mechanism for the initiation of parturition (birth) is unclear. Birth is preceded by increased levels of fetal glucocorticoids, which act on the placenta to increase estrogen and decrease progesterone. Stretching of the cervix stimulates the release of oxytocin from the posterior pituitary gland. Oxytocin and estrogen stimulate the release of prostaglandins, and prostaglandins and oxytocin increase uterine contractions. This positive feedback mechanism results in the birth of the fetus.

*Lactation*: During pregnancy, levels of the hormone prolactin increase, but its effect on the mammary glands is inhibited by estrogen and progesterone. After parturition, the levels of these hormones decrease, and prolactin is able to stimulate the production of milk. Suckling stimulates the release of oxytocin, which results in the ejection of milk.

## INTEGUMENTARY SYSTEM

The integumentary system, which consists of the skin including the sebaceous glands, sweat glands, hair, and nails, serves a variety of functions associated with protection, secretion, and communication. In the functions associated with protection, the integumentary system protects the body from **pathogens** including bacteria, viruses, and various chemicals. In the functions associated with secretion, **sebaceous glands** secrete **sebum** (oil) that waterproofs the skin, and **sweat glands** are associated with the body's homeostatic relationship of **thermoregulation**. Sweat glands also serve as excretory organs and help rid the body of metabolic wastes. In the functions associated with communication, **sensory receptors** distributed throughout the skin send information to the brain regarding pain, touch, pressure, and temperature. In addition to protection, secretion, and communication, the skin manufactures **vitamin D** and can absorb certain chemicals such as specific medications.

> **Review Video: Integumentary System**
> Visit mometrix.com/academy and enter code: 655980

### LAYERS OF THE SKIN

The layers of the skin from the surface of the skin inward are the epidermis and dermis. The subcutaneous layer lying below the dermis is also part of the integumentary system. The **epidermis** is the most superficial layer of the skin. The epidermis, which consists entirely of **epithelial cells**, does not contain any blood vessels. The deepest portion of the epidermis is the **stratum basale**, which is a single layer of cells that continually undergo division. As more and more cells are produced, older cells are pushed toward the surface. Most epidermal cells are keratinized. **Keratin** is a waxy protein that helps to waterproof the skin. As the cells die, they are sloughed off. The **dermis** lies directly beneath the epidermis. The dermis consists mostly of connective tissue. The dermis contains blood vessels, sensory receptors, hair follicles, sebaceous glands, and sweat glands. The dermis also contains **elastin** and **collagen fibers**. The **subcutaneous layer** or **hypodermis** is actually not a layer of the skin. The subcutaneous layer consists of connective tissue, which binds the skin to the underlying muscles. Fat deposits in the subcutaneous layer help to cushion and insulate the body.

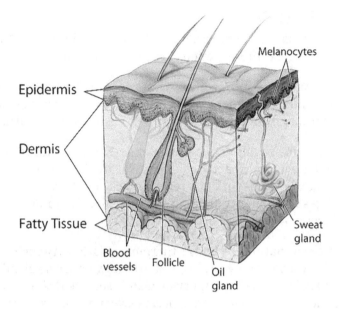

The types of cells found in the epidermis and dermis:

| Cell Type | Location | Description |
|---|---|---|
| Keratinocytes | Epidermis | The most common type of cell in the epidermis.<br>Arise from stem cells in the stratum basale<br>They flatten and die as they move toward the surface of the skin<br>Produce keratin - a fibrous protein that hardens the cell and helps make the skin water resistant |
| Melanocytes | Epidermis | Produces melanin - a pigment that gives skin its color and protects against UV radiation |
| Langerhans cells | Epidermis | Antigen-presenting cells of the immune system (phagocytes)<br>More common in stratum spinosum than other layers of epidermis |
| Merkel cells | Epidermis | Cutaneous receptors, detect light touch. Located in stratum basale |
| Fibroblasts | Dermis | Secrete collagen, elastin, glycosaminoglycans, and other components of the extracellular matrix |
| Adipocytes | Dermis | Fat cells |
| Macrophages | Dermis | Phagocytic cells that engulf potential pathogens |
| Mast cells | Dermis | Antigen-presenting cells that play a role in the inflammatory response (release histamine) |

### SKIN'S INVOLVEMENT IN TEMPERATURE HOMEOSTASIS

The skin is involved in **temperature homeostasis** or thermoregulation through the activation of the sweat glands. By **thermoregulation**, the body maintains a stable body temperature as one component of a stable internal environment. The temperature of the body is controlled by a negative feedback system consisting of a receptor, control center, and effector. The **receptors** are sensory cells located in the dermis of the skin. The **control center** is the **hypothalamus**, which is located in the brain. The **effectors** include the *sweat glands, blood vessels, and muscles* (shivering). The evaporation of sweat across the surface of the skin cools the body to maintain its tolerance range. **Vasodilation** of the blood vessels near the surface of the skin also releases heat into the environment to lower body temperature. Shivering is associated with the muscular system.

## SEBACEOUS GLANDS VS. SWEAT GLANDS

Sebaceous glands and sweat glands are exocrine glands found in the skin. **Exocrine glands** secrete substances into **ducts**. In this case, the secretions are through the ducts to the surface of the skin.

**Sebaceous glands** are **holocrine glands**, which secrete sebum. **Sebum** is an oily mixture of lipids and proteins. Sebaceous glands are connected to hair follicles and secrete sebum through the hair pore. Sebum inhibits water loss from the skin and protects against bacterial and fungal infections.

**Sweat glands** are either eccrine glands or apocrine glands. **Eccrine glands** are not connected to hair follicles. They are activated by elevated body temperature. Eccrine glands are located throughout the body and can be found on the forehead, neck, and back. Eccrine glands secrete a salty solution of electrolytes and water containing sodium chloride, potassium, bicarbonate, glucose, and antimicrobial peptides.

Eccrine glands are activated as part of the body's thermoregulation. **Apocrine glands** secrete an oily solution containing fatty acids, triglycerides, and proteins. Apocrine glands are located in the armpits, groin, palms, and soles of the feet. Apocrine glands secrete this oily sweat when a person experiences stress or anxiety. Bacteria feed on apocrine sweat and expel aromatic fatty acids, producing body odor.

## ENDOCRINE SYSTEM

The endocrine system is responsible for secreting the **hormones** and other molecules that help regulate the entire body in both the short and the long term. There is a close working relationship between the endocrine system and the nervous system. The **hypothalamus** and the **pituitary gland** coordinate to serve as a **neuroendocrine control center**.

Hormone secretion is triggered by a variety of signals, including hormonal signs, chemical reactions, and environmental cues. Only cells with particular **receptors** can benefit from hormonal influence. This is the "key in the lock" model for hormonal action. **Steroid hormones** trigger gene activation and protein synthesis in some target cells. **Protein hormones** change the activity of existing enzymes in target cells. Hormones such as **insulin** work quickly when the body signals an urgent need. Slower acting hormones afford longer, gradual, and sometimes permanent changes in the body.

The eight major endocrine glands and their functions are:

- **Adrenal cortex** – Monitors blood sugar level; helps in lipid and protein metabolism.
- **Adrenal medulla** – Controls cardiac function; raises blood sugar and controls the size of blood vessels.
- **Thyroid gland** – Helps regulate metabolism and functions in growth and development.
- **Parathyroid** – Regulates calcium levels in the blood.
- **Pancreas islets** – Raises and lowers blood sugar; active in carbohydrate metabolism.
- **Thymus gland** – Plays a role in immune responses.
- **Pineal gland** – Has an influence on daily biorhythms and sexual activity.
- **Pituitary gland** – Plays an important role in growth and development.

Endocrine glands are intimately involved in a myriad of reactions, functions, and secretions that are crucial to the well-being of the body.

> **Review Video: Endocrine System**
> Visit mometrix.com/academy and enter code: 678939

## HORMONES OF THE HYPOTHALAMUS AND PITUITARY

The **hypothalamus** is the link between the nervous system and the endocrine system. It is located in the brain, superior to the pituitary and inferior to the thalamus. The hypothalamus communicates with the pituitary by secreting "releasing hormones" (RH) and "inhibiting hormones" (IH). Hormones of the hypothalamus include:

| Hormone | Action |
|---|---|
| GnRH - gonadotropin RH | Stimulates anterior pituitary to release LH and FSH |
| GHRH - growth hormone RH | Stimulates anterior pituitary to release GH |
| GHIH - growth hormone IH (somatostatin) | Inhibits the release of GH from the anterior pituitary |
| TRH - thyrotropin RH | Stimulates anterior pituitary to release thyrotropin (TSH) |
| PRH - prolactin RH | Stimulates anterior pituitary to release prolactin |
| PIH - prolactin IH (dopamine) | Inhibits the release of prolactin from the anterior pituitary |
| CRH - corticotropin RH | Stimulates anterior pituitary to release ACTH |
| Oxytocin | Targets the uterus - stimulates contractions. Targets the mammary glands - milk secretion |
| ADH - antidiuretic hormone (vasopressin) | Targets the kidneys and blood vessels - increases water retention |

The **pituitary** is nicknamed the "master gland" because many of the hormones it secretes act on other endocrine glands. It is located within the sella turcica of the sphenoid bone, beneath the hypothalamus. This pea-sized gland hangs from a thin stalk called the infundibulum, and it consists of an anterior and posterior lobe - each with a different function.

| Source | Hormone | Action |
|---|---|---|
| **Pituitary gland (anterior)** | TSH - thyroid stimulating hormone (thyrotropin) | Targets the thyroid - stimulates the secretion of thyroid hormones |
| | ACTH - adrenocorticotropic hormone | Targets the adrenal cortex - stimulates the release of glucocorticoids and mineralocorticoids |
| | GH - growth hormone | Targets muscle and bone - stimulates growth |
| | FSH - follicle stimulating hormone | Targets the gonads - stimulates the maturation of sperm cells and ovarian follicles |
| | LH - luteinizing hormone | Targets the gonads - stimulates the production of sex hormones; surge stimulates ovulation in females |
| | PRL - prolactin | Targets the mammary glands - stimulates production of milk |

| Source | Hormone | Action |
|---|---|---|
| **Pituitary gland (posterior)** | Oxytocin (produced in hypothalamus; stored and released by posterior pituitary) | Targets the uterus - stimulates contractions Targets the mammary glands - stimulates milk secretion |
| | ADH - antidiuretic hormone (vasopressin) (produced in hypothalamus; stored and released by posterior pituitary) | Targets the kidneys and blood vessels - increases water retention |

## HORMONE SOURCES OF THE HEAD AND NECK

| Source/Description | Hormone | Action |
|---|---|---|
| **Pineal gland** Situated between the two hemispheres of the brain where the two halves of the thalamus join. | Melatonin | Targets the brain - regulates daily rhythm (wake and sleep) |
| **Thyroid gland** Butterfly-shaped gland; the point of attachment between the two lobes is called the isthmus. The isthmus is on the anterior portion of the trachea, with the lobes wrapping partially around the trachea. | $T_3$ - triiodothyronine | Targets most cells - stimulates cellular metabolism |
| | $T_4$ - thyroxine | Targets most cells - stimulates cellular metabolism |
| | Calcitonin | Targets bone and kidneys - lowers blood calcium |
| **Parathyroid gland** Four small glands that are embedded in the posterior aspect of the thyroid. | PTH - Parathyroid hormone | Targets bone and kidneys - raises blood calcium |

## HORMONE SOURCES OF THE ABDOMEN

| Source/Description | Hormone | Action |
|---|---|---|
| **Thymus gland** Located between the sternum and the heart, embedded in the mediastinum. It slowly decreases in size after puberty. | Thymosin | Targets lymphatic tissues - stimulates the production of T-cells |
| **Pancreas** The head of the pancreas is situated in the curve of the duodenum and the tail points toward the left side of the body. The pancreas is mostly posterior to the stomach. | Insulin | Targets the liver, muscle, and adipose tissue - decreases blood glucose |
| | Glucagon | Targets the liver - increases blood glucose |
| | GHIH - growth hormone IH (somatostatin) | Inhibits the secretion of insulin and glucagon |
| **Adrenal medulla** Located on top of the kidneys. The adrenal medulla is the inner part of the gland. | Epinephrine and norepinephrine | Target heart, blood vessels, liver, and lungs - increase heart rate, increase blood sugar (fight or flight response) |
| **Adrenal cortex** | Mineralocorticoids (aldosterone) | Target the kidneys - increase the retention of $Na^+$ and excretion of $K^+$ |

| Source/Description | Hormone | Action |
|---|---|---|
| The adrenal cortex is the outer portion of the adrenal gland. | Glucocorticoids | Target most tissues - released in response to long-term stressors, increase blood glucose (but not as quickly as glucagon) |
| | Androgens | Target most tissues - stimulate development of secondary sex characteristics |
| **GI tract** | Gastrin | Targets the stomach - stimulates the release of HCl |
| | Secretin | Targets the pancreas and liver - stimulates the release of digestive enzymes and bile |
| | CCK - cholecystokinin | Targets the pancreas and liver - stimulates the release of digestive enzymes and bile |
| **Kidneys** | Erythropoietin | Targets the bone marrow - stimulates the production of red blood cells |
| | Calcitriol | Targets the intestines - increases the reabsorption of $Ca^{2+}$ |
| **Heart** | ANP - atrial natriuretic peptide | Targets the kidneys and adrenal cortex - reduces reabsorption of $Na^+$, lowers blood pressure |
| **Adipose Tissue** | Leptin | Targets the brain - suppresses appetite |

## HORMONE SOURCES OF THE REPRODUCTIVE SYSTEM

| Source/Description | Hormone | Action |
|---|---|---|
| **Ovaries** The ovaries rest in depressions in the pelvic cavity on each side of the uterus. (Note that ovaries produce testosterone in small amounts.) | Estrogen | Target the uterus, ovaries, mammary glands, brain, and other tissues - stimulate uterine lining growth, regulate menstrual cycle, facilitate the development of secondary sex characteristics |
| | Progesterone | Targets mainly the uterus and mammary glands - stimulates uterine lining growth, regulates menstrual cycle, required for maintenance of pregnancy |
| | Inhibin | Targets the anterior pituitary - inhibits the release of FSH |
| **Placenta** Attached to the wall of the uterus during pregnancy | Estrogen, progesterone, and inhibin | (See above) |
| | Human chorionic gonadotropin (hCG) | Targets the ovaries - stimulates the production of estrogen and progesterone |
| **Testes** Located within the scrotum, behind the penis. | Testosterone | Targets the testes and many other tissues - promotes spermatogenesis, secondary sex characteristics |
| | Inhibin | (See above) |

## URINARY SYSTEM

The urinary system is capable of eliminating excess substances while preserving the substances needed by the body to function. The **urinary system** consists of the kidneys, urinary ducts, and bladder.

> **Review Video: Urinary System**
> Visit mometrix.com/academy and enter code: 601053

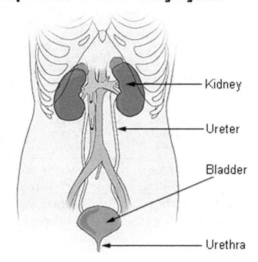

### KIDNEYS

The kidneys are bean-shaped structures that are located at the back of the abdominal cavity just under the diaphragm. Each **kidney** consists of three layers: the renal cortex (outer layer), renal medulla (inner layer), and renal pelvis (innermost portion).

The **renal cortex** is composed of approximately one million **nephrons**, which are the tiny, individual filters of the kidneys. Each nephron contains a cluster of capillaries called a **glomerulus** surrounded by the cup-shaped **Bowman's capsule**, which leads to a tubule.

The kidneys receive blood from the **renal arteries**, which branch off the aorta. In general, the kidneys filter the blood, reabsorb needed materials, and secrete wastes and excess water in the urine. More specifically, blood flows from the renal arteries into **arterioles** into the glomerulus, where it is filtered. The **glomerular filtrate** enters the **proximal convoluted tubule** where water, glucose, ions, and other organic molecules are reabsorbed back into the bloodstream.

Additional substances such as urea and drugs are removed from the blood in the **distal convoluted tubule**. Also, the pH of the blood can be adjusted in the distal convoluted tubule by the secretion of **hydrogen ions**. Finally, the unabsorbed materials flow out from the collecting tubules located in the **renal medulla** to the **renal pelvis** as urine. Urine is drained from the kidneys through the ureters to the **urinary bladder**, where it is stored until expulsion from the body through the **urethra**.

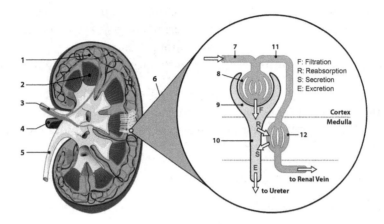

*KIDNEY STRUCTURE*

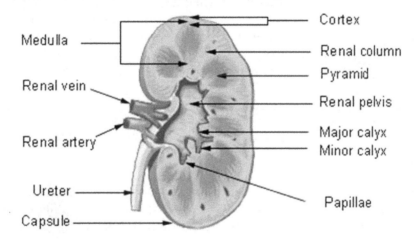

## IMMUNE SYSTEM

The immune system protects the body against invading **pathogens** including bacteria, viruses, fungi, and protists. The immune system includes the **lymphatic system** (lymph, lymph capillaries, lymph vessel, and lymph nodes) as well as the **red bone marrow** and numerous **leukocytes**, or white blood cells. Tissue fluid enters the **lymph capillaries**, which combine to form **lymph vessels**. Skeletal muscle contractions move the lymph one way through the lymphatic system to lymphatic ducts, which dump back into the venous blood supply into the **lymph nodes**, which are situated along the lymph vessels, and filter the lymph of pathogens and other matter. The lymph nodes are concentrated in the neck, armpits, and groin areas. Outside the lymphatic vessel system lies the **lymphatic tissue** including the tonsils, adenoids, thymus, spleen, and Peyer's patches. The **tonsils**, located in the pharynx, protect against pathogens entering the body through the mouth and throat. The **thymus** serves as a maturation chamber for the immature T cells that are formed in the bone marrow. The **spleen** cleans the blood of dead cells and pathogens. **Peyer's patches**, which are located in the small intestine, protect the digestive system from pathogens.

The body's general immune defenses include:

- **Skin** – An intact epidermis and dermis form a formidable barrier against bacteria.
- **Ciliated Mucous Membranes** – Cilia sweep pathogens out of the respiratory tract.
- **Glandular Secretions** – Secretions from exocrine glands destroy bacteria.
- **Gastric Secretions** – Gastric acid destroys pathogens.
- **Normal Bacterial Populations** – Compete with pathogens in the gut and vagina.

In addition, **phagocytes** and inflammation responses mobilize white blood cells and chemical reactions to stop infection. These responses include localized redness, tissue repair, and fluid-seeping healing agents. Additionally, **plasma proteins** act as the complement system to repel bacteria and pathogens.

Three types of white blood cells form the foundation of the body's immune system:

- **Macrophages** – Phagocytes that alert T cells to the presence of foreign substances.
- **T Lymphocytes** – These directly attack cells infected by viruses and bacteria.
- **B Lymphocytes** – These cells target specific bacteria for destruction.

**Memory cells**, **suppressor T cells**, and **helper T cells** also contribute to the body's defense. Immune responses can be **antibody-mediated** when the response is to an antigen, or **cell-mediated** when the response is to already infected cells. These responses are controlled and measured counterattacks that recede when the foreign agents are destroyed. Once an invader has attacked the body, if it returns it is immediately recognized and a secondary immune response occurs. This secondary response is rapid and powerful, much more so than the original response. These memory lymphocytes circulate throughout the body for years, alert to a possible new attack.

---

**Review Video: Immune System**
Visit mometrix.com/academy and enter code: 622899

---

### TYPES OF LEUKOCYTES

Leukocytes, or white blood cells, are produced in the red bone marrow. Leukocytes can be classified as **monocytes** (macrophages and dendritic cells), **granulocytes** (neutrophils, basophils, and eosinophils), **T lymphocytes**, **B lymphocytes**, or **natural killer cells**.

**Macrophages** found traveling in the lymph or fixed in lymphatic tissue are the largest, long-living phagocytes that engulf and destroy pathogens. **Dendritic cells** present antigens (foreign particles) to T cells. **Neutrophils** are short-living phagocytes that respond quickly to invaders. **Basophils** alert the body of invasion. **Eosinophils** are large, long-living phagocytes that defend against multicellular invaders.

**T lymphocytes** or T cells include helper T cells, killer T cells, suppressor T cells, and memory T cells. **Helper T cells** help the body fight infections by producing antibodies and other chemicals. **Killer T cells** destroy cells that are infected with a virus or pathogen and tumor cells. **Suppressor T cells** stop or "suppress" the other T cells when the battle is over. **Memory T cells** remain in the blood on alert in case the invader attacks again. **B lymphocytes**, or B cells, produce antibodies.

### ANTIGEN AND TYPICAL IMMUNE RESPONSE

Antigens are substances that stimulate the **immune system**. Antigens are typically proteins on the surfaces of bacteria, viruses, and fungi.

Substances such as drugs, toxins, and foreign particles can also be antigens. The human body recognizes the antigens of its own cells, but it will attack cells or substances with unfamiliar antigens.

Specific **antibodies** are produced for each antigen that enters the body. In a typical immune response, when a pathogen or foreign substance enters the body, it is engulfed by a **macrophage**, which presents fragments of the antigen on its surface. A **helper T cell** joins the macrophage, and the killer (cytotoxic) T cells and B cells are activated. **Killer T cells** search out and destroy cells presenting the same antigens. **B cells** differentiate into plasma cells and memory cells.

**Plasma cells** produce antibodies specific to that pathogen or foreign substance. **Antibodies** bind to antigens on the surface of pathogens and mark them for destruction by other phagocytes. **Memory cells** remain in the blood stream to protect against future infections from the same pathogen.

### Active and Passive Immunity

At birth, an **innate immune system** protects an individual from pathogens. When an individual encounters infection or has an immunization, the individual develops an **adaptive immunity** that reacts to pathogens. So, this adaptive immunity is acquired. Active and passive immunities can be acquired naturally or artificially.

A **naturally acquired active immunity** is natural because the individual is exposed and builds immunity to a pathogen *without an immunization*. An **artificially acquired active immunity** is artificial because the individual is exposed and builds immunity to a pathogen *by a vaccine*.

A **naturally acquired passive immunity** is natural because it happens *during pregnancy* as antibodies move from the mother's bloodstream to the bloodstream of the fetus. The antibodies can also be transferred from a mother's breast milk. During infancy, these antibodies provide temporary protection until childhood.

An **artificially acquired passive immunity** is an *immunization* that is given in recent outbreaks or emergency situations. This immunization provides quick and short-lived protection to disease by the use of antibodies that can come from another person or animal.

## Skeletal System
### Axial Skeleton and the Appendicular Skeleton

The human skeletal system, which consists of 206 bones along with numerous tendons, ligaments, and cartilage, is divided into the axial skeleton and the appendicular skeleton. The **axial skeleton** consists of 80 bones and includes the vertebral column, rib cage, sternum, skull, and hyoid bone. The **vertebral column** consists of 33 vertebrae classified as cervical vertebrae, thoracic vertebrae, lumbar vertebrae, and sacral vertebrae. The **rib cage** includes 12 paired ribs, 10 pairs of true ribs and 2 pairs of floating ribs, and the **sternum**, which consists of the manubrium, corpus sterni, and xiphoid process. The **skull** includes the cranium and facial bones. The **ossicles** are bones in the middle ear. The **hyoid bone** provides an attachment point for the tongue muscles. The **axial skeleton** protects vital organs including the brain, heart, and lungs. The **appendicular skeleton** consists of 126 bones including the pectoral girdle, pelvic girdle, and appendages. The **pectoral girdle** consists of the scapulae (shoulders) and clavicles (collarbones). The **pelvic girdle** consists of two pelvic (hip) bones, which attach to the sacrum. The **upper appendages** (arms) include the humerus, radius, ulna, carpals, metacarpals, and phalanges. The **lower appendages** (legs) include the femur, patella, fibula, tibia, tarsals, metatarsals, and phalanges.

## ADULT HUMAN SKELETON

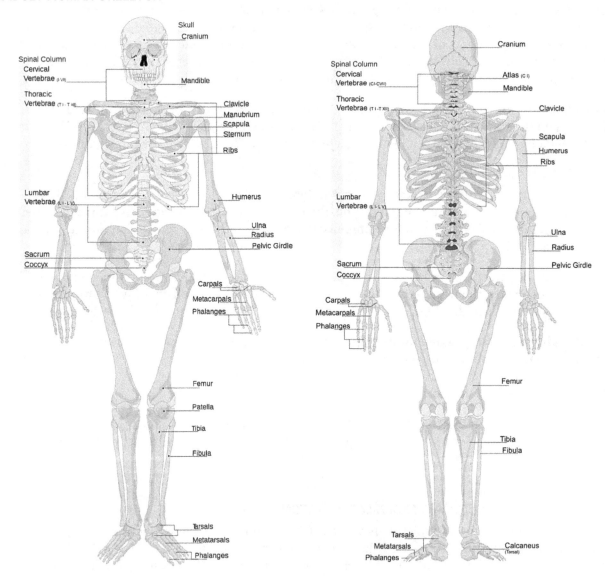

## JOINT STRUCTURES

**Joints** are the locations where two or more elements of the skeleton connect. They can be classified according to range of motion, as well as the material that holds the joint together.

**Functional classification**

| Class | Description | Range of Motion | Examples |
|---|---|---|---|
| **Synarthrosis** | Either fibrous or cartilaginous | Immovable | Skull sutures, teeth/mandible |
| **Amphiarthrosis** | Either fibrous or cartilaginous | Slight | Intervertebral discs, distal tibiofibular joint |
| **Diarthrosis** | Always synovial | Free movement | Wrist, knee, shoulder |

**Structural classification**

| Class | Description | Types, Range of Motion | Examples |
|-------|-------------|------------------------|----------|
| Fibrous | Held together by fibrous connective tissue | **Suture**: immovable | skull |
| | | **Gomphosis**: immovable | teeth/mandible |
| | | **Syndesmosis**: slightly movable | distal tibiofibular joint |
| Cartilaginous | Held together by cartilage | **Synchondrosis**: hyaline cartilage, nearly immovable | first rib/sternum |
| | | **Symphysis**: fibrocartilage, slightly movable | intervertebral discs, pubic symphysis |
| Synovial | The most common type of joint; characterized by a joint cavity filled with synovial fluid | **Pivot**: allows rotation | atlantoaxial joint |
| | | **Hinge**: allows movement in one plane | knee |
| | | **Saddle**: allows pivoting in two planes and axial rotation | first metacarpal/trapezium |
| | | **Gliding**: allows sliding | carpals |
| | | **Condyloid**: allows pivoting in two planes but no axial rotation | radiocarpal joint |
| | | **Ball and socket**: have the highest range of motion | hip |

## FUNCTIONS OF THE SKELETAL SYSTEM

The skeletal system serves many functions including providing structural support, providing movement, providing protection, producing blood cells, and storing substances such as fat and minerals. The skeletal system provides the body with structure and support for the muscles and organs. The axial skeleton transfers the weight from the upper body to the lower appendages. The skeletal system provides movement with **joints** and the muscular system. Bones provide attachment points for muscles. Joints including **hinge joints**, **ball-and-socket joints**, **pivot joints**, **ellipsoid joints**, **gliding joints**, and **saddle joints**. Each muscle is attached to two bones: the origin and the insertion. The **origin** remains immobile, and the **insertion** is the bone that moves as the muscle contracts and relaxes. The skeletal system serves to protect the body. The **cranium** protects the brain. The **vertebrae** protect the spinal cord. The **rib cage** protects the heart and lungs. The **pelvis** protects the reproductive organs. The **red marrow** manufactures red and white blood cells. All bone marrow is red at birth, but adults have approximately one-half red bone marrow and one-half yellow bone marrow. **Yellow bone marrow** stores fat. Also, the skeletal system provides a reservoir to store the minerals **calcium** and **phosphorus**.

The skeletal system has an important role in the following body functions:

- **Movement** – The action of skeletal muscles on bones moves the body.
- **Mineral Storage** – Bones serve as storage facilities for essential mineral ions.
- **Support** – Bones act as a framework and support system for the organs.
- **Protection** – Bones surround and protect key organs in the body.
- **Blood Cell Formation** – Red blood cells are produced in the marrow of certain bones.

Bones are classified as long, short, flat, or irregular. They are a connective tissue with a base of pulp containing **collagen** and living cells. Bone tissue is constantly regenerating itself as the mineral composition changes. This allows for special needs during growth periods and maintains calcium levels for the body. Bone regeneration can deteriorate in old age, particularly among women, leading to **osteoporosis**.

The flexible and curved **backbone** is supported by muscles and ligaments. **Intervertebral discs** are stacked one above another and provide cushioning for the backbone. Trauma or shock may cause these discs to **herniate** and cause pain. The sensitive **spinal cord** is enclosed in a cavity which is well protected by the bones of the vertebrae.

Joints are areas of contact adjacent to bones. **Synovial joints** are the most common, and are freely moveable. These may be found at the shoulders and knees. **Cartilaginous joints** fill the spaces between some bones and restrict movement. Examples of cartilaginous joints are those between vertebrae. **Fibrous joints** have fibrous tissue connecting bones and no cavity is present.

### COMPACT AND SPONGY BONE

**Compact Bone & Spongy (Cancellous) Bone**

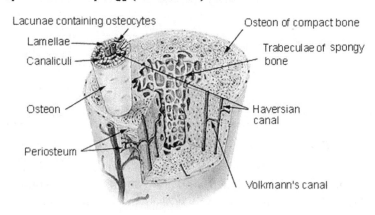

Two types of connective bone tissue include compact bone and spongy bone.

**Compact**, or **cortical**, bone, which consists of tightly packed cells, is strong, dense, and rigid. Running vertically throughout compact bone are the **Haversian canals**, which are surrounded by concentric circles of bone tissue called **lamellae**. The spaces between the lamellae are called the **lacunae**. These lamellae and canals along with their associated arteries, veins, lymph vessels, and nerve endings are referred to collectively as the **Haversian system**.

The Haversian system provides a reservoir for calcium and phosphorus for the blood. Also, bones have a thin outside layer of compact bone, which gives them their characteristic smooth, white appearance.

**Spongy**, or **cancellous**, bone consists of **trabeculae**, which are a network of girders with open spaces filled with red bone marrow.

Compared to compact bone, spongy bone is lightweight and porous, which helps reduce the bone's overall weight. The red marrow manufactures red and white blood cells. In long bones, the **diaphysis** consists of compact bone surrounding the marrow cavity and spongy bone containing red marrow in the **epiphyses**. Bones have varying amounts of compact bone and spongy bone depending on their classification.

# Life and Physical Sciences

## MACROMOLECULES

Macromolecules are large and complex, and play an important role in cell structure and function. The four basic organic macromolecules produced by anabolic reactions are **carbohydrates** (polysaccharides), **nucleic acids**, **proteins**, and **lipids**. The four basic building blocks involved in catabolic reactions are **monosaccharides** (glucose), **amino acids**, **fatty acids** (glycerol), and **nucleotides**.

An **anabolic reaction** is one that builds larger and more complex molecules (macromolecules) from smaller ones. **Catabolic reactions** are the opposite. Larger molecules are broken down into smaller, simpler molecules. Catabolic reactions *release energy*, while anabolic ones *require energy*.

**Endothermic reactions** are chemical reactions that *absorb* heat and **exothermic reactions** are chemical reactions that *release* heat.

> **Review Video: Macromolecules**
> Visit mometrix.com/academy and enter code: 220156

### CARBOHYDRATE

Carbohydrates are the primary source of energy and are responsible for providing energy as they can be easily converted to **glucose**. It is the oxidation of carbohydrates that provides the cells with most of their energy. Glucose can be further broken down by respiration or fermentation by **glycolysis**. They are involved in the metabolic energy cycles of photosynthesis and respiration.

Structurally, carbohydrates usually take the form of some variation of $CH_2O$ as they are made of carbon, hydrogen, and oxygen. Carbohydrates (**polysaccharides**) are broken down into sugars or glucose.

The simple sugars can be grouped into monosaccharides (glucose, fructose, and galactose) and disaccharides. These are both types of carbohydrates. Monosaccharides have one monomer of sugar and disaccharides have two. Monosaccharides ($CH_2O$) have one carbon for every water molecule.

A **monomer** is a small molecule. It is a single compound that forms chemical bonds with other monomers to make a polymer. A **polymer** is a compound of large molecules formed by repeating monomers. Carbohydrates, proteins, and nucleic acids are groups of macromolecules that are polymers.

> **Review Video: Carbohydrates**
> Visit mometrix.com/academy and enter code: 601714

### LIPIDS

**Lipids** are molecules that are soluble in nonpolar solvents, but are hydrophobic, meaning they do not bond well with water or mix well with water solutions. Lipids have numerous **C–H bonds**. In this way, they are similar to **hydrocarbons** (substances consisting only of carbon and hydrogen). The major roles of lipids include *energy storage and structural functions*. Examples of lipids include fats, phospholipids, steroids, and waxes. **Fats** (which are triglycerides) are made of long chains of fatty acids (three fatty acids bound to a glycerol). **Fatty acids** are chains with reduced carbon at one end and a carboxylic acid group at the other. An example is soap, which contains the sodium salts of free fatty acids. **Phospholipids** are lipids that have a phosphate group rather than a fatty acid.

**Glycerides** are another type of lipid. Examples of glycerides are fat and oil. Glycerides are formed from fatty acids and glycerol (a type of alcohol).

> **Review Video: Lipids**
> Visit mometrix.com/academy and enter code: 269746

## PROTEINS

Proteins are macromolecules formed from amino acids. They are **polypeptides**, which consist of many (10 to 100) peptides linked together. The peptide connections are the result of condensation reactions. A **condensation reaction** results in a loss of water when two molecules are joined together. A **hydrolysis reaction** is the opposite of a condensation reaction. During hydrolysis, water is added. –H is added to one of the smaller molecules and OH is added to another molecule being formed. A **peptide** is a compound of two or more amino acids. **Amino acids** are formed by the partial hydrolysis of protein, which forms an **amide bond**. This partial hydrolysis involves an amine group and a carboxylic acid. In the carbon chain of amino acids, there is a **carboxylic acid group** (–COOH), an **amine group** ($–NH_2$), a **central carbon atom** between them with an attached hydrogen, and an attached **"R" group** (side chain), which is different for different amino acids. It is the "R" group that determines the properties of the protein.

> **Review Video: Proteins**
> Visit mometrix.com/academy and enter code: 903713

## ENZYMES

Enzymes are proteins with strong **catalytic** power. They greatly accelerate the speed at which specific reactions approach equilibrium. Although enzymes do not start chemical reactions that would not eventually occur by themselves, they do make these reactions happen *faster and more often*. This acceleration can be substantial, sometimes making reactions happen a million times faster. Each type of enzyme deals with **reactants**, also called **substrates**. Each enzyme is highly selective, only interacting with substrates that are a match for it at an active site on the enzyme. This is the "key in the lock" analogy: a certain enzyme only fits with certain substrates. Even with a matching substrate, sometimes an enzyme must reshape itself to fit well with the substrate, forming a strong bond that aids in catalyzing a reaction before it returns to its original shape. An unusual quality of enzymes is that they are not permanently consumed in the reactions they speed up. They can be used again and again, providing a constant source of energy accelerants for cells. This allows for a tremendous increase in the number and rate of reactions in cells.

## NUCLEIC ACIDS

Nucleic acids are macromolecules that are composed of **nucleotides**. **Hydrolysis** is a reaction in which water is broken down into **hydrogen cations** (H or H⁺) and **hydroxide anions** (OH or OH⁻). This is part of the process by which nucleic acids are broken down by enzymes to produce shorter strings of RNA and DNA (oligonucleotides). **Oligonucleotides** are broken down into smaller sugar nitrogenous units called **nucleosides**. These can be digested by cells since the sugar is divided from the nitrogenous base. This, in turn, leads to the formation of the five types of nitrogenous bases, sugars, and the preliminary substances involved in the synthesis of new RNA and DNA. DNA and RNA have a helix shape.

**Macromolecular nucleic acid polymers**, such as RNA and DNA, are formed from nucleotides, which are monomeric units joined by **phosphodiester bonds**. Cells require energy in the form of ATP to synthesize proteins from amino acids and replicate DNA. **Nitrogen fixation** is used to synthesize nucleotides for DNA and amino acids for proteins. Nitrogen fixation uses the enzyme nitrogenase in the reduction of dinitrogen gas ($N_2$) to ammonia ($NH_3$).

**Nucleic acids** store information and energy and are also important catalysts. It is the **RNA** that catalyzes the transfer of **DNA genetic information** into protein coded information. ATP is an RNA nucleotide. **Nucleotides** are used to form the nucleic acids. Nucleotides are made of a five-carbon sugar, such as ribose or deoxyribose, a nitrogenous base, and one or more phosphates. Nucleotides consisting of more than one phosphate can also store energy in their bonds.

> **Review Video: Nucleic Acids**
> Visit mometrix.com/academy and enter code: 503931

# DNA

**Chromosomes** consist of **genes**, which are single units of genetic information. Genes are made up of deoxyribonucleic acid (DNA). DNA is a nucleic acid located in the cell nucleus. There is also DNA in the **mitochondria**. DNA replicates to pass on genetic information. The DNA in almost all cells is the same. It is also involved in the biosynthesis of proteins.

The model or structure of DNA is described as a **double helix**. A helix is a curve, and a double helix is two congruent curves connected by horizontal members. The model can be likened to a spiral staircase. It is right-handed. The British scientist Rosalind Elsie Franklin is credited with taking the x-ray diffraction image in 1952 that was used by Francis Crick and James Watson to formulate the double-helix model of DNA and speculate about its important role in carrying and transferring genetic information.

> **Review Video: DNA**
> Visit mometrix.com/academy and enter code: 639552

## DNA STRUCTURE

DNA has a double helix shape, resembles a twisted ladder, and is compact. It consists of **nucleotides**. Nucleotides consist of a **five-carbon sugar** (pentose), a **phosphate group**, and a **nitrogenous base**. Two bases pair up to form the rungs of the ladder. The "side rails" or backbone consists of the covalently bonded sugar and phosphate. The bases are attached to each other with hydrogen bonds, which are easily dismantled so replication can occur. Each base is attached to a phosphate and to a sugar. There are four types of nitrogenous bases: **adenine** (A), **guanine** (G), **cytosine** (C), and **thymine** (T). There are about 3 billion bases in human DNA. The bases are mostly the same in everybody, but their order is different. It is the order of these bases that creates diversity in people. *Adenine (A) pairs with thymine (T)*, and *cytosine (C) pairs with guanine (G)*.

## PURINES AND PYRIMIDINES

The five bases in DNA and RNA can be categorized as either pyrimidine or purine according to their structure. The **pyrimidine bases** include *cytosine, thymine, and uracil*. They are six-sided and have a single ring shape. The **purine bases** are *adenine and guanine*, which consist of two attached rings. One ring has five sides and the other has six. When combined with a sugar, any of the five bases become **nucleosides**. Nucleosides formed from purine bases end in "osine" and those formed from pyrimidine bases end in "idine." **Adenosine** and **thymidine** are examples of nucleosides. Bases are the most basic components, followed by nucleosides, nucleotides, and then DNA or RNA.

## CODONS

Codons are groups of three nucleotides on the messenger RNA, and can be visualized as three rungs of a ladder. A **codon** has the code for a single amino acid. There are 64 codons but 20 amino acids. More than one combination, or triplet, can be used to synthesize the necessary amino acids. For example, AAA (adenine-adenine-adenine) or AAG (adenine-adenine-guanine) can serve as codons for lysine. These groups of three occur in strings, and might be thought of as frames. For example, AAAUCUUCGU, if read in groups of three from the beginning, would be AAA, UCU, UCG, which are codons for lysine, serine, and serine, respectively. If the same sequence was read in groups of three starting from the second position, the groups would be AAU (asparagine), CUU (proline), and so on. The resulting amino acids would be completely different. For this reason, there are **start and stop codons** that indicate the beginning and ending of a sequence (or frame). **AUG** (methionine) is the start codon. **UAA, UGA**, and **UAG**, also known as ocher, opal, and amber, respectively, are stop codons.

> **Review Video: Codons**
> Visit mometrix.com/academy and enter code: 978172

## DNA REPLICATION

Pairs of chromosomes are composed of DNA, which is tightly wound to conserve space. When replication starts, it unwinds. The steps in **DNA replication** are controlled by enzymes. The enzyme **helicase** instigates the deforming of hydrogen bonds between the bases to split the two strands. The splitting starts at the A-T bases (adenine and thymine) as there are only two hydrogen bonds. The cytosine-guanine base pair has three bonds. The term **"origin of replication"** is used to refer to where the splitting starts. The portion of the DNA that is unwound to be replicated is called the **replication fork**. Each strand of DNA is transcribed by an mRNA. It copies the DNA onto itself, base by base, in a complementary manner. The exception is that uracil replaces thymine.

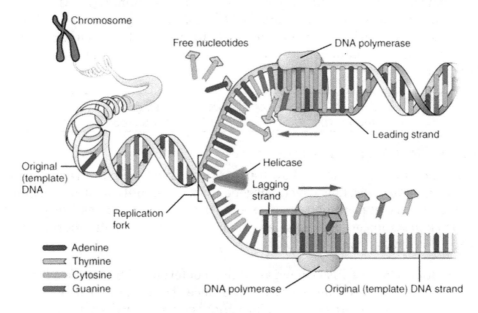

# RNA

## TYPES OF RNA

RNA acts as a *helper* to DNA and carries out a number of other functions. Types of RNA include ribosomal RNA (rRNA), transfer RNA (tRNA), and messenger RNA (mRNA). Viruses can use RNA to carry their genetic material to DNA. **Ribosomal RNA** is not believed to have changed much over time. For this reason, it can be used to study relationships in organisms. **Messenger RNA** carries a copy of a strand of DNA and transports it from the nucleus to the cytoplasm. **Transcription** is the process in which RNA polymerase copies DNA into RNA. DNA unwinds itself and serves as a template while RNA is being assembled. The DNA molecules are copied to RNA. **Translation** is the process whereby ribosomes use transcribed RNA to put together the needed protein. **Transfer RNA** is a molecule that helps in the translation process, and is found in the cytoplasm.

### DIFFERENCES BETWEEN RNA AND DNA

RNA and DNA differ in terms of structure and function. RNA has a different sugar than DNA. It has **ribose** rather than **deoxyribose** sugar. The RNA nitrogenous bases are adenine (A), guanine (G), cytosine (C), and uracil (U). **Uracil** is found only in RNA and **thymine** in found only in DNA. RNA consists of a single strand and DNA has two strands. If straightened out, DNA has two side rails. RNA only has one "backbone," or strand of sugar and phosphate group components. RNA uses the fully hydroxylated sugar **pentose**, which includes an extra oxygen compared to deoxyribose, which is the sugar used by DNA. RNA supports the functions carried out by DNA. It aids in gene expression, replication, and transportation.

> **Review Video: DNA vs. RNA**
> Visit mometrix.com/academy and enter code: 184871

### MENDEL'S LAWS

Mendel's laws are the law of segregation (the first law), the law of independent assortment (the second law), and the law of dominance (the third law). The **law of segregation** states that there are two **alleles** and that half of the total number of alleles are contributed by each parent organism. The **law of independent assortment** states that traits are passed on randomly and are not influenced by other traits. The exception to this is linked traits. A **Punnett square** can illustrate how alleles combine from the contributing genes to form various **phenotypes**. One set of a parent's genes are put in columns, while the genes from the other parent are placed in rows. The allele combinations are shown in each cell. The **law of dominance** states that when two different alleles are present in a pair, the **dominant** one is expressed. A Punnett square can be used to predict the outcome of crosses.

> **Review Video: Punnett Square**
> Visit mometrix.com/academy and enter code: 853855

### GENE, GENOTYPE, PHENOTYPE, AND ALLELE

A gene is a portion of DNA that identifies how traits are expressed and passed on in an organism. A gene is part of the **genetic code**. Collectively, all genes form the **genotype** of an individual. The genotype includes genes that may not be expressed, such as **recessive genes**. The **phenotype** is the physical, visual manifestation of genes. It is determined by the basic genetic information and how genes have been affected by their environment.

An **allele** is a variation of a gene. Also known as a trait, it determines the manifestation of a gene. This manifestation results in a specific physical appearance of some facet of an organism, such as eye color or height. For example, the genetic information for eye color is a gene. The gene variations responsible for blue, green, brown, or black eyes are called alleles. **Locus** (pl. loci) refers to the location of a gene or alleles.

> **Review Video: Genotype vs Phenotype**
> Visit mometrix.com/academy and enter code: 922853

## DOMINANT AND RECESSIVE

Gene traits are represented in pairs with an upper-case letter for the dominant trait (A) and a lower-case letter for the recessive trait (a). Genes occur in pairs (AA, Aa, or aa). There is one gene on each chromosome half supplied by each parent organism. Since half the genetic material is from each parent, the offspring's traits are represented as a combination of these. A dominant trait only requires one gene of a gene pair for it to be expressed in a phenotype, whereas a recessive trait requires both genes in order to be manifested. For example, if the mother's genotype is Dd and the father's is dd, the possible combinations are Dd and dd. The dominant trait will be manifested if the genotype is DD or Dd. The recessive trait will be manifested if the genotype is dd. Both DD and dd are homozygous pairs. Dd is heterozygous.

## MONOHYBRID AND HYBRID CROSSES

**Genetic crosses** are the possible combinations of alleles, and can be represented using Punnett squares. A **monohybrid cross** refers to a cross involving only one trait. Typically, the ratio is 3:1 (DD, Dd, Dd, dd), which is the ratio of dominant gene manifestation to recessive gene manifestation. This ratio occurs when both parents have a pair of dominant and recessive genes. If one parent has a pair of dominant genes (DD) and the other has a pair of recessive (dd) genes, the recessive trait cannot be expressed in the next generation because the resulting crosses all have the Dd genotype.

A **dihybrid cross** refers to one involving more than one trait, which means more combinations are possible. The ratio of genotypes for a dihybrid cross is 9:3:3:1 when the traits are not linked. The ratio for incomplete dominance is 1:2:1, which corresponds to dominant, mixed, and recessive phenotypes.

### MONOHYBRID CROSS EXAMPLE

A monohybrid cross is a genetic cross for a single trait that has two alleles. A monohybrid cross can be used to show which allele is **dominant** for a single trait. The first monohybrid cross typically occurs between two **homozygous** parents. Each parent is homozygous for a separate allele for a particular trait. For example, in pea plants, green pods (G) are dominant over yellow pods (g). In a genetic cross of two pea plants that are homozygous for pod color, the $F_1$ generation will be 100% heterozygous green pods.

|   | **g** | **g** |
|---|---|---|
| **G** | Gg | Gg |
| **G** | Gg | Gg |

If the plants with the heterozygous green pods are crossed, the $F_2$ generation should be 50% heterozygous green, 25% homozygous green, and 25% homozygous yellow.

|   | **G** | **g** |
|---|---|---|
| **G** | GG | Gg |
| **g** | Gg | gg |

### DIHYBRID CROSS EXAMPLE

A dihybrid cross is a genetic cross for **two traits** that each have two alleles. For example, in pea plants, green pods (G) are dominant over yellow pods (g), and yellow seeds (Y) are dominant over green seeds (y). In a genetic cross of two pea plants that are homozygous for pod color and seed color, the $F_1$ generation will be 100% heterozygous green pods and yellow seeds (GgYy). If these $F_1$

plants are crossed, the resulting F$_2$ generation is shown below. There are nine genotypes for green-pod, yellow-seed plants: one GGYY, two GGYy, two GgYY, and four GgYy. There are three genotypes for green-pod, green-seed plants: one GGyy and two Ggyy. There are three genotypes for yellow-pod, yellow-seed plants: one ggYY and two ggYy. There is only one genotype for yellow-pod, green-seed plants: ggyy. This cross has a 9:3:3:1 ratio.

|        | GY   | Gy   | gY   | gy   |
|--------|------|------|------|------|
| **GY** | GGYY | GGYy | GgYY | GgYy |
| **Gy** | GGYy | GGyy | GgYy | Ggyy |
| **gY** | GgYY | GgYy | ggYY | ggYy |
| **gy** | GgYy | Ggyy | ggYy | ggyy |

## NON-MENDELIAN CONCEPTS
### CO-DOMINANCE

Co-dominance refers to the expression of *both alleles* so that both traits are shown. Cows, for example, can have hair colors of red, white, or red and white (not pink). In the latter color, both traits are fully expressed. The ABO human blood typing system is also co-dominant.

> **Review Video: Mendelian & Non-Mendelian Concepts**
> Visit mometrix.com/academy and enter code: 113159

### INCOMPLETE DOMINANCE

Incomplete dominance is when both the **dominant** and **recessive** genes are expressed, resulting in a phenotype that is a mixture of the two. The fact that snapdragons can be red, white, or pink is a good example. The dominant red gene (RR) results in a red flower because of large amounts of red pigment. White (rr) occurs because both genes call for no pigment. Pink (Rr) occurs because one gene is for red and one is for no pigment. The colors blend to produce pink flowers. A cross of pink flowers (Rr) can result in red (RR), white (rr), or pink (Rr) flowers.

### POLYGENIC INHERITANCE

Polygenic inheritance goes beyond the simplistic Mendelian concept that one gene influences one trait. It refers to traits that are influenced by *more than one gene*, and takes into account environmental influences on development.

### MULTIPLE ALLELES

Each gene is made up of only two alleles, but in some cases, there are more than two possibilities for what those two alleles might be. For example, in blood typing, there are three alleles (A, B, O), but each person has only two of them. A gene with more than two possible alleles is known as a multiple allele. A gene that can result in two or more possible forms or expressions is known as a polymorphic gene.

## BASIC ATOMIC STRUCTURE
### PIECES OF AN ATOM

All matter consists of atoms. Atoms consist of a **nucleus** and **electrons**. The nucleus consists of **protons** and **neutrons**. The properties of these are measurable; they have mass and an electrical charge. The nucleus is **positively charged** due to the presence of protons. Electrons are **negatively charged** and orbit the nucleus. The nucleus has considerably more mass than the surrounding electrons. Atoms can bond together to make **molecules**. Atoms that have an equal number of protons and electrons are electrically **neutral**. If the number of protons and electrons in an atom is not equal, the atom has a positive or negative charge and is an **ion**.

> **Review Video: Structure of Atoms**
> Visit mometrix.com/academy and enter code: 905932

## MODELS OF ATOMS

Atoms are extremely small. A hydrogen atom is about $5 \times 10^{-8}$ mm in diameter. According to some estimates, five trillion hydrogen atoms could fit on the head of a pin. **Atomic radius** refers to the average distance between the nucleus and the outermost electron. Models of atoms that include the proton, nucleus, and electrons typically show the electrons very close to the nucleus and revolving around it, similar to how the Earth orbits the sun. However, another model relates the Earth as the nucleus and its atmosphere as electrons, which is the basis of the term "**electron cloud.**" Another description is that electrons swarm around the nucleus. It should be noted that these atomic models are not to scale. A more accurate representation would be a nucleus with a diameter of about 2 cm in a stadium. The electrons would be in the bleachers. This model is similar to the not-to-scale solar system model.

## ATOMIC NUMBER

The atomic number of an element refers to the **number of protons** in the nucleus of an atom. It is a unique identifier. It can be represented as Z. Atoms with a neutral charge have an atomic number that is equal to the **number of electrons**.

## ATOMIC MASS

Atomic mass is also known as the **mass number**. The atomic mass is the *total number of protons and neutrons* in the nucleus of an atom. It is referred to as "A." The atomic mass (A) is equal to the number of protons (Z) plus the number of neutrons (N). This can be represented by the equation A = Z + N. The mass of electrons in an atom is basically insignificant because it is so small. Atomic weight may sometimes be referred to as "**relative atomic mass**," but should not be confused with atomic mass. Atomic weight is the ratio of the average mass per atom of a sample (which can include various isotopes of an element) to 1/12 of the mass of an atom of carbon-12.

## ISOTOPES

**Isotopes** are atoms of the same element that vary in their number of neutrons. Isotopes of the same element have the same number of protons and thus the same atomic number. They are denoted by the element symbol, preceded in superscript and subscript by the mass number and atomic number, respectively. For instance, the notations for protium, deuterium, and tritium are, respectively: $_{1}^{1}H$, $_{1}^{2}H$, and $_{1}^{3}H$.

Isotopes that have not been observed to decay are **stable**, or non-radioactive, isotopes. It is not known whether some stable isotopes may have such long decay times that observing decay is not possible. Currently, 80 elements have one or more stable isotopes. There are 256 known stable isotopes in total. Carbon, for example, has three isotopes. Two (carbon-12 and carbon-13) are stable and one (carbon-14) is radioactive. **Radioactive isotopes** have unstable nuclei and can undergo spontaneous nuclear reactions, which results in particles or radiation being emitted. It cannot be predicted when a specific nucleus will decay, but large groups of identical nuclei decay at predictable rates. Knowledge about rates of decay can be used to *estimate the age of materials* that contain radioactive isotopes.

> **Review Video:** <u>Isotopes</u>
> Visit mometrix.com/academy and enter code: 294271

## ELECTRONS

Electrons are subatomic particles that orbit the nucleus at various levels commonly referred to as **layers**, **shells**, or **clouds**. The orbiting electron or electrons account for only a fraction of the atom's mass. They are much smaller than the nucleus, are negatively charged, and exhibit wave-like characteristics. Electrons are part of the **lepton** family of elementary particles. Electrons can occupy orbits that are varying distances away from the nucleus, and tend to occupy the lowest energy level they can. If an atom has all its electrons in the lowest available positions, it has a **stable** electron arrangement. The outermost electron shell of an atom in its uncombined state is known as the **valence shell**. The electrons there are called **valence electrons**, and it is their number that determines **bonding behavior**. Atoms tend to react in a manner that will allow them to fill or empty their valence shells.

### CHEMICAL BONDS AND ELECTRON SHELLS

Chemical bonds involve a negative-positive attraction between an electron or electrons and the nucleus of an atom or nuclei of more than one atom. The attraction keeps the atom cohesive, but also enables the formation of bonds among other atoms and molecules. Each of the four **energy levels** (or shells) of an atom has a maximum number of electrons they can contain. Each level must be completely filled before electrons can be added to the **valence level**. The farther away from the nucleus an electron is, the more energy it has. The first shell, or K-shell, can hold a maximum of 2 electrons; the second, the L-shell, can hold 8; the third, the M-shell, can hold 18; the fourth, the N-shell, can hold 32. The shells can also have **subshells**. Chemical bonds form and break between atoms when atoms gain, lose, or share an electron in the outer valence shell. **Polar bond** refers to a covalent type of bond with a separation of charge. One end is negative and the other is positive. The hydrogen-oxygen bond in water is one example of a polar bond.

### IONS

Most atoms are **neutral** since the positive charge of the protons in the nucleus is balanced by the negative charge of the surrounding electrons. Electrons are transferred between atoms when they come into contact with each other. This creates a molecule or atom in which the number of electrons does not equal the number of protons, which gives it a positive or negative charge. A **negative ion** is created when an atom gains electrons, while a **positive ion** is created when an atom loses electrons. An **ionic bond** is formed between ions with opposite charges. The resulting compound is neutral. **Ionization** refers to the process by which neutral particles are ionized into charged particles. Gases and plasmas can be partially or fully ionized through ionization.

### CHEMICAL BONDS BETWEEN ATOMS

Atoms of the same element may bond together to form **molecules** or **crystalline solids**. When two or more different types of atoms bind together chemically, a **compound** is made. The physical properties of compounds reflect the nature of the interactions among their molecules. These interactions are determined by the structure of the molecule, including the atoms they consist of and the distances and angles between them.

A union between the electron structures of atoms is called **chemical bonding**. An atom may gain, surrender, or share its electrons with another atom it bonds with. Listed below are three types of chemical bonding.

- **Ionic bonding** – When an atom gains or loses electrons it becomes negatively or positively charged, turning it into an ion. An ionic bond is a relationship between two *oppositely charged ions*.
- **Covalent bonding** – Atoms that share electrons have what is called a covalent bond. Electrons shared equally have a *non-polar bond*, while electrons shared unequally have a *polar bond*.
- **Hydrogen bonding** – The atom of a molecule interacts with a hydrogen atom in the same area. Hydrogen bonds can also form between two different parts of the same molecule, as in the structure of DNA and other large molecules.

A **cation** or positive ion is formed when an atom loses one or more electrons. An **anion** or negative ion is formed when an atom gains one or more electrons.

## IONIC BONDING

The transfer of electrons from one atom to another is called **ionic bonding**. Atoms that lose or gain electrons are referred to as **ions**. The gain or loss of electrons will result in an ion having a positive or negative charge. Here is an example:

> Take an atom of sodium (Na) and an atom of chlorine (Cl). The sodium atom has a total of 11 electrons (including one electron in its outer shell). The chlorine has 17 electrons (including 7 electrons in its outer shell). From this, the atomic number, or number of protons, of sodium can be calculated as 11 because the number of protons equals the number of electrons in an atom. When sodium chloride (NaCl) is formed, one electron from sodium transfers to chlorine. Ions have charges. They are written with a plus (+) or minus (−) symbol. Ions in a compound are attracted to each other because they have *opposite charges*.

$$Na{\cdot} + \underset{\times\,\times}{\overset{\times\,\times}{\times Cl\,\times}} \longrightarrow [Na]^+ [{:}Cl\,{\times}]^-$$

electron transfer from
sodium to chlorine

## COVALENT BONDING

Covalent bonding is characterized by the sharing of one or more pairs of electrons between two atoms or between an atom and another **covalent bond**. This produces an attraction to repulsion stability that holds these molecules together.

Atoms have the tendency to share electrons with each other so that all outer electron shells are filled. The resultant bonds are always stronger than the **intermolecular hydrogen bond** and are similar in strength to ionic bonds.

Covalent bonding occurs most frequently between atoms with similar **electronegativities**. **Nonmetals** are more likely to form covalent bonds than metals since it is more difficult for nonmetals to liberate an electron. **Electron sharing** takes place when one species encounters another species with similar electronegativity. Covalent bonding of metals is important in both *process chemistry* and *industrial catalysis.*

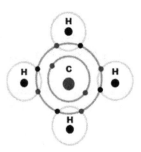

### ELECTRONEGATIVITY

Electronegativity is a measure of how capable an atom is of attracting a pair of bonding electrons. It refers to the fact that one atom exerts slightly more force in a bond than another, creating a **dipole**. If the electronegative difference between two atoms is small, the atoms will form a **polar covalent bond**. If the difference is large, the atoms will form an **ionic bond**. When there is no electronegativity, a **pure nonpolar covalent bond** is formed.

> **Review Video: Electronegativity**
> Visit mometrix.com/academy and enter code: 823348

### COMPOUNDS

An **element** is the most basic type of matter. It has unique properties and cannot be broken down into other elements. The smallest unit of an element is the **atom**. A chemical combination of two or more types of elements is called a **compound**.

Compounds often have properties that are very different from those of their constituent elements. The smallest independent unit of an element or compound is known as a **molecule**. Most elements are found somewhere in nature in single-atom form, but a few elements only exist naturally in pairs. These are called **diatomic elements**, of which some of the most common are hydrogen, nitrogen, and oxygen.

Elements and compounds are represented by **chemical symbols**, one or two letters, most often the first in the element name. More than one atom of the same element in a compound is represented with a subscript number designating how many atoms of that element are present. Water, for instance, contains two hydrogens and one oxygen. Thus, the chemical formula is $H_2O$. Methane contains one carbon and four hydrogens, so its formula is $CH_4$.

## PERIODIC TABLE

| 1 IA | | | | | | | | | | | | | | | | | 18 VIIIA |
|------|------|------|------|------|------|------|------|------|------|------|------|------|------|------|------|------|------|
| 1 **H** 1.01 | 2 IIA | | | | | | | | | | | 13 IIIA | 14 IVA | 15 VA | 16 VIA | 17 VIIA | 2 **He** 4.00 |
| 3 **Li** 6.94 | 4 **Be** 9.01 | | | | | | | | | | | 5 **B** 10.81 | 6 **C** 12.01 | 7 **N** 14.01 | 8 **O** 16.00 | 9 **F** 19.00 | 10 **Ne** 20.18 |
| 11 **Na** 22.99 | 12 **Mg** 24.31 | 3 IIIB | 4 IVB | 5 VB | 6 VIB | 7 VIIB | 8 | 9 VIIIB | 10 | 11 IB | 12 IIB | 13 **Al** 26.98 | 14 **Si** 28.09 | 15 **P** 30.97 | 16 **S** 32.07 | 17 **Cl** 35.45 | 18 **Ar** 39.95 |
| 19 **K** 39.1 | 20 **Ca** 40.08 | 21 **Sc** 44.96 | 22 **Ti** 47.88 | 23 **V** 50.94 | 24 **Cr** 52.00 | 25 **Mn** 54.94 | 26 **Fe** 55.85 | 27 **Co** 58.93 | 28 **Ni** 58.69 | 29 **Cu** 63.55 | 30 **Zn** 65.39 | 31 **Ga** 69.72 | 32 **Ge** 72.61 | 33 **As** 74.92 | 34 **Se** 78.96 | 35 **Br** 79.90 | 36 **Kr** 83.80 |
| 37 **Rb** 85.47 | 38 **Sr** 87.62 | 39 **Y** 88.91 | 40 **Zr** 91.22 | 41 **Nb** 92.91 | 42 **Mo** 95.94 | 43 **Tc** (98) | 44 **Ru** 101.07 | 45 **Rh** 102.91 | 46 **Pd** 106.42 | 47 **Ag** 107.87 | 48 **Cd** 112.41 | 49 **In** 114.82 | 50 **Sn** 118.71 | 51 **Sb** 121.76 | 52 **Te** 127.6 | 53 **I** 126.9 | 54 **Xe** 131.29 |
| 55 **Cs** 132.9 | 56 **Ba** 137.3 | 57 **La\*** 138.9 | 72 **Hf** 178.5 | 73 **Ta** 180.9 | 74 **W** 183.9 | 75 **Re** 186.2 | 76 **Os** 190.2 | 77 **Ir** 192.2 | 78 **Pt** 195.1 | 79 **Au** 197.0 | 80 **Hg** 200.6 | 81 **Tl** 204.4 | 82 **Pb** 207.2 | 83 **Bi** 209 | 84 **Po** (209) | 85 **At** (210) | 86 **Rn** (222) |
| 87 **Fr** (223) | 88 **Ra** (226) | 89 **Ac^** (227) | 104 **Rf** (261) | 105 **Db** (262) | 106 **Sg** (263) | 107 **Bh** (264) | 108 **Hs** (265) | 109 **Mt** (268) | 110 **Ds** (271) | 111 **Rg** (272) | | | | | | | |

| * | 58 **Ce** 140.1 | 59 **Pr** 140.9 | 60 **Nd** 144.2 | 61 **Pm** (145) | 62 **Sm** 150.4 | 63 **Eu** 152.0 | 64 **Gd** 157.3 | 65 **Tb** 158.9 | 66 **Dy** 162.5 | 67 **Ho** 164.9 | 68 **Er** 167.3 | 69 **Tm** 168.9 | 70 **Yb** 173.0 | 71 **Lu** 175.0 |
|---|---|---|---|---|---|---|---|---|---|---|---|---|---|---|
| ^ | 90 **Th** 232.0 | 91 **Pa** (231) | 92 **U** 238.0 | 93 **Np** (237) | 94 **Pu** (244) | 95 **Am** (243) | 96 **Cm** (247) | 97 **Bk** (247) | 98 **Cf** (251) | 99 **Es** (252) | 100 **Fm** (257) | 101 **Md** (258) | 102 **No** (259) | 103 **Lr** (260) |

The **periodic table** is a tabular arrangement of the elements and is organized according to **periodic law**. The properties of the elements depend on their **atomic structure** and vary with **atomic number**. It shows periodic trends of physical and chemical properties and identifies families of elements with similar properties. In the periodic table, the elements are arranged by atomic number in horizontal rows called **periods** and vertical columns called **groups** or **families**. They are further categorized as metals, metalloids, or nonmetals. The majority of known elements are metals; there are seventeen nonmetals and eight metalloids. **Metals** are situated at the left end of the periodic table, **nonmetals** to the right and **metalloids** between the two.

A typical periodic table shows the elements' symbols and atomic number, the number of protons in the atomic nucleus. Some more detailed tables also list **atomic mass**, **electronegativity**, and other data. The position of an element in the table reveals its group, its block, and whether it is a representative, transition, or inner transition element. Its position also shows the element as a metal, nonmetal, or metalloid.

For the representative elements, the last digit of the **group number** reveals the number of outer-level electrons. Roman numerals for the A groups also reveal the number of outer level electrons within the group. The position of the element in the table reveals its **electronic configuration** and how it differs in atomic size from neighbors in its period or group. In this example, Boron has an atomic number of 5 and an atomic weight of 10.811. It is found in group 13, in which all atoms of the group have 3 valence electrons; the group's Roman numeral representation is IIIA.

### IMPORTANT FEATURES AND STRUCTURE

The most important feature of the table is its arrangement according to **periodicity**, or the predictable trends observable in atoms. The arrangement enables classification, organization, and prediction of important elemental properties.

The table is organized in horizontal rows called **Periods**, and vertical columns called **Groups** or **Families**. Groups of elements share predictable characteristics, the most important of which is that their outer energy levels have the same configuration of electrons. For example, the highest group is group 18, the noble gases. Each element in this group has a full complement of electrons in its outer level, making the reactivity low. Elements in periods also share some common properties, but most classifications rely more heavily on groups.

## CHEMICAL REACTIVITY

Reactivity refers to the tendency of a substance to engage in **chemical reactions**. If that tendency is high, the substance is said to be highly reactive, or to have **high reactivity**. Because the basis of a chemical reaction is the transfer of electrons, reactivity depends upon the presence of uncommitted electrons which are available for transfer. **Periodicity** allows us to predict an element's reactivity based on its position on the periodic table. High numbered groups on the right side of the table have a fuller complement of electrons in their outer levels, making them less likely to react. Noble gases, on the far right of the table, each have eight electrons in the outer level, with the exception of He, which has two. Because atoms tend to lose or gain electrons to reach an ideal of eight in the outer level, these elements have very low reactivity.

## GROUPS AND PERIODS IN TERMS OF REACTIVITY

Reading left to right within a period, each element contains one more electron than the one preceding it. (Note that H and He are in the same period, though nothing is between them and they are in different groups.) As electrons are added, their attraction to the nucleus increases, meaning that as we read to the right in a period, each atom's electrons are more densely compacted, more strongly bound to the nucleus, and less likely to be pulled away in reactions. As we read down a group, each successive atom's outer electrons are less tightly bound to the nucleus, thus increasing their reactivity, because the principal energy levels are increasingly full as we move downward within the group. **Principal energy levels** shield the outer energy levels from nuclear attraction, allowing the valence electrons to react. For this reason, noble gases farther down the group can react under certain circumstances.

## METALS, NONMETALS, AND METALLOIDS IN THE PERIODIC TABLE

The metals are located on the left side and center of the periodic table, and the nonmetals are located on the right side of the periodic table. The metalloids or semimetals form a zigzag line between the metals and nonmetals. Metals include the **alkali metals** such as lithium, sodium, and potassium and the **alkaline earth metals** such as beryllium, magnesium, and calcium. Metals also include the **transition metals** such as iron, copper, and nickel and the **inner transition metals** such as thorium, uranium, and plutonium. **Nonmetals** include the **chalcogens** such as oxygen and sulfur, the **halogens** such as fluorine and chlorine, and the **noble gases** such as helium and argon. Carbon, nitrogen, and phosphorus are also nonmetals. **Metalloids** or **semimetals** include boron, silicon, germanium, antimony, and polonium.

## CHARACTERISTIC PROPERTIES OF SUBSTANCES
### INTENSIVE AND EXTENSIVE PROPERTIES

Physical properties are categorized as either intensive or extensive. **Intensive properties** *do not* depend on the amount of matter or quantity of the sample. This means that intensive properties will not change if the sample size is increased or decreased. Intensive properties include color, hardness, melting point, boiling point, density, ductility, malleability, specific heat, temperature, concentration, and magnetization.

**Extensive properties** *do* depend on the amount of matter or quantity of the sample. Therefore, extensive properties do change if the sample size is increased or decreased. If the sample size is increased, the property increases. If the sample size is decreased, the property decreases. Extensive properties include volume, mass, weight, energy, entropy, number of moles, and electrical charge.

## PHYSICAL PROPERTIES OF MATTER

Physical properties are any property of matter that can be **observed** or **measured**. These include properties such as color, elasticity, mass, volume, and temperature. **Mass** is a measure of the amount of substance in an object. **Weight** is a measure of the gravitational pull of Earth on an object. **Volume** is a measure of the amount of space occupied. There are many formulas to determine volume. For example, the volume of a cube is the length of one side cubed ($a^3$) and the volume of a rectangular prism is length times width times height ($l \times w \times h$). The volume of an irregular shape can be determined by how much water it displaces. **Density** is a measure of the amount of mass per unit volume. The formula to find density is mass divided by volume ($D = m/V$). It is expressed in terms of mass per cubic unit, such as grams per cubic centimeter ($g/cm^3$). **Specific gravity** is a measure of the ratio of a substance's density compared to the density of water.

### DENSITY

The density of an object is equal to its *mass divided by its volume* ($d = m/v$). It is important to note the difference between an *object's density* and a *material's density*. Water has a density of one gram per cubic centimeter, while steel has a density approximately eight times that. Despite having a much higher material density, an object made of steel may still float. A hollow steel sphere, for instance, will float easily because the density of the object includes the air contained within the sphere.

### SPECIFIC HEAT CAPACITY

Specific heat capacity, also known as **specific heat**, is the *heat capacity per unit mass*. Each element and compound has its own specific heat. For example, it takes different amounts of heat energy to raise the temperature of the same amounts of magnesium and lead by one degree. The equation for relating heat energy to specific heat capacity is $Q = mc\Delta T$, where m represents the mass of the object, and c represents its specific heat capacity.

> **Review Video: Specific Heat Capacity**
> Visit mometrix.com/academy and enter code: 736791

## CONDUCTION

Heat always flows from a region of higher temperature to a region of lower temperature. If two regions are at the same temperature, there is a **thermal equilibrium** between them and there will be **no net heat transfer** between them. **Conduction** is a form of heat transfer that requires contact. Since heat is a measure of kinetic energy, most commonly vibration, at the atomic level, it may be transferred from one location to another or one object to another by contact.

## CHEMICAL PROPERTIES OF MATTER

If a chemical change must be carried out in order to observe and measure a property, then the property is a **chemical property**. For example, when hydrogen gas is burned in oxygen, it forms water. This is a chemical property of hydrogen because after burning, a different chemical substance – water – is all that remains. The hydrogen cannot be recovered from the water by means of a physical change such as freezing or boiling.

> **Review Video: Chemical and Physical Properties of Matter**
> Visit mometrix.com/academy and enter code: 717349

## PROPERTIES OF WATER

The important properties of water ($H_2O$) are *high polarity, hydrogen bonding, cohesiveness, adhesiveness, high specific heat, high latent heat, and high heat of vaporization*. It is **essential to life** as we know it, as water is one of the main if not the main constituent of many living things. Water is a liquid at room temperature. The high specific heat of water means it resists the breaking of its hydrogen bonds and resists heat and motion, which is why it has a relatively high boiling point and high vaporization point. It also resists temperature change. In its solid state, water floats. (Most substances are heavier in their solid forms.) Water is **cohesive**, which means it is attracted to itself. It is also **adhesive**, which means it readily attracts other molecules. If water tends to adhere to another substance, the substance is said to be **hydrophilic**. Because of its cohesive and adhesive properties, water makes a good solvent. Substances, particularly those with polar ions and molecules, readily dissolve in water.

> **Review Video: Properties of Water**
> Visit mometrix.com/academy and enter code: 279526

## HYDROGEN BONDS

Hydrogen bonds are weaker than covalent and ionic bonds, and refer to the type of attraction in an **electronegative atom** such as oxygen, fluorine, or nitrogen. Hydrogen bonds can form within a single molecule or between molecules. A water molecule is **polar**, meaning it is partially positively charged on one end (the hydrogen end) and partially negatively charged on the other (the oxygen end). This is because the hydrogen atoms are arranged around the oxygen atom in a close tetrahedron. Hydrogen is **oxidized** (its number of electrons is reduced) when it bonds with oxygen to form water. Hydrogen bonds tend not only to be weak but also short-lived. They also tend to be numerous. Hydrogen bonds give water many of its important properties, including its high specific heat and high heat of vaporization, its solvent qualities, its adhesiveness and cohesiveness, its hydrophobic qualities, and its ability to float in its solid form. Hydrogen bonds are also an important component of *proteins, nucleic acids, and DNA*.

## PASSIVE TRANSPORT MECHANISMS: DIFFUSION AND OSMOSIS

Transport mechanisms allow for the movement of substances through membranes. **Passive transport mechanisms** include simple and facilitated diffusion and osmosis. They do not require energy from the cell. **Diffusion** occurs when particles are transported from areas of higher concentration to areas of lower concentration. When equilibrium is reached, diffusion stops. Examples are gas exchange (carbon dioxide and oxygen) during photosynthesis and the transport of oxygen from air to blood and from blood to tissue. **Facilitated diffusion** occurs when specific molecules are transported by a specific carrier protein. **Carrier proteins** vary in terms of size, shape, and charge. Glucose and amino acids are examples of substances transported by carrier proteins.

**Osmosis** is the diffusion of water through a semi-permeable membrane from an area of lower solute concentration to one of higher solute concentration. Examples of osmosis include the absorption of water by plant roots and the alimentary canal. Plants lose and gain water through osmosis. A plant cell that swells because of water retention is said to be **turgid**.

> **Review Video: Passive Transport: Diffusion and Osmosis**
> Visit mometrix.com/academy and enter code: 642038

## STATES OF MATTER

Matter refers to substances that *have mass and occupy space* (or volume). The traditional definition of matter describes it as having three states: solid, liquid, and gas. These different states are caused by differences in the distances and angles between molecules or atoms, which result in differences in the energy that binds them. **Solid** structures are rigid or nearly rigid and have strong bonds. Molecules or atoms of **liquids** move around and have weak bonds, although they are not weak enough to readily break. Molecules or atoms of **gases** move almost independently of each other, are typically far apart, and do not form bonds. The current definition of matter describes it as having four states. The fourth is **plasma**, which is an ionized gas that has some electrons that are described as free because they are not bound to an atom or molecule. However, the TEAS will only be concerned with solids, liquids, and gases.

The table below outlines the characteristic properties of the three states of matter:

| State of matter | Volume/shape | Density | Compressibility | Molecular motion |
|---|---|---|---|---|
| Gas | Assumes volume and shape of its container | Low | High | Very free motion |
| Liquid | Volume remains constant but it assumes shape of its container | High | Virtually none | Move past each other freely |
| Solid | Definite volume and shape | High | Virtually none | Vibrate around fixed positions |

The three states of matter can be traversed by the addition or removal of **heat**. For example, when a solid is heated to its melting point, it can begin to form a liquid. However, in order to transition from solid to liquid, additional heat must be added at the melting point to overcome the **latent heat of fusion**. Upon further heating to its boiling point, the liquid can begin to form a gas, but again, additional heat must be added at the boiling point to overcome the **latent heat of vaporization**.

In the solid state, water is less dense than in the liquid state. This can be observed quite simply by noting that an ice cube floats at the surface of a glass of water. Were this not the case, ice would not form on the surface of lakes and rivers in those regions of the world where the climate produces temperatures below the freezing point. If water behaved as other substances do, lakes and rivers would freeze from the bottom up, which would be detrimental to many forms of aquatic life.

The lower density of ice occurs because of a combination of the unique structure of the water molecule and hydrogen bonding. In the case of ice, each oxygen atom is bound to four hydrogen atoms, two covalently and two by hydrogen bonds. This forms an ordered roughly **tetrahedral** structure that prevents the molecules from getting close to each other. As such, there are empty spaces in the structure that account for the low density of ice.

> **Review Video: States of Matter**
> Visit mometrix.com/academy and enter code: 742449

### CHANGES IN STATES OF MATTER

A substance that is undergoing a change from a solid to a liquid is said to be **melting**. If this change occurs in the opposite direction, from liquid to solid, this change is called **freezing**. A liquid which is being converted to a gas is undergoing **vaporization**. The reverse of this process is known as **condensation**. Direct transitions from gas to solid and solid to gas are much less common in everyday life, but they can occur given the proper conditions. Solid to gas conversion is known as **sublimation**, while the reverse is called **deposition**.

*Evaporation*: Evaporation is the change of state in a substance from a liquid to a gaseous form at a temperature below its boiling point (the temperature at which all of the molecules in a liquid are changed to gas through vaporization). Some of the molecules at the surface of a liquid always maintain enough **heat energy** to escape the cohesive forces exerted on them by neighboring molecules. At higher temperatures, the molecules in a substance move more rapidly, increasing their number with enough energy to break out of the liquid form. The rate of evaporation is higher when more of the surface area of a liquid is exposed (as in a large water body, such as an ocean). The amount of moisture already in the air also affects the rate of evaporation—if there is a significant amount of water vapor in the air around a liquid, some evaporated molecules will return to the liquid. The speed of the evaporation process is also decreased by increased **atmospheric pressure**.

*Condensation*: Condensation is the phase change in a substance from a gaseous to liquid form; it is the opposite of evaporation or vaporization. When temperatures decrease in a gas, such as water vapor, the material's component molecules move more slowly. The decreased motion of the molecules enables **intermolecular cohesive forces** to pull the molecules closer together and, in water, establish hydrogen bonds. Condensation can also be caused by an increase in the pressure exerted on a gas, which results in a decrease in the substance's volume (it reduces the distance between particles). In the **hydrologic cycle**, this process is initiated when warm air containing water vapor rises and then cools. This occurs due to convection in the air, meteorological fronts, or lifting over high land formations.

## OVERVIEW OF CHEMICAL REACTIONS

Chemical reactions measured in human time can take place quickly or slowly. They can take a fraction of a second or billions of years. The **rates** of chemical reactions are determined by how frequently reacting atoms and molecules interact. Rates are also influenced by the temperature and various properties (such as shape) of the reacting materials. **Catalysts** accelerate chemical reactions, while **inhibitors** decrease reaction rates. Some types of reactions release energy in the form of heat and light. Some types of reactions involve the transfer of either electrons or hydrogen ions between reacting ions, molecules, or atoms. In other reactions, chemical bonds are broken down by heat or light to form **reactive radicals** with electrons that will readily form new bonds. Processes such as the formation of ozone and greenhouse gases in the atmosphere and the burning and processing of fossil fuels are controlled by radical reactions.

> **Review Video: <u>Chemical Reactions</u>**
> Visit mometrix.com/academy and enter code: 579876

## READING AND BALANCING CHEMICAL EQUATIONS

Chemical equations describe chemical reactions. The **reactants** are on the left side before the arrow and the **products** are on the right side after the arrow. The arrow indicates the **reaction** or change. The **coefficient**, or stoichiometric coefficient, is the number before the element, and indicates the ratio of reactants to products in terms of moles. The equation for the formation of water from hydrogen and oxygen, for example, is $2H_{2(g)} + O_{2(g)} \rightarrow 2H_2O_{(l)}$. The 2 preceding hydrogen and water is the coefficient, which means there are 2 moles of hydrogen and 2 of water. There is 1 mole of oxygen, which does not have to be indicated with the number 1. In parentheses, *g* stands for gas, *l* stands for liquid, *s* stands for solid, and *aq* stands for aqueous solution (a substance dissolved in water). **Charges** are shown in superscript for individual ions, but not for ionic compounds.

**Polyatomic ions** are separated by parentheses so the ion will not be confused with the number of ions.

An **unbalanced equation** is one that does not follow the **law of conservation of mass**, which states that matter can only be changed, not created. If an equation is unbalanced, the numbers of atoms indicated by the stoichiometric coefficients on each side of the arrow will not be equal. Start by writing the formulas for each species in the reaction. Count the atoms on each side and determine if the number is equal. **Coefficients** must be whole numbers. Fractional amounts, such as half a molecule, are not possible. Equations can be **balanced** by multiplying the coefficients by a constant that will produce the smallest possible whole number coefficient. $H_2 + O_2 \rightarrow H_2O$ is an example of an unbalanced equation. The balanced equation is $2H_2 + O_2 \rightarrow 2H_2O$, which indicates that it takes two moles of hydrogen and one of oxygen to produce two moles of water.

> **Review Video: How to Balance a Chemical Equation**
> Visit mometrix.com/academy and enter code: 341228

## LAW OF CONSERVATION OF MASS

The Law of Conservation of Mass in a chemical reaction is commonly stated as follows:

*In a chemical reaction, matter is neither created nor destroyed.*

What this means is that there will always be the same **total mass** of material after a reaction as before. This allows for predicting how molecules will combine by balanced equations in which the number of each type of atom is the same on either side of the equation. For example, two hydrogen molecules combine with one oxygen molecule to form water. This is a balanced chemical equation because the number of each type of atom is the same on both sides of the arrow. It has to balance because the reaction obeys the Law of Conservation of Mass.

## REACTIONS

### BASIC MECHANISMS

Chemical reactions normally occur when electrons are transferred from one atom or molecule to another. Reactions and reactivity depend on the **octet rule**, which describes the tendency of atoms to gain or lose electrons until their outer energy levels contain eight. The changes in a reaction may be in **composition** or **configuration** of a compound or substance, and result in one or more products being generated which were not present in isolation before the reaction occurred. For instance, when oxygen reacts with methane ($CH_4$), water and carbon dioxide are the products; one set of substances ($CH_4 + O$) was transformed into a new set of substances ($CO_2 + H_2O$).

Reactions depend on the presence of a **reactant**, or substance undergoing change, a **reagent**, or partner in the reaction less transformed than the reactant (such as a catalyst), and **products**, or the final result of the reaction. **Reaction conditions**, or environmental factors, are also important components in reactions. These include conditions such as temperature, pressure, concentration, whether the reaction occurs in solution, the type of solution, and presence or absence of catalysts. Chemical reactions are usually written in the following format: Reactants → Products.

## FIVE BASIC CHEMICAL REACTIONS

### COMBINATION REACTIONS

Combination, or synthesis, reactions: In a combination reaction, two or more reactants combine to make one product. This can be seen in the equation $A + B \rightarrow AB$. These reactions are also called **synthesis** or **addition reactions**. An example is burning hydrogen in air to produce water. The equation is $2H_2$ (g) + $O_2$ (g) → $2H_2O$ (l). Another example is when water and sulfur trioxide react to form sulfuric acid. The equation is $H_2O + SO_3$ → $H_2SO_4$.

### DECOMPOSITION REACTIONS

Decomposition (or desynthesis, decombination, or deconstruction) reactions; in a decomposition reaction, a reactant is broken down into two or more products. This can be seen in the equation AB → A + B. When a compound or substance separates into these simpler substances, the **byproducts** are often substances that are different from the original. Decomposition can be viewed as the *opposite* of combination reactions. These reactions are also called analysis reactions. Most decomposition reactions are **endothermic**. Heat needs to be added for the chemical reaction to occur. **Thermal decomposition** is caused by heat. **Electrolytic decomposition** is due to electricity. An example of this type of reaction is the decomposition of water into hydrogen and oxygen gas. The equation is $2H_2O$ → $2H_2 + O_2$. Separation processes can be **mechanical** or **chemical**, and usually involve reorganizing a mixture of substances without changing their chemical nature. The separated products may differ from the original mixture in terms of chemical or physical properties. Types of separation processes include **filtration**, **crystallization**, **distillation**, and **chromatography**. Basically, decomposition *breaks down* one compound into two or more compounds or substances that are different from the original; separation *sorts* the substances from the original mixture into like substances.

### SINGLE REPLACEMENT REACTIONS

**Single substitution, displacement, or replacement reactions occur when one reactant** is displaced by another to form the final product (A + BC → B + AC). Single substitution reactions can be **cationic** or **anionic**. When a piece of copper (Cu) is placed into a solution of silver nitrate ($AgNO_3$), the solution turns blue. The copper appears to be replaced with a silvery-white material. The equation is $2AgNO_3 + Cu$ → $Cu(NO_3)_2 + 2Ag$. When this reaction takes place, the copper dissolves and the silver in the silver nitrate solution precipitates (becomes a solid), thus resulting in copper nitrate and silver. Copper and silver have switched places in the nitrate.

> **Review Video: Single-Replacement Reactions**
> Visit mometrix.com/academy and enter code: 742449

### DOUBLE REPLACEMENT REACTIONS

**Double displacement, double replacement, substitution, metathesis, or ion exchange reactions occur when ions** or bonds are exchanged by two compounds to form different compounds (AC + BD → AD + BC). An example of this is that silver nitrate and sodium chloride form two different products (silver chloride and sodium nitrate) when they react. The formula for this reaction is $AgNO_3 + NaCl$ → $AgCl + NaNO_3$.

Double replacement reactions are **metathesis reactions**. In a double replacement reaction, the chemical reactants exchange ions but the oxidation state stays the same. One of the indicators of this is the formation of a **solid precipitate**. In acid/base reactions, an **acid** is a compound that can donate a proton, while a **base** is a compound that can accept a proton. In these types of reactions, the acid and base react to form a salt and water. When the proton is donated, the base becomes **water** and the remaining ions form a **salt**. One method of determining whether a reaction is an oxidation/reduction or a metathesis reaction is that the oxidation number of atoms does not change during a metathesis reaction.

## COMBUSTION REACTIONS

Combustion, or burning, is a sequence of chemical reactions involving **fuel** and an **oxidant** that produces heat and sometimes light. There are many types of combustion, such as rapid, slow, complete, turbulent, microgravity, and incomplete. Fuels and oxidants determine the **compounds** formed by a combustion reaction. For example, when rocket fuel consisting of hydrogen and oxygen combusts, it results in the formation of water vapor. When air and wood burn, resulting compounds include nitrogen, unburned carbon, and carbon compounds. Combustion is an **exothermic** process, meaning it releases energy. Exothermic energy is commonly released as heat, but can take other forms, such as light, electricity, or sound.

> **Review Video: Combustion**
> Visit mometrix.com/academy and enter code: 592219

## CATALYSTS

Catalysts, substances that help *change the rate of reaction* without changing their form, can increase reaction rate by decreasing the number of steps it takes to form products. The **mass** of the catalyst should be the same at the beginning of the reaction as it is at the end. The **activation energy** is the minimum amount required to get a reaction started. Activation energy causes particles to collide with sufficient energy to start the reaction. A **catalyst** enables more particles to react, which lowers the activation energy. Examples of catalysts in reactions are manganese oxide ($MnO_2$) in the decomposition of hydrogen peroxide, iron in the manufacture of ammonia using the Haber process, and concentrate of sulfuric acid in the nitration of benzene.

## PH

The **potential of hydrogen** (pH) is a measurement of the *concentration of hydrogen ions* in a substance in terms of the number of moles of $H^+$ per liter of solution. All substances fall between 0 and 14 on the pH scale. A lower pH indicates a higher $H^+$ concentration, while a higher pH indicates a lower $H^+$ concentration.

Pure water has a **neutral pH**, which is 7. Anything with a pH lower than pure water (<7) is considered **acidic**. Anything with a pH higher than pure water (>7) is a **base**. Drain cleaner, soap, baking soda, ammonia, egg whites, and sea water are common bases. Urine, stomach acid, citric acid, vinegar, hydrochloric acid, and battery acid are acids. A **pH indicator** is a substance that acts as a detector of hydrogen or hydronium ions. It is **halochromic**, meaning it changes color to indicate that hydrogen or hydronium ions have been detected.

> **Review Video: pH**
> Visit mometrix.com/academy and enter code: 187395

## BASES

Basic chemicals are usually in aqueous solution and have the following traits: a bitter taste; a soapy or slippery texture to the touch; the capacity to restore the blue color of litmus paper which had previously been turned red by an acid; the ability to produce salts in reaction with acids. The word **alkaline** is used to describe bases.

In contrast to acids, which yield **hydrogen ions** ($H^+$) when dissolved in solution, bases yield **hydroxide ions** ($OH^-$); the same models used to describe acids can be inverted and used to describe bases—Arrhenius, Bronsted-Lowry, and Lewis.

Some **nonmetal oxides** (such as $Na_2O$) are classified as bases even though they do not contain hydroxides in their molecular form. However, these substances easily produce hydroxide ions when reacted with water, which is why they are classified as bases.

## ACIDS

Acids are a unique class of compounds characterized by consistent properties. The most significant property of an acid is not readily observable and is what gives acids their unique behaviors: the **ionization of H atoms**, or their tendency to dissociate from their parent molecules and take on an electrical charge. **Carboxylic acids** are also characterized by ionization, but of the O atoms. Some other properties of acids are easy to observe without any experimental apparatus. These properties include the following:

- They have a sour taste
- They change the color of litmus paper to red
- They produce gaseous $H_2$ in reaction with some metals
- They produce salt precipitates in reaction with bases

Other properties, while no more complex, are less easily observed. For instance, most inorganic acids are easily soluble in water and have high boiling points.

## STRONG OR WEAK ACIDS AND BASES

The characteristic properties of acids and bases derive from the tendency of atoms to **ionize** by donating or accepting charged particles. The strength of an acid or base is a reflection of the degree to which its atoms ionize in solution. For example, if all of the atoms in an acid ionize, the acid is said to be **strong**. When only a few of the atoms ionize, the acid is **weak**. Acetic acid ($HC_2H_3O_2$) is a weak acid because only its $O_2$ atoms ionize in solution. Another way to think of the strength of an acid or base is to consider its **reactivity**. Highly reactive acids and bases are strong because they tend to form and break bonds quickly and most of their atoms ionize in the process.

> **Review Video: <u>Strong and Weak Acids and Bases</u>**
> Visit mometrix.com/academy and enter code: 268930

## SALTS

Some properties of **salts** are that they are formed from acid base reactions, are ionic compounds consisting of metallic and nonmetallic ions, dissociate in water, and are comprised of tightly bonded ions. Some common salts are sodium chloride (NaCl), sodium bisulfate, potassium dichromate ($K_2Cr_2O_7$), and calcium chloride ($CaCl_2$). Calcium chloride is used as a drying agent, and may be used to absorb moisture when freezing mixtures. Potassium nitrate ($KNO_3$) is used to make fertilizer and in the manufacture of explosives. Sodium nitrate ($NaNO_3$) is also used in the making of fertilizer. Baking soda (sodium bicarbonate) is a salt, as are Epsom salts [magnesium sulfate ($MgSO_4$)]. Salt and water can react to form a base and an acid. This is called a **hydrolysis reaction**.

# Scientific Reasoning

## METRIC SYSTEM

Using the metric system is generally accepted as the preferred method for taking measurements. Having a universal standard allows individuals to interpret measurements more easily, regardless of where they are located.

The basic units of measurement are: the **meter**, which measures length; the **liter**, which measures volume; and the **gram**, which measures mass. The metric system starts with a **base unit** and increases or decreases in units of 10. The prefix and the base unit combined are used to indicate an amount.

For example, deka is 10 times the base unit. A dekameter is 10 meters; a dekaliter is 10 liters; and a dekagram is 10 grams. The prefix hecto refers to 100 times the base amount; kilo is 1,000 times the base amount. The prefixes that indicate a fraction of the base unit are deci, which is 1/10 of the base unit; centi, which is 1/100 of the base unit; and milli, which is 1/1000 of the base unit.

## SI UNITS OF MEASUREMENT

SI uses the **second** (s) to measure time. Fractions of seconds are usually measured in metric terms using prefixes such as millisecond (1/1,000 of a second) or nanosecond (1/1,000,000,000 of a second). Increments of time larger than a second are measured in minutes and hours, which are multiples of 60 and 24. An example of this is a swimmer's time in the 800-meter freestyle being described as 7:32.67, meaning 7 minutes, 32 seconds, and 67 one-hundredths of a second. One second is equal to 1/60 of a minute, 1/3,600 of an hour, and 1/86,400 of a day.

Other SI base units are the **ampere** (A) (used to measure electric current), the **kelvin** (K) (used to measure thermodynamic temperature), the **candela** (cd) (used to measure luminous intensity), and the **mole** (mol) (used to measure the amount of a substance at a molecular level). **Meter** (m) is used to measure length and **kilogram** (kg) is used to measure mass.

## METRIC PREFIXES FOR MULTIPLES AND SUBDIVISIONS

The prefixes for multiples are as follows:

- deka (da), $10^1$ (deka is the American spelling, but deca is also used)
- hecto (h), $10^2$
- kilo (k), $10^3$
- mega (M), $10^6$
- giga (G), $10^9$
- tera (T), $10^{12}$

The prefixes for subdivisions are as follows:

- deci (d), $10^{-1}$
- centi (c), $10^{-2}$
- milli (m), $10^{-3}$
- micro (μ), $10^{-6}$
- nano (n), $10^{-9}$
- pico (p), $10^{-12}$

The rule of thumb is that prefixes greater than $10^3$ are capitalized when abbreviating. Abbreviations do not need a period after them. A decimeter (dm) is a tenth of a meter, a deciliter (dL) is a tenth of a liter, and a decigram (dg) is a tenth of a gram. Pluralization is understood. For example, when referring to 5 mL of water, no "s" needs to be added to the abbreviation.

## LAB GLASSWARE

### GRADUATED CYLINDERS AND BURETTES

Graduated cylinders are used for precise measurements and are considered more accurate than flasks or beakers. They are made of either **polypropylene** (which is shatter-resistant and resistant to chemicals but cannot be heated) or **polymethylpentene** (which is known for its clarity). They are lighter to ship and less fragile than glass.

To read a graduated cylinder, it should be placed on a flat surface and read at eye level. The surface of a liquid in a graduated cylinder forms a lens-shaped curve. The measurement should be taken from the bottom of the curve. A ring may be placed at the top of tall, narrow cylinders to help avoid breakage if they are tipped over.

A **burette**, or buret, is a piece of lab glassware used to accurately dispense liquid. It looks similar to a narrow graduated cylinder, but includes a stopcock and tip. It may be filled with a funnel or pipette.

### FLASKS, BEAKERS, AND PIPETTES

Two types of flasks commonly used in lab settings are **Erlenmeyer flasks** and **volumetric flasks**, which can also be used to accurately measure liquids. Erlenmeyer flasks and **beakers** can be used for mixing, transporting, and reacting, but are not appropriate for accurate measurements.

A **pipette** can be used to accurately measure small amounts of liquid. Liquid is drawn into the pipette through the bulb and a finger is then quickly placed at the top of the container. The liquid measurement is read exactly at the **meniscus**. Liquid can be released from the pipette by lifting the finger. There are also plastic disposal pipettes. A **repipette** is a hand-operated pump that dispenses solutions.

## BALANCES

Unlike laboratory glassware that measures volume, **balances** such as triple-beam balances, spring balances, and electronic balances measure **mass** and **force**. An **electronic balance** is the most accurate, followed by a **triple-beam balance** and then a **spring balance**.

One part of a triple-beam balance is the **plate**, which is where the item to be weighed is placed. There are also three **beams** that have hatch marks indicating amounts and hold the weights that rest in the notches. The front beam measures weights between 0 and 10 grams, the middle beam measures weights in 100-gram increments, and the far beam measures weights in 10-gram increments.

The sum of the weight of each beam is the total weight of the object. A triple-beam balance also includes a **set screw** to calibrate the equipment and a mark indicating the object and counterweights are in balance. Analytical balances are accurate to within 0.0001 g.

## REVIEW A SCIENTIFIC EXPLANATION WITH LOGIC AND EVIDENCE

### DATA COLLECTION

A valid experiment must be measurable. **Data tables** should be formed, and meticulous, detailed data should be collected for every trial. First, the researcher must determine exactly what data are needed and why those data are needed. The researcher should know in advance what will be done with those data at the end of the experimental research. The data should be *repeatable, reproducible, and accurate*. The researcher should be sure that the procedure for data collection will be reliable and consistent. The researcher should validate the measurement system by performing **practice tests** and making sure that all of the equipment is correctly **calibrated** and periodically retesting the procedure and equipment to ensure that all data being collected are still valid.

## SCIENTIFIC PROCESS SKILLS

Perhaps the most important skill in science is that of **observation**. Scientists must be able to take accurate data from their experimental setup or from nature without allowing bias to alter the results. Another important skill is **hypothesizing**. Scientists must be able to combine their knowledge of theory and of other experimental results to logically determine what should occur in their own tests.

The **data-analysis process** requires the twin skills of ordering and categorizing. Gathered data must be arranged in such a way that it is readable and readily shows the key results. A skill that may be integrated with the previous two is comparing. Scientists should be able to **compare** their own results with other published results. They must also be able to **infer**, or draw logical conclusions, from their results. They must be able to **apply** their knowledge of theory and results to create logical experimental designs and determine cases of special behavior.

Lastly, scientists must be able to **communicate** their results and their conclusions. The greatest scientific progress is made when scientists are able to review and test one another's work and offer advice or suggestions.

## SCIENTIFIC STATEMENTS

**Hypotheses** are educated guesses about what is likely to occur, and are made to provide a starting point from which to begin design of the experiment. They may be based on results of previously observed experiments or knowledge of theory, and follow logically forth from these.

**Assumptions** are statements that are taken to be fact without proof for the purpose of performing a given experiment. They may be entirely true, or they may be true only for a given set of conditions under which the experiment will be conducted. Assumptions are necessary to simplify experiments; indeed, many experiments would be impossible without them.

**Scientific models** are mathematical statements that describe a physical behavior. Models are only as good as our knowledge of the actual system. Often models will be discarded when new discoveries are made that show the model to be inaccurate. While a model can never perfectly represent an actual system, it is useful for simplifying a system to allow for better understanding of its behavior.

**Scientific laws** are statements of natural behavior that have stood the test of time and have been found to produce accurate and repeatable results in all testing. A **theory** is a statement of behavior that consolidates all current observations. Theories are similar to laws in that they describe natural behavior, but are more recently developed and are more susceptible to being proved wrong. Theories may eventually become laws if they stand up to scrutiny and testing.

## EVENTS AND OBJECTS

### EVENTS

A **cause** is an act or event that makes something happen, and an **effect** is the thing that happens as a result of the cause. A cause-and-effect relationship is not always explicit, but there are some terms in English that signal causes, such as *since*, *because*, and *due to*. Terms that signal effects include *consequently, therefore, this lead(s) to*.

A *single* cause can have *multiple* effects (e.g., *Single cause*: Because you left your homework on the table, your dog engulfs the assignment. *Multiple effects*: As a result, you receive a failing grade; your parents do not allow you to visit your friends; you miss out on the new movie and holding the hand of a potential significant other).

A *single* effect can have *multiple* causes (e.g., *Single effect*: Alan has a fever. *Multiple causes*: An unexpected cold front came through the area, and Alan forgot to take his multi-vitamin to avoid being sick.)

An *effect* can in turn be the cause of *another effect*, in what is known as a **cause-and-effect chain**. (e.g., As a result of her disdain for procrastination, Lynn prepared for her exam. This led to her passing her test with high marks. Hence, her resume was accepted and her application was approved.)

## SCALE

From the largest objects in outer space to the smallest pieces of the human body, there are objects that can come in many different sizes and shapes. Many of those objects need to be measured in different ways. So, it is important to know which **unit of measurement** is needed to record the length or width and the weight of an object.

An example is taking the measurements of a patient. When measuring the total height of a patient or finding the length of an extremity, the accepted measure is given in meters. However, when one is asked for the diameter of a vein, the accepted measure is given in millimeters. Another example would be measuring the weight of a patient which would be given in kilograms, while the measurement of a human heart would be given in grams. The same idea for scale holds true with time as well. When measuring the lifespan of a patient, the accepted measure is given in days, months, or years. However, when measuring the number of breaths that a patient takes, the accepted measure is given in terms of minutes (e.g., breaths per minute).

## SCIENTIFIC INQUIRY
### SCIENTIFIC METHOD

The scientific method of inquiry is a general method by which ideas are tested and either confirmed or refuted by experimentation. The first step in the scientific method is **formulating the problem** that is to be addressed. It is essential to define clearly the limits of what is to be observed, since that allows for a more focused analysis.

Once the problem has been defined, it is necessary to form a **hypothesis**. This educated guess should be a possible solution to the problem that was formulated in the first step.

The next step is to test that hypothesis by **experimentation**. This often requires the scientist to design a complete experiment. The key to making the best possible use of an experiment is observation. Observations may be **quantitative**, that is, when a numeric measurement is taken, or they may be **qualitative**, that is, when something is evaluated based on feeling or preference. This measurement data will then be examined to find trends or patterns that are present.

From these trends, the scientist will draw **conclusions** or make **generalizations** about the results, intended to predict future results. If these conclusions support the original hypothesis, the experiment is complete and the scientist will publish his conclusions to allow others to test them by repeating the experiment. If they do not support the hypothesis, the results should then be used to develop a new hypothesis, which can then be verified by a new or redesigned experiment.

## EXPERIMENTAL DESIGN

Designing relevant experiments that allow for meaningful results is not a simple task. Every stage of the experiment must be carefully planned to ensure that the right data can be safely and accurately taken.

Ideally, an experiment should be **controlled** so that all of the conditions except the ones being manipulated are held **constant**. This helps to ensure that the results are not skewed by unintended consequences of shifting conditions. A good example of this is a placebo group in a drug trial. All other conditions are the same, but that group is not given the medication.

In addition to proper control, it is important that the experiment be designed with **data collection** in mind. For instance, if the quantity to be measured is temperature, there must be a temperature device such as a thermocouple integrated into the experimental setup. While the data are being collected, they should periodically be checked for obvious errors. If there are data points that are orders of magnitude from the expected value, then it might be a good idea to make sure that no experimental errors are being made, either in data collection or condition control.

Once all the data have been gathered, they must be **analyzed**. The way in which this should be done depends on the type of data and the type of trends observed. It may be useful to fit curves to the data to determine if the trends follow a common mathematical form. It may also be necessary to perform a statistical analysis of the results to determine what effects are significant. Data should be clearly presented.

## CONTROLS

A valid experiment must be carefully **controlled**. All variables except the one being tested must be carefully maintained. This means that all conditions must be kept exactly the same except for the independent variable.

Additionally, a set of data is usually needed for a **control group**. The control group represents the "normal" state or condition of the variable being manipulated. Controls can be negative or positive. **Positive controls** are the variables that the researcher expects to have an effect on the outcome of the experiment. A positive control group can be used to verify that an experiment is set up properly. **Negative control groups** are typically thought of as placebos. A negative control group should verify that a variable has no effect on the outcome of the experiment.

The better an experiment is controlled, the more valid the conclusions from that experiment will be. A researcher is more likely to draw a valid conclusion if all variables other than the one being manipulated are being controlled.

## VARIABLES

Every experiment has several **variables**; however, only one variable should be purposely changed and tested. This variable is the **manipulated** or **independent variable**. As this variable is manipulated or changed, another variable, called the **responding** or **dependent variable**, is observed and recorded.

All other variables in the experiment must be carefully controlled and are usually referred to as **constants**. For example, when testing the effect of temperature on solubility of a solute, the independent variable is the temperature, and the dependent variable is the solubility. All other factors in the experiment such as pressure, amount of stirring, type of solvent, type of solute, and particle size of the solute are the constants.

> **Review Video: <u>Identifying Variables</u>**
> Visit mometrix.com/academy and enter code: 627181

# English and Language Usage

## Conventions of Standard English: Spelling

### GENERAL SPELLING RULES

#### WORDS ENDING WITH A CONSONANT

Usually, the final consonant is **doubled** on a word before adding a suffix. This is the rule for single syllable words, words ending with one consonant, and multi-syllable words with the last syllable accented. The following are examples:

- *beg* becomes *begging* (single syllable)
- *shop* becomes *shopped* (single syllable)
- *add* becomes *adding* (already ends in double consonant, do not add another *d*)
- *deter* becomes *deterring* (multi-syllable, accent on last syllable)
- *regret* becomes *regrettable* (multi-syllable, accent on last syllable)
- *compost* becomes *composting* (do not add another *t* because the accent is on the first syllable)

#### WORDS ENDING WITH Y OR C

The general rule for words ending in *y* is to keep the *y* when adding a suffix if the **y is preceded by a vowel**. If the word **ends in a consonant and y** the *y* is changed to an *i* before the suffix is added (unless the suffix itself begins with *i*). The following are examples:

- *pay* becomes *paying* (keep the *y*)
- *bully* becomes *bullied* (change to *i*)
- *bully* becomes *bullying* (keep the *y* because the suffix is –*ing*)

If a word ends with *c* and the suffix begins with an *e, i,* or *y*, the letter *k* is usually added to the end of the word. The following are examples:

- panic becomes panicky
- mimic becomes mimicking

#### WORDS CONTAINING IE OR EI, AND/OR ENDING WITH E

Most words are spelled with an *i* before *e*, except when they follow the letter *c*, **or** sound like *a*. For example, the following words are spelled correctly according to these rules:

- piece, friend, believe (*i* before *e*)
- receive, ceiling, conceited (except after *c*)
- weight, neighborhood, veil (sounds like *a*)

To add a suffix to words ending with the letter *e*, first determine if the *e* is silent. If it is, the *e* will be kept if the added suffix begins with a consonant. If the suffix begins with a vowel, the *e* is dropped. The following are examples:

- *age* becomes *ageless* (keep the *e*)
- *age* becomes *aging* (drop the *e*)

An exception to this rule occurs when the word ends in *ce* or *ge* and the suffix *able* or *ous* is added; these words will retain the letter *e*. The following are examples:

- courage becomes courageous
- notice becomes noticeable

### WORDS ENDING WITH ISE OR IZE

A small number of words end with *ise*. Most of the words in the English language with the same sound end in *ize*. The following are examples:

- advertise, advise, arise, chastise, circumcise, and comprise
- compromise, demise, despise, devise, disguise, enterprise, excise, and exercise
- franchise, improvise, incise, merchandise, premise, reprise, and revise
- supervise, surmise, surprise, and televise

Words that end with *ize* include the following:

- accessorize, agonize, authorize, and brutalize
- capitalize, caramelize, categorize, civilize, and demonize
- downsize, empathize, euthanize, idolize, and immunize
- legalize, metabolize, mobilize, organize, and ostracize
- plagiarize, privatize, utilize, and visualize

(Note that some words may technically be spelled with *ise*, especially in British English, but it is more common to use *ize*. Examples include *symbolize/symbolise* and *baptize/baptise*.)

### WORDS ENDING WITH CEED, SEDE, OR CEDE

There are only three words in the English language that end with *ceed*: *exceed, proceed,* and *succeed*. There is only one word in the English language that ends with *sede*: *supersede*. Most other words that sound like *sede* or *ceed* end with *cede*. The following are examples:

- concede, recede, and precede

### WORDS ENDING IN ABLE OR IBLE

For words ending in *able* or *ible*, there are no hard and fast rules. The following are examples:

- adjustable, unbeatable, collectable, deliverable, and likeable
- edible, compatible, feasible, sensible, and credible

There are more words ending in *able* than *ible*; this is useful to know if guessing is necessary.

### WORDS ENDING IN ANCE OR ENCE

The suffixes *ence, ency,* and *ent* are used in the following cases:

- the suffix is preceded by the letter *c* but sounds like *s* – *innocence*
- the suffix is preceded by the letter *g* but sounds like *j* – *intelligence, negligence*

The suffixes *ance, ancy,* and *ant* are used in the following cases:

- the suffix is preceded by the letter *c* but sounds like *k* – *significant, vacant*
- the suffix is preceded by the letter *g* with a hard sound – *elegant, extravagance*

If the suffix is preceded by other letters, there are no clear rules. For example: *finance, abundance,* and *assistance* use the letter *a*, while *decadence, competence,* and *excellence* use the letter *e*.

### WORDS ENDING IN TION, SION, OR CIAN

Words ending in *tion, sion,* or *cian* all sound like *shun* or *zhun*. There are no rules for which ending is used for words. The following are examples:

- action, agitation, caution, fiction, nation, and motion
- admission, expression, mansion, permission, and television
- electrician, magician, musician, optician, and physician (note that these words tend to describe occupations)

### WORDS WITH THE AI OR IA COMBINATION

When deciding if *ai* or *ia* is correct, the combination of *ai* usually sounds like one vowel sound, as in *Britain*, while the vowels in *ia* are pronounced separately, as in *guardian*. The following are examples:

- captain, certain, faint, hair, malaise, and praise (*ai* makes one sound)
- bacteria, beneficiary, diamond, humiliation, and nuptial (*ia* makes two sounds)

## RULES FOR PLURALS

### NOUNS ENDING IN CH, SH, S, X, OR Z

When a noun ends in the letters *ch, sh, s, x,* or *z*, an *es* instead of a singular *s* is added to the end of the word to make it plural. The following are examples:

- church becomes churches
- bush becomes bushes
- bass becomes basses
- mix becomes mixes
- buzz becomes buzzes

This is the rule with proper names as well; the Ross family would become the Rosses.

### NOUNS ENDING IN Y OR AY/EY/IY/OY/UY

If a noun ends with a **consonant and y**, the plural is formed by replacing the *y* with *ies*. For example, *fly* becomes *flies* and *puppy* becomes *puppies*. If a noun ends with a **vowel and y**, the plural is formed by adding an *s*. For example, *alley* becomes *alleys* and *boy* becomes *boys*.

### NOUNS ENDING IN F OR FE

Most nouns ending in *f* or *fe* are pluralized by replacing the *f* with *v* and adding *es*. The following are examples:

- knife becomes knives; self becomes selves; wolf becomes wolves.

An exception to this rule is the word *roof*; *roof* becomes *roofs*.

### NOUNS ENDING IN O

Most nouns ending with a **consonant and o** are pluralized by adding *es*. The following are examples:

- hero becomes heroes; tornado becomes tornadoes; potato becomes potatoes

Most nouns ending with a **vowel and *o*** are pluralized by adding *s*. The following are examples:

- portfolio becomes portfolios; radio becomes radios; cameo becomes cameos.

An exception to these rules is seen with musical terms ending in *o*. These words are pluralized by adding *s* even if they end in a consonant and *o*. The following are examples: *soprano* becomes *sopranos; banjo* becomes *banjos; piano* becomes *pianos.*

### LETTERS, NUMBERS, AND SYMBOLS

Letters and numbers become plural by adding an apostrophe and *s*. The following are examples:

- The *L's* are the people whose names begin with the letter *L*.
- They broke the teams down into groups of *3's*.
- The sorority girls were all *KD's*.

### COMPOUND NOUNS

A **compound noun** is a noun that is made up of two or more words; they can be written with hyphens. For example, *mother-in-law* or *court-martial* are compound nouns. To make them plural, an *s* or *es* is added to the noun portion of the word. The following are examples: *mother-in-law* becomes *mothers-in-law; court-martial* becomes *courts-martial.*

### EXCEPTIONS

Some words do not fall into any specific category for making the singular form plural. They are **irregular**. Certain words become plural by changing the vowels within the word. The following are examples:

- woman becomes women; goose becomes geese; foot becomes feet

Some words change in unusual ways in the plural form. The following are examples:

- mouse becomes mice; ox becomes oxen; person becomes people

Some words are the same in both the singular and plural forms. The following are examples:

- *Salmon, deer*, and *moose* are the same whether singular or plural.

## COMMONLY MISSPELLED WORDS

| | | | |
|---|---|---|---|
| accidentally | accommodate | accompanied | accompany |
| achieved | acknowledgment | across | address |
| aggravate | aisle | ancient | anxiety |
| apparently | appearance | arctic | argument |
| arrangement | attendance | auxiliary | awkward |
| bachelor | barbarian | beggar | beneficiary |
| biscuit | brilliant | business | cafeteria |
| calendar | campaign | candidate | ceiling |
| cemetery | changeable | changing | characteristic |
| chauffeur | colonel | column | commit |
| committee | comparative | compel | competent |
| competition | conceive | congratulations | conqueror |
| conscious | coolly | correspondent | courtesy |
| curiosity | cylinder | deceive | deference |

| | | | |
|---|---|---|---|
| deferred | definite | describe | desirable |
| desperate | develop | diphtheria | disappear |
| disappoint | disastrous | discipline | discussion |
| disease | dissatisfied | dissipate | drudgery |
| ecstasy | efficient | eighth | eligible |
| embarrass | emphasize | especially | exaggerate |
| exceed | exhaust | exhilaration | existence |
| explanation | extraordinary | familiar | fascinate |
| February | fiery | finally | forehead |
| foreign | foreigner | foremost | forfeit |
| ghost | glamorous | government | grammar |
| grateful | grief | grievous | handkerchief |
| harass | height | hoping | hurriedly |
| hygiene | hypocrisy | imminent | incidentally |
| incredible | independent | indigestible | inevitable |
| innocence | intelligible | intentionally | intercede |
| interest | irresistible | judgment | legitimate |
| liable | library | likelihood | literature |
| maintenance | maneuver | manual | mathematics |
| mattress | miniature | mischievous | misspell |
| momentous | mortgage | neither | nickel |
| niece | ninety | noticeable | notoriety |
| obedience | obstacle | occasion | occurrence |
| omitted | operate | optimistic | organization |
| outrageous | pageant | pamphlet | parallel |
| parliament | permissible | perseverance | persuade |
| physically | physician | possess | possibly |
| practically | prairie | preceding | prejudice |
| prevalent | professor | pronunciation | pronouncement |
| propeller | protein | psychiatrist | psychology |
| quantity | questionnaire | rally | recede |
| receive | recognize | recommend | referral |
| referred | relieve | religious | resistance |
| restaurant | rhetoric | rhythm | ridiculous |
| sacrilegious | salary | scarcely | schedule |
| secretary | sentinel | separate | severely |
| sheriff | shriek | similar | soliloquy |
| sophomore | species | strenuous | studying |
| suffrage | supersede | suppress | surprise |
| symmetry | temperament | temperature | tendency |
| tournament | tragedy | transferred | truly |
| twelfth | tyranny | unanimous | unpleasant |
| usage | vacuum | valuable | vein |
| vengeance | vigilance | villain | Wednesday |
| weird | wholly | | |

## COMMONLY CONFUSED WORDS
### WHICH, THAT, AND WHO

*Which* is used for things only.

> Example: John's dog, *which was called Max*, is large and fierce.

*That* is used for people or things.

> Example: Is this the only book *that Louis L'Amour wrote?*

> Example: Is Louis L'Amour the author *that wrote Western novels?*

*Who* is used for people only.

> Example: Mozart was the composer *who wrote those operas.*

### HOMOPHONES

Homophones are words that sound alike (or similar), but they have different **spellings** and **definitions**.

### TO, TOO, AND TWO

**To** can be an adverb or a preposition for showing direction, purpose, and relationship. See your dictionary for the many other ways use *to* in a sentence.

> Examples: I went to the store. | I want to go with you.

**Too** is an adverb that means *also, as well, very, or more than enough.*

> Examples: I can walk a mile too. | You have eaten too much.

**Two** is the second number in the series of numbers (e.g., one (1), two, (2), three (3)...)

> Example: You have two minutes left.

### THERE, THEIR, AND THEY'RE

**There** can be an adjective, adverb, or pronoun. Often, *there* is used to show a place or to start a sentence.

> Examples: I went there yesterday. | There is something in his pocket.

**Their** is a pronoun that is used to show ownership.

> Examples: He is their father. | This is their fourth apology this week.

**They're** is a contraction of *they are.*

> Example: Did you know that they're in town?

## KNEW AND NEW

**Knew** is the past tense of *know*.

> Example: I knew the answer.

**New** is an adjective that means something is current, has not been used, or modern.

> Example: This is my new phone.

## THEN AND THAN

**Then** is an adverb that indicates sequence or order:

> Example: I'm going to run to the library and then come home.

**Than** is special-purpose word used only for comparisons:

> Example: Susie likes chips better than candy.

## ITS AND IT'S

**Its** is a pronoun that shows ownership.

> Example: The guitar is in its case.

**It's** is a contraction of *it is*.

> Example: It's an honor and a privilege to meet you.

Note: The *h* in honor is silent, so the sound of the vowel *o* must have the article *an*.

## YOUR AND YOU'RE

**Your** is a pronoun that shows ownership.

> Example: This is your moment to shine.

**You're** is a contraction of *you are*.

> Example: Yes, you're correct.

## AFFECT AND EFFECT

There are two main reasons that **affect** and **effect** are so often confused: 1) both words can be used as either a noun or a verb, and 2) unlike most homophones, their usage and meanings are closely related to each other. Here is a quick rundown of the four usage options:

**Affect (n):** feeling, emotion, or mood that is displayed

> Example: The patient had a flat *affect.* (i.e., his face showed little or no emotion)

**Affect (v):** to alter, to change, to influence

> Example: The sunshine *affects* the plant's growth.

**Effect (n):** a result, a consequence

> Example: What *effect* will this weather have on our schedule?

**Effect (v):** to bring about, to cause to be

> Example: These new rules will *effect* order in the office.

The noun form of *affect* is rarely used outside of technical medical descriptions, so if a noun form is needed on the test, you can safely select *effect.* The verb form of *effect* is not as rare as the noun form of *affect,* but it's still not all that likely to show up on your test. If you need a verb and you can't decide which to use based on the definitions, choosing *affect* is your best bet.

## HOMOGRAPHS

Homographs are words that share the same spelling, and they have multiple meanings. To figure out which meaning is being used, you should be looking for context clues. The context clues give hints to the meaning of the word. For example, the word *spot* has many meanings. It can mean "a place" or "a stain or blot." In the sentence "After my lunch, I saw a spot on my shirt," the word *spot* means "a stain or blot." The context clues of "After my lunch…" and "on my shirt" guide you to this decision.

## BANK

> (noun): an establishment where money is held for savings or lending

> (verb): to collect or pile up

## CONTENT

> (noun): the topics that will be addressed within a book

> (adjective): pleased or satisfied

## FINE

> (noun): an amount of money that acts a penalty for an offense

> (adjective): very small or thin

## INCENSE

> (noun): a material that is burned in religious settings and makes a pleasant aroma

> (verb): to frustrate or anger

## LEAD

(noun): the first or highest position

(verb): to direct a person or group of followers

## OBJECT

(noun): a lifeless item that can be held and observed

(verb): to disagree

## PRODUCE

(noun): fruits and vegetables

(verb): to make or create something

## REFUSE

(noun): garbage or debris that has been thrown away

(verb): to not allow

## SUBJECT

(noun): an area of study

(verb): to force or subdue

## TEAR

(noun): a fluid secreted by the eyes

(verb): to separate or pull apart

# Conventions of Standard English: Punctuation

## END PUNCTUATION

### PERIODS

Use a period to end all sentences except direct questions, exclamations.

### DECLARATIVE SENTENCE

A declarative sentence gives information or makes a statement.

> Examples: I can fly a kite. | The plane left two hours ago.

### IMPERATIVE SENTENCE

An imperative sentence gives an order or command.

> Examples: You are coming with me. | Bring me that note.

### PERIODS FOR ABBREVIATIONS

> Examples: 3 P.M. | 2 A.M. | Mr. Jones | Mrs. Stevens | Dr. Smith | Bill Jr. | Pennsylvania Ave.

Note: an abbreviation is a shortened form of a word or phrase.

### QUESTION MARKS

Question marks should be used following a direct question. A polite request can be followed by a period instead of a question mark.

> **Direct Question**: What is for lunch today? | How are you? | Why is that the answer?

> **Polite Requests**: Can you please send me the item tomorrow. | Will you please walk with me on the track.

### EXCLAMATION MARKS

Exclamation marks are used after a word group or sentence that shows much feeling or has special importance. Exclamation marks should not be overused. They are saved for proper **exclamatory interjections**.

> Example: We're going to the finals! | You have a beautiful car! | That's crazy!

---

**Review Video: Exclamation Points**
Visit mometrix.com/academy and enter code: 199367

---

## COMMAS

The comma is a punctuation mark that can help you understand connections in a sentence. Not every sentence needs a comma. However, if a sentence needs a comma, you need to put it in the right place. A comma in the wrong place (or an absent comma) will make a sentence's meaning unclear. These are some of the rules for commas:

1. Use a comma **before a coordinating conjunction** joining independent clauses
   Example: Bob caught three fish, and I caught two fish.

2. Use a comma after an introductory phrase or an adverbial clause

   Examples:

   > *After the final out,* we went to a restaurant to celebrate.
   > *Studying the stars,* I was surprised at the beauty of the sky.

3. Use a comma between items in a series.

   Example: I will bring the turkey, the pie, and the coffee.

4. Use a comma **between coordinate adjectives** not joined with *and*

   Incorrect: The kind, brown dog followed me home.
   Correct: The *kind, loyal* dog followed me home.
   Not all adjectives are **coordinate** (i.e., equal or parallel). There are two simple ways to know if your adjectives are coordinate. One, you can join the adjectives with *and*: *The kind and loyal dog*. Two, you can change the order of the adjectives: *The loyal, kind dog*.

5. Use commas for **interjections** and **after *yes* and *no*** responses

   Examples:

   > **Interjection**: Oh, I had no idea. | Wow, you know how to play this game.
   > **Yes and No**: *Yes,* I heard you. | *No,* I cannot come tomorrow.

6. Use commas to separate nonessential modifiers and nonessential appositives

   Examples:

   > **Nonessential Modifier**: John Frank, who is coaching the team, was promoted today.
   > **Nonessential Appositive**: Thomas Edison, an American inventor, was born in Ohio.

7. Use commas to set off nouns of direct address, interrogative tags, and contrast

   Examples:

   > **Direct Address**: You, *John,* are my only hope in this moment.
   > **Interrogative Tag**: This is the last time, *correct*?
   > **Contrast**: You are my friend, *not my enemy.*

8. Use commas with dates, addresses, geographical names, and titles

   Examples:

   > **Date**: *July 4, 1776,* is an important date to remember.
   > **Address**: He is meeting me at *456 Delaware Avenue, Washington, D.C.,* tomorrow morning.
   > **Geographical Name**: *Paris, France,* is my favorite city.
   > **Title**: John Smith, *Ph. D.,* will be visiting your class today.

9. Use commas to **separate expressions like *he said*** and ***she said*** if they come between a sentence of a quote

   Examples:

   > "I want you to know," he began, "that I always wanted the best for you."
   > "You can start," Jane said, "with an apology."

---

**Review Video: Commas**
Visit mometrix.com/academy and enter code: 786797

---

## SEMICOLONS

The semicolon is used to connect major sentence pieces of equal value. Some rules for semicolons include:

1. Use a semicolon **between closely connected independent clauses** that are not connected with a coordinating conjunction.

   Examples:

   > She is outside; we are inside.
   > You are right; we should go with your plan.

2. Use a semicolon **between independent clauses linked with a transitional word.**

   Examples:

   > I think that we can agree on this; *however,* I am not sure about my friends.
   > You are looking in the wrong places; *therefore,* you will not find what you need.

3. Use a semicolon **between items in a series that has internal punctuation.**

   Example: I have visited New York, New York; Augusta, Maine; and Baltimore, Maryland.

   > **Review Video: Semicolon Usage**
   > Visit mometrix.com/academy and enter code: 370605

## COLONS

The colon is used to call attention to the words that follow it. A colon must come after a **complete independent clause**. The rules for colons are as follows:

1. Use a colon after an independent clause to **make a list**

   Example: I want to learn many languages: Spanish, German, and Italian.

2. Use a colon for **explanations** or to **give a quote**

   Examples:

   > **Quote**: He started with an idea: "We are able to do more than we imagine."
   > **Explanation**: There is one thing that stands out on your resume: responsibility.

3. Use a colon **after the greeting in a formal letter**, to **show hours and minutes**, and to **separate a title and subtitle**

   Examples:

   > **Greeting in a formal letter**: Dear Sir: | To Whom It May Concern:
   > **Time**: It is 3:14 P.M.
   > **Title**: The essay is titled "America: A Short Introduction to a Modern Country"

   > **Review Video: Colons**
   > Visit mometrix.com/academy and enter code: 868673

## PARENTHESES

Parentheses are used for additional information. Also, they can be used to put labels for letters or numbers in a series. Parentheses should be not be used very often. If they are overused, parentheses can be a distraction instead of a help.

Examples:

**Extra Information**: The rattlesnake (see Image 2) is a dangerous snake of North and South America.

**Series**: Include in the email (1) your name, (2) your address, and (3) your question for the author.

---

**Review Video: Parentheses**
Visit mometrix.com/academy and enter code: 947743

---

## QUOTATION MARKS

Use quotation marks to close off **direct quotations** of a person's spoken or written words. Do not use quotation marks around indirect quotations. An indirect quotation gives someone's message without using the person's exact words. Use **single quotation marks** to close off a quotation inside a quotation.

**Direct Quote**: Nancy said, "I am waiting for Henry to arrive."

**Indirect Quote**: Henry said that he is going to be late to the meeting.

**Quote inside a Quote**: The teacher asked, "Has everyone read 'The Gift of the Magi'?"

Quotation marks should be used around the titles of **short works**: newspaper and magazine articles, poems, short stories, songs, television episodes, radio programs, and subdivisions of books or web sites.

Examples:

"Rip van Winkle" (short story by Washington Irving)

"O Captain! My Captain!" (poem by Walt Whitman)

Although it is not standard usage, quotation marks are sometimes used to highlight **irony**, or the use of words to mean something other than their dictionary definition. This type of usage should be employed sparingly, if at all.

Examples:

The boss warned Frank that he was walking on "thin ice."

(Frank is not walking on real ice. Instead, Frank is being warned to avoid mistakes.)

The teacher thanked the young man for his "honesty."

(In this example, the quotation marks around *honesty* show that the teacher does not believe the young man's explanation.)

---

**Review Video: Quotation Marks**
Visit mometrix.com/academy and enter code: 884918

---

Periods and commas are put **inside** quotation marks. Colons and semicolons are put **outside** the quotation marks. Question marks and exclamation points are placed inside quotation marks when they are part of a quote. When the question or exclamation mark goes with the whole sentence, the mark is left outside of the quotation marks.

Examples:

*Period and comma*: We read "The Gift of the Magi," "The Skylight Room," and "The Cactus."

*Semicolon*: They watched "The Nutcracker"; then, they went home.

*Exclamation mark that is a part of a quote*: The crowd cheered, "Victory!"

*Question mark that goes with the whole sentence*: Is your favorite short story "The Tell-Tale Heart"?

## APOSTROPHES

An apostrophe is used to show **possession** or the **deletion of letters in contractions**. An apostrophe is not needed with the possessive pronouns *his, hers, its, ours, theirs, whose*, and *yours*.

**Singular Nouns**: David's car | a book's theme | my brother's board game

**Plural Nouns with -*s***: the scissors' handle | boys' basketball

**Plural Nouns without -*s***: Men's department | the people's adventure

> **Review Video: Apostrophes**
> Visit mometrix.com/academy and enter code: 213068
>
> **Review Video: Punctuation Errors in Possessive Pronouns**
> Visit mometrix.com/academy and enter code: 221438

## HYPHENS

Hyphens are used to **separate compound words**. Use hyphens in the following cases:

1. **Compound numbers** between 21 and 99 when written out in words
   Example: This team needs *twenty-five* points to win the game.

2. **Written-out fractions** that are used as **adjectives**
   Correct: The recipe says that we need a *three-fourths* cup of butter.
   Incorrect: *One-fourth* of the road is under construction.

3. Compound words used as **adjectives that come before a noun**
   Correct: The *well-fed* dog took a nap.
   Incorrect: The dog was *well-fed* for his nap.

4. Compound words that would be **hard to read** or **easily confused with other words**
   Examples: Semi-irresponsible | Anti-itch | Re-sort

Note: This is not a complete set of the rules for hyphens. A dictionary is the best tool for knowing if a compound word needs a hyphen.

> **Review Video: Hyphens**
> Visit mometrix.com/academy and enter code: 981632

## DASHES

Dashes are used to show a **break** or a **change in thought** in a sentence or to act as parentheses in a sentence. When typing, use two hyphens to make a dash. Do not put a space before or after the dash. The following are the rules for dashes:

1. To set off **parenthetical statements** or an **appositive with internal punctuation**

   Example: The three trees—oak, pine, and magnolia—are coming on a truck tomorrow.

2. To show a **break or change in tone or thought**

   Example: The first question—how silly of me—does not have a correct answer.

## ELLIPSIS MARKS

The ellipsis mark has three periods (…) to show when **words have been removed** from a quotation. If a full sentence or more is removed from a quoted passage, you need to use four periods to show the removed text and the end punctuation mark. The ellipsis mark should not be used at the beginning of a quotation. The ellipsis mark should also not be used at the end of a quotation unless some words have been deleted from the end of the final sentence.

Example:

"Then he picked up the groceries…paid for them…later he went home."

## BRACKETS

There are two main reasons to use brackets:

1. When **placing parentheses inside of parentheses**

   Example: The hero of this story, Paul Revere (a silversmith and industrialist [see Ch. 4]), rode through towns of Massachusetts to warn of advancing British troops.

2. When adding **clarification or detail** to a quotation that is **not part of the quotation**
   Example:

   The father explained, "My children are planning to attend my alma mater [State University]."

---

**Review Video: Brackets**
Visit mometrix.com/academy and enter code: 727546

---

# Conventions of Standard English: Grammar

## THE EIGHT PARTS OF SPEECH

### NOUNS

When you talk about a person, place, thing, or idea, you are talking about **nouns**. The two main types of nouns are **common** and **proper** nouns. Also, nouns can be abstract (i.e., general) or concrete (i.e., specific).

**Common nouns** are the class or group of people, places, and things (Note: Do not capitalize common nouns). Examples of common nouns:

> *People*: boy, girl, worker, manager
>
> *Places*: school, bank, library, home
>
> *Things*: dog, cat, truck, car

**Proper nouns** are the names of a specific person, place, or thing (Note: Capitalize all proper nouns). Examples of proper nouns:

> *People*: Abraham Lincoln, George Washington, Martin Luther King, Jr.
>
> *Places*: Los Angeles, California / New York / Asia
>
> *Things*: Statue of Liberty, Earth*, Lincoln Memorial

> *Note: When you talk about the planet that we live on, you capitalize *Earth*. When you mean the dirt, rocks, or land, you lowercase *earth*.

**General nouns** are the names of conditions or ideas. **Specific nouns** name people, places, and things that are understood by using your senses.

General nouns:

> *Condition*: beauty, strength
>
> *Idea*: truth, peace

Specific nouns:

> *People*: baby, friend, father
>
> *Places*: town, park, city hall
>
> *Things*: rainbow, cough, apple, silk, gasoline

**Collective nouns** are the names for a person, place, or thing that may act as a whole. The following are examples of collective nouns: *class, company, dozen, group, herd, team,* and *public*.

## PRONOUNS

Pronouns are words that are used to stand in for a noun. A pronoun may be classified as personal, intensive, relative, interrogative, demonstrative, indefinite, and reciprocal.

**Personal:** *Nominative* is the case for nouns and pronouns that are the subject of a sentence. *Objective* is the case for nouns and pronouns that are an object in a sentence. *Possessive* is the case for nouns and pronouns that show possession or ownership.

### SINGULAR

|  | Nominative | Objective | Possessive |
| --- | --- | --- | --- |
| **First Person** | I | me | my, mine |
| **Second Person** | you | you | your, yours |
| **Third Person** | he, she, it | him, her, it | his, her, hers, its |

### PLURAL

|  | Nominative | Objective | Possessive |
| --- | --- | --- | --- |
| **First Person** | we | us | our, ours |
| **Second Person** | you | you | your, yours |
| **Third Person** | they | them | their, theirs |

**Intensive**: I myself, you yourself, he himself, she herself, the (thing) itself, we ourselves, you yourselves, they themselves

**Relative**: which, who, whom, whose

**Interrogative**: what, which, who, whom, whose

**Demonstrative**: this, that, these, those

**Indefinite**: all, any, each, everyone, either/neither, one, some, several

**Reciprocal**: each other, one another

> **Review Video: Nouns and Pronouns**
> Visit mometrix.com/academy and enter code: 312073

## VERBS

If you want to write a sentence, then you need a verb in your sentence. Without a verb, you have no sentence. The verb of a sentence explains action or being. In other words, the verb shows the subject's movement or the movement that has been done to the subject.

### TRANSITIVE AND INTRANSITIVE VERBS

A transitive verb is a verb whose action (e.g., drive, run, jump) points to a receiver (e.g., car, dog, kangaroo). Intransitive verbs do not point to a receiver of an action. In other words, the action of the verb does not point to a subject or object.

**Transitive**: He plays the piano. | The piano was played by him.

**Intransitive**: He plays. | John writes well.

A dictionary will let you know whether a verb is transitive or intransitive. Some verbs can be transitive and intransitive.

## ACTION VERBS AND LINKING VERBS

An action verb is a verb that shows what the subject is doing in a sentence. In other words, an action verb shows action. A sentence can be complete with one word: an action verb. Linking verbs are intransitive verbs that show a condition (i.e., the subject is described but does no action).

**Linking verbs** link the subject of a sentence to a noun or pronoun, or they link a subject with an adjective. You always need a verb if you want a complete sentence. However, linking verbs are not able to complete a sentence.

Common linking verbs include *appear, be, become, feel, grow, look, seem, smell, sound,* and *taste*. However, any verb that shows a condition and has a noun, pronoun, or adjective that describes the subject of a sentence is a linking verb.

**Action**: He sings. | Run! | Go! | I talk with him every day. | She reads.

**Linking**:

> Incorrect: I am.

> Correct: I am John. | I smell roses. | I feel tired.

Note: Some verbs are followed by words that look like prepositions, but they are a part of the verb and a part of the verb's meaning. These are known as phrasal verbs and examples include *call off, look up,* and *drop off*.

> **Review Video: Action Verbs and Linking Verbs**
> Visit mometrix.com/academy and enter code: 743142

## VOICE

Transitive verbs come in active or passive voice. If the subject does an action or receives the action of the verb, then you will know whether a verb is active or passive. When the subject of the sentence is doing the action, the verb is **active voice**. When the subject receives the action, the verb is **passive voice**.

> **Active**: Jon drew the picture. (The subject *Jon* is doing the action of *drawing a picture*.)

> **Passive**: The picture is drawn by Jon. (The subject *picture* is receiving the action from Jon.)

## VERB TENSES

A verb tense shows the different form of a verb to point to the time of an action. The present and past tense are shown by changing the verb's form. An action in the present *I talk* can change form for the past: *I talked*. However, for the other tenses, an auxiliary (i.e., helping) verb is needed to show the change in form. These helping verbs include *am, are, is* | *have, has, had* | *was, were, will* (or *shall*).

| | |
|---|---|
| Present: I talk | Present perfect: I have talked |
| Past: I talked | Past perfect: I had talked |
| Future: I will talk | Future perfect: I will have talked |

**Present**: The action happens at the current time.

>   Example: He *walks* to the store every morning.

To show that something is happening right now, use the progressive present tense: I *am walking*.

**Past**: The action happened in the past.

>   Example: He *walked* to the store an hour ago.

**Future**: The action is going to happen later.

>   Example: I *will walk* to the store tomorrow.

**Present perfect**: The action started in the past and continues into the present.

>   Example: I *have walked* to the store three times today.

**Past perfect**: The second action happened in the past. The first action came before the second.

>   Example: Before I walked to the store (Action 2), I *had walked* to the library (Action 1).

**Future perfect**: An action that uses the past and the future. In other words, the action is complete before a future moment.

>   Example: When she comes for the supplies (future moment), I *will have walked* to the store (action completed in the past).

### CONJUGATING VERBS

When you need to change the form of a verb, you are **conjugating** a verb. The key parts of a verb are first person singular, present tense (dream); first person singular, past tense (dreamed); and the past participle (dreamed). Note: the past participle needs a helping verb to make a verb tense. For example, I *have dreamed* of this day. | I *am dreaming* of this day.

**Present Tense: Active Voice**

|                | Singular          | Plural     |
| -------------- | ----------------- | ---------- |
| **First Person**  | I dream           | We dream   |
| **Second Person** | You dream         | You dream  |
| **Third Person**  | He, she, it dreams | They dream |

### MOOD

There are three moods in English: the indicative, the imperative, and the subjunctive.

The **indicative mood** is used for facts, opinions, and questions.

>   Fact: You can do this.

>   Opinion: I think that you can do this.

>   Question: Do you know that you can do this?

The **imperative** is used for orders or requests.

> Order: You are going to do this!

> Request: Will you do this for me?

The **subjunctive mood** is for wishes and statements that go against fact.

> Wish: I wish that I were going to do this.

> Statement against fact: If I were you, I would do this. (This goes against fact because I am not you. You have the chance to do this, and I do not have the chance.)

The mood that causes trouble for most people is the subjunctive mood. If you have trouble with any of the moods, then be sure to practice.

> **Review Video: Verb Tenses**
> Visit mometrix.com/academy and enter code: 269472

### ADJECTIVES

An adjective is a word that is used to modify a noun or pronoun. An adjective answers a question: *Which one? What kind of?* or *How many?* Usually, adjectives come before the words that they modify, but they may also come after a linking verb.

> Which one? The *third* suit is my favorite.

> What kind? This suit is *navy blue*.

> How many? Can I look over the *four* neckties for the suit?

### ARTICLES

Articles are adjectives that are used to mark nouns. There are only three: the **definite** (i.e., limited or fixed amount) article *the*, and the **indefinite** (i.e., no limit or fixed amount) articles *a* and *an*. Note: *An* comes before words that start with a vowel sound (i.e., vowels include *a, e, i, o, u,* and *y*). For example, "Are you going to get an **u**mbrella?"

> **Definite**: I lost *the* bottle that belongs to me.

> **Indefinite**: Does anyone have *a* bottle to share?

### COMPARISON WITH ADJECTIVES

Some adjectives are relative and other adjectives are absolute. Adjectives that are **relative** can show the comparison between things. Adjectives that are **absolute** can show comparison. However, they show comparison in a different way. Let's say that you are reading two books. You think that one book is perfect, and the other book is not exactly perfect. It is not possible for the book to be more perfect than the other. Either you think that the book is perfect, or you think that the book is not perfect.

The adjectives that are relative will show the different **degrees** of something or someone to something else or someone else. The three degrees of adjectives include positive, comparative, and superlative.

The **positive** degree is the normal form of an adjective.

Example: This work is *difficult*. | She is *smart*.

The **comparative** degree compares one person or thing to another person or thing.

Example: This work is *more difficult* than your work. | She is *smarter* than me.

The **superlative** degree compares more than two people or things.

Example: This is the *most difficult* work of my life. | She is the *smartest* lady in school.

---

**Review Video: What is an Adjective?**
Visit mometrix.com/academy and enter code: 470154

---

### ADVERBS

An adverb is a word that is used to **modify** a verb, adjective, or another adverb. Usually, adverbs answer one of these questions: *When?, Where?, How?,* and *Why?* . The negatives *not* and *never* are known as adverbs. Adverbs that modify adjectives or other adverbs **strengthen** or **weaken** the words that they modify.

Examples:

He walks quickly through the crowd.

The water flows smoothly on the rocks.

Note: While many adverbs end in *-ly*, you need to remember that not all adverbs end in *-ly*. Also, some words that end in *-ly* are adjectives, not adverbs. Some examples include: *early, friendly, holy, lonely, silly,* and *ugly*. To know if a word that ends in *-ly* is an adjective or adverb, you need to check your dictionary.

Examples:

He is *never* angry.

You talk *too* loudly.

### COMPARISON WITH ADVERBS

The rules for comparing adverbs are the same as the rules for adjectives.

The **positive** degree is the standard form of an adverb.

Example: He arrives soon. | She speaks softly to her friends.

The **comparative** degree compares one person or thing to another person or thing.

Example: He arrives sooner than Sarah. | She speaks more softly than him.

The **superlative** degree compares more than two people or things.

Example: He arrives soonest of the group. | She speaks most softly of any of her friends.

> **Review Video: Adverbs**
> Visit mometrix.com/academy and enter code: 713951

## PREPOSITIONS

A preposition is a word placed before a noun or pronoun that shows the relationship between an object and another word in the sentence.

*Common prepositions*:

| | | | | |
|---|---|---|---|---|
| about | before | during | on | under |
| after | beneath | for | over | until |
| against | between | from | past | up |
| among | beyond | in | through | with |
| around | by | of | to | within |
| at | down | off | toward | without |

Examples:

The napkin is *in* the drawer.

The Earth rotates *around* the Sun.

The needle is *beneath* the haystack.

Can you find me *among* the words?

> **Review Video: What is a Preposition?**
> Visit mometrix.com/academy and enter code: 946763

## CONJUNCTIONS

Conjunctions join words, phrases, or clauses, and they show the connection between the joined pieces. **Coordinating** conjunctions connect equal parts of sentences. **Correlative** conjunctions show the connection between pairs. **Subordinating** conjunctions join subordinate (i.e., dependent) clauses with independent clauses.

### COORDINATING CONJUNCTIONS

The coordinating conjunctions include: *and, but, yet, or, nor, for,* and *so*

Examples:

The rock was small, but it was heavy.

She drove in the night, and he drove in the day.

## CORRELATIVE CONJUNCTIONS

The correlative conjunctions are: *either...or* | *neither...nor* | *not only...but also*

Examples:

> *Either* you are coming *or* you are staying.

> He ran *not only* three miles *but also* swam 200 yards.

> **Review Video: Coordinating and Correlative Conjunctions**
> Visit mometrix.com/academy and enter code: 390329

## SUBORDINATING CONJUNCTIONS

Common subordinating conjunctions include:

| | | |
|---|---|---|
| after | since | whenever |
| although | so that | where |
| because | unless | wherever |
| before | until | whether |
| in order that | when | while |

Examples:

> I am hungry *because* I did not eat breakfast.

> He went home *when* everyone left.

> **Review Video: Subordinating Conjunctions**
> Visit mometrix.com/academy and enter code: 958913

## *INTERJECTIONS*

An interjection is a word for **exclamation** (i.e., great amount of feeling) that is used alone or as a piece to a sentence. Often, they are used at the beginning of a sentence for an **introduction**. Sometimes, they can be used in the middle of a sentence to show a **change** in thought or attitude.

Common Interjections: Hey! | Oh, | Ouch! | Please! | Wow!

# Conventions of Standard English: Sentence Structure

## SUBJECTS AND PREDICATES

### SUBJECTS

Every sentence has two things: a subject and a verb. The **subject** of a sentence names who or what the sentence is all about. The subject may be directly stated in a sentence, or the subject may be the implied *you*.

The **complete subject** includes the simple subject and all of its modifiers. To find the complete subject, ask *Who* or *What* and insert the verb to complete the question. The answer is the complete subject. To find the **simple subject**, remove all of the modifiers (adjectives, prepositional phrases, etc.) in the complete subject. Being able to locate the subject of a sentence helps with many problems, such as those involving sentence fragments and subject-verb agreement.

Examples:

> The small red car is the one that he wants for Christmas.

> (The complete subject is *the small red car.*)

> The young artist is coming over for dinner.

> (The complete subject is *the young artist.*)

> **Review Video: Subjects**
> Visit mometrix.com/academy and enter code: 444771

In **imperative** sentences, the verb's subject is understood (e.g., [You] Run to the store), but not actually present in the sentence. Normally, the subject comes before the verb. However, the subject comes after the verb in sentences that begin with *There are* or *There was*.

Direct:

> John knows the way to the park.

> (Who knows the way to the park? Answer: John)

> The cookies need ten more minutes.

> (What needs ten minutes? Answer: The cookies)

> By five o' clock, Bill will need to leave.

> (Who needs to leave? Answer: Bill)

Remember: The subject can come after the verb.

> There are five letters on the table for him.

> (What is on the table? Answer: Five letters)

> There were coffee and doughnuts in the house.

> (What was in the house? Answer: Coffee and doughnuts)

Implied:

> Go to the post office for me.

> (Who is going to the post office? Answer: You are.)

> Come and sit with me, please?

> (Who needs to come and sit? Answer: You do.)

## PREDICATES

In a sentence, you always have a predicate and a subject. The subject tells what the sentence is about, and the **predicate** explains or describes the subject.

Think about the sentence: *He sings*. In this sentence, we have a subject (He) and a predicate (sings). This is all that is needed for a sentence to be complete. Would we like more information? Of course, we would like to know more. However, if this all the information that you are given, you have a complete sentence.

Now, let's look at another sentence:

> *John and Jane sing on Tuesday nights at the dance hall.*

What is the subject of this sentence?

> **Answer**: John and Jane.

What is the predicate of this sentence?

> **Answer**: Everything else in the sentence (sing on Tuesday nights at the dance hall).

## SUBJECT-VERB AGREEMENT

Verbs **agree** with their subjects in number. In other words, *singular* subjects need *singular* verbs. *Plural* subjects need *plural* verbs. Singular is for one person, place, or thing. Plural is for more than one person, place, or thing. Subjects and verbs must also agree in person: first, second, or third. The present tense ending *-s* is used on a verb if its subject is third person singular; otherwise, the verb takes no ending.

> **Review Video: Subject-Verb Agreement**
> Visit mometrix.com/academy and enter code: 479190

## NUMBER AGREEMENT EXAMPLES:

> Single Subject and Verb: *Dan calls home.*

> (Dan is one person. So, the singular verb *calls* is needed.)

> Plural Subject and Verb: *Dan and Bob call home.*

> (More than one person needs the plural verb *call*.)

## PERSON AGREEMENT EXAMPLES:

First Person: I *am* walking.

Second Person: You *are* walking.

Third Person: He *is* walking.

## COMPLICATIONS WITH SUBJECT-VERB AGREEMENT

### WORDS BETWEEN SUBJECT AND VERB

Words that come between the simple subject and the verb may serve as an effective distraction, but they have no bearing on subject-verb agreement.

Examples:

The joy of my life returns home tonight.

(**Singular Subject**: joy. **Singular Verb**: returns)

The phrase *of my life* does not influence the verb *returns*.

The question that still remains unanswered is "Who are you?"

(**Singular Subject**: question. **Singular Verb**: is)

Don't let the phrase "*that still remains...*" trouble you. The subject *question* goes with *is*.

### COMPOUND SUBJECTS

A compound subject is formed when two or more nouns joined by *and*, *or*, or *nor* jointly act as the subject of the sentence.

#### JOINED BY AND

When a compound subject is joined by *and*, it is treated as a plural subject and requires a plural verb.

Examples:

You and Jon are invited to come to my house.

(**Plural Subject**: You and Jon. **Plural Verb**: are)

The pencil and paper belong to me.

(**Plural Subject**: pencil and paper. **Plural Verb**: belong)

#### JOINED BY OR/NOR

For a compound subject joined by *or* or *nor*, the verb must agree in number with the part of the subject that is closest to the verb (italicized in the examples below).

Examples:

Today or *tomorrow is* the day.

(**Subject**: Today / tomorrow. **Verb**: is)

Stan or *Phil wants* to read the book.

(**Subject**: Stan / Phil. **Verb**: wants)

Neither the books nor the *pen is* on the desk.

(**Subject**: Books / Pen. **Verb**: is)

Either the blanket or *pillows arrive* this afternoon.

(**Subject**: Blanket / Pillows. **Verb**: arrive)

### INDEFINITE PRONOUNS AS SUBJECT

An indefinite pronoun is a pronoun that does not refer to a specific noun. Indefinite pronouns may be only singular, be only plural, or change depending on how they are used.

#### ALWAYS SINGULAR

Pronouns such as *each*, *either*, *everybody*, *anybody*, *somebody*, and *nobody* are always singular.

Examples:

*Each* of the runners *has* a different bib number.

(**Singular Subject**: Each. **Singular Verb**: has)

*Is either* of you ready for the game?

(**Singular Subject**: Either. **Singular Verb**: is)

Note: The words *each* and *either* can also be used as adjectives (e.g., *each* person is unique). When one of these adjectives modifies the subject of a sentence, it is always a singular subject.

*Everybody grows* a day older every day.

(**Singular Subject**: Everybody. **Singular Verb**: grows)

*Anybody is* welcome to bring a tent.

(**Singular Subject**: Anybody. **Singular Verb**: is)

#### ALWAYS PLURAL

Pronouns such as *both*, *several*, and *many* are always plural.

Examples:

*Both* of the siblings *were* too tired to argue.

(**Plural Subject**: Both. **Plural Verb**: were)

*Many have* tried, but none have succeeded.

(**Plural Subject**: Many. **Plural Verb**: have tried)

### DEPEND ON CONTEXT

Pronouns such as *some*, *any*, *all*, *none*, *more*, and *most* can be either singular or plural depending on what they are representing in the context of the sentence.

Examples:

> *All* of my dog's food *was* still there in his bowl
>
> (**Singular Subject**: All. **Singular Verb**: was)
>
> By the end of the night, *all* of my guests *were* already excited about coming to my next party.
>
> (**Plural Subject**: All. **Plural Verb**: were)

### OTHER CASES INVOLVING PLURAL OR IRREGULAR FORM

Some nouns are **singular in meaning but plural in form**: news, mathematics, physics, and economics.

> The *news is* coming on now.
>
> *Mathematics is* my favorite class.

Some nouns are plural in form and meaning, and have **no singular equivalent**: scissors and pants.

> Do these *pants come* with a shirt?
>
> The *scissors are* for my project.

Mathematical operations are **irregular** in their construction, but are normally considered to be **singular in meaning**.

> *One plus one is* two.
>
> *Three times three is* nine.

Note: Look to your **dictionary** for help when you aren't sure whether a noun with a plural form has a singular or plural meaning.

## COMPLEMENTS

A complement is a noun, pronoun, or adjective that is used to give more information about the subject or verb in the sentence.

### DIRECT OBJECTS

A direct object is a noun or pronoun that takes or receives the **action** of a verb. (Remember: a complete sentence does not need a direct object, so not all sentences will have them. A sentence needs only a subject and a verb.) When you are looking for a direct object, find the verb and ask *who* or *what*.

Examples:

> I took the blanket. (Who or what did I take? *The blanket*)

> Jane read books. (Who or what does Jane read? *Books*)

### INDIRECT OBJECTS

An indirect object is a word or group of words that show how an action had an **influence** on someone or something. If there is an indirect object in a sentence, then you always have a direct object in the sentence. When you are looking for the indirect object, find the verb and ask *to/for whom or what*.

Examples:

> We taught the old dog a new trick.

> (To/For Whom or What was taught? *The old dog*)

> I gave them a math lesson.

> (To/For Whom or What was given? *Them*)

> **Review Video: Direct and Indirect Objects**
> Visit mometrix.com/academy and enter code: 817385

### PREDICATE NOMINATIVES AND PREDICATE ADJECTIVES

As we looked at previously, verbs may be classified as either action verbs or linking verbs. A linking verb is so named because it links the subject to words in the predicate that describe or define the subject. These words are called predicate nominatives (if nouns or pronouns) or predicate adjectives (if adjectives).

Examples:

> My father is a *lawyer*.

> (Father is the **subject**. Lawyer is the **predicate nominative**.)

> Your mother is *patient*.

> (Mother is the **subject**. Patient is the **predicate adjective**.)

### PRONOUN USAGE

The **antecedent** is the noun that has been replaced by a pronoun. A pronoun and its antecedent **agree** when they have the same number (singular or plural) and gender (male, female, or neuter).

Examples:

> **Singular agreement**: *John* came into town, and *he* played for us.

> (The word *he* replaces *John*.)

> **Plural agreement**: *John and Rick* came into town, and *they* played for us.

> (The word *they* replaces *John and Rick*.)

To determine which is the correct pronoun to use in a compound subject or object, try each pronoun **alone** in place of the compound in the sentence. Your knowledge of pronouns will tell you which one is correct.

Example:

Bob and (I, me) will be going.

Test: (1) *I will be going* or (2) *Me will be going*. The second choice cannot be correct because *me* cannot be used as the subject of a sentence. Instead, *me* is used as an object.

**Answer**: Bob and I will be going.

When a pronoun is used with a noun immediately following (as in "we boys"), try the sentence **without the added noun**.

Example:

(We/Us) boys played football last year.

Test: (1) *We played football last ye*ar or (2) *Us played football last year*. Again, the second choice cannot be correct because *us* cannot be used as a subject of a sentence. Instead, *us* is used as an object.

**Answer**: We boys played football last year.

| |
|---|
| **Review Video: Pronoun Usage**<br>Visit mometrix.com/academy and enter code: 666500 |

A pronoun should point clearly to the **antecedent**. Here is how a pronoun reference can be unhelpful if it is not directly stated or puzzling.

**Unhelpful**: Ron and Jim went to the store, and *he* bought soda.

(Who bought soda? Ron or Jim?)

**Helpful**: Jim went to the store, and *he* bought soda.

(The sentence is clear. Jim bought the soda.)

Some pronouns change their form by their placement in a sentence. A pronoun that is a subject in a sentence comes in the **subjective case**. Pronouns that serve as objects appear in the **objective case**. Finally, the pronouns that are used as possessives appear in the **possessive case**.

Examples:

**Subjective case**: *He* is coming to the show.

(The pronoun *He* is the subject of the sentence.)

**Objective case**: Josh drove *him* to the airport.

(The pronoun *him* is the object of the sentence.)

**Possessive case**: The flowers are *mine*.

(The pronoun *mine* shows ownership of the flowers.)

The word *who* is a subjective-case pronoun that can be used as a **subject**. The word *whom* is an objective-case pronoun that can be used as an **object**. The words *who* and *whom* are common in subordinate clauses or in questions.

Examples:

**Subject**: He knows who wants to come.

(*Who* is the subject of the verb *wants*.)

**Object**: He knows the man whom we want at the party.

(*Whom* is the object of *we want*.)

## CLAUSES

A clause is a group of words that contains both a subject and a predicate (verb). There are two types of clauses: independent and dependent. An **independent clause** contains a complete thought, while a **dependent (or subordinate) clause** does not. A dependent clause includes a subject and a verb, and may also contain objects or complements, but it cannot stand as a complete thought without being joined to an independent clause. Dependent clauses function within sentences as adjectives, adverbs, or nouns.

Example:

**Independent Clause**: I am running

**Dependent Clause**: because I want to stay in shape

The clause *I am running* is an independent clause: it has a subject and a verb, and it gives a complete thought. The clause *because I want to stay in shape* is a dependent clause: it has a subject and a verb, but it does not express a complete thought. It adds detail to the independent clause to which it is attached.

**Combined**: I am running because I want to stay in shape.

> **Review Video: Clauses**
> Visit mometrix.com/academy and enter code: 940170

### TYPES OF DEPENDENT CLAUSES
#### ADJECTIVE CLAUSES

An **adjective clause** is a dependent clause that modifies a noun or a pronoun. Adjective clauses begin with a relative pronoun (*who, whose, whom, which,* and *that*) or a relative adverb (*where, when,* and *why*).

Also, adjective clauses come after the noun that the clause needs to explain or rename. This is done to have a clear connection to the independent clause.

Examples:

I learned the reason *why I won the award*.

This is the place *where I started my first job*.

An adjective clause can be an essential or nonessential clause. An essential clause is very important to the sentence. **Essential clauses** explain or define a person or thing. **Nonessential clauses** give more information about a person or thing but are not necessary to define them. Nonessential clauses are set off with commas while essential clauses are not.

Examples:

**Essential**: A person *who works hard at first* can often rest later in life.

**Nonessential**: Neil Armstrong, *who walked on the moon*, is my hero.

### ADVERB CLAUSES

An **adverb clause** is a dependent clause that modifies a verb, adjective, or adverb. In sentences with multiple dependent clauses, adverb clauses are usually placed immediately before or after the independent clause. An adverb clause is introduced with words such as *after, although, as, before, because, if, since, so, unless, when, where,* and *while*.

Examples:

*When you walked outside*, I called the manager.

I will go with you *unless you want to stay*.

### NOUN CLAUSES

A **noun clause** is a dependent clause that can be used as a subject, object, or complement. Noun clauses begin with words such as *how, that, what, whether, which, who,* and *why*. These words can also come with an adjective clause. Unless the noun clause is being used as the subject of the sentence, it should come after the verb of the independent clause.

Examples:

The real mystery is *how you avoided serious injury*.

*What you learn from each other* depends on your honesty with others.

### *SUBORDINATION*

When two related ideas are not of equal importance, the ideal way to combine them is to make the more important idea an independent clause, and the less important idea a dependent or subordinate clause. This is called **subordination**.

Example:

**Separate ideas**: The team had a perfect regular season. The team lost the championship.

**Subordinated**: Despite having a perfect regular season, *the team lost the championship*.

## PHRASES

A phrase is a group of words that functions as a single part of speech, usually a noun, adjective, or adverb. A phrase is not a complete thought, but it adds **detail** or **explanation** to a sentence, or **renames** something within the sentence.

### PREPOSITIONAL PHRASES

One of the most common types of phrases is the prepositional phrase. A **prepositional phrase** begins with a preposition and ends with a noun or pronoun that is the object of the preposition. Normally, the prepositional phrase functions as an **adjective** or an **adverb** within the sentence.

Examples:

The picnic is *on the blanket*.

I am sick *with a fever* today.

*Among the many flowers*, John found a four-leaf clover.

### VERBAL PHRASES

A verbal is a word or phrase that is formed from a verb but does not function as a verb. Depending on its particular form, it may be used as a noun, adjective, or adverb. A verbal does **not** replace a verb in a sentence.

Examples:

Correct: *Walk* a mile daily.

(*Walk* is the verb of this sentence. The subject is the implied *you*.)

Incorrect: *To walk* a mile.

(*To walk* is a type of verbal. This is not a sentence since there is no functional verb)

There are three types of verbals: **participles**, **gerunds**, and **infinitives**. Each type of verbal has a corresponding **phrase** that consists of the verbal itself along with any complements or modifiers.

### PARTICIPLES

A **participle** is a type of verbal that always functions as an adjective. The present participle always ends with -*ing*. Past participles end with -*d*, -*ed*, -*n*, or -*t*.

Examples: Verb: *dance* | Present Participle: *dancing* | Past Participle: *danced*

**Participial phrases** most often come right before or right after the noun or pronoun that they modify.

Examples:

*Shipwrecked on an island*, the boys started to fish for food.

*Having been seated for five hours*, we got out of the car to stretch our legs.

*Praised for their work*, the group accepted the first-place trophy.

## GERUNDS

A **gerund** is a type of verbal that always functions as a noun. Like present participles, gerunds always end with -*ing*, but they can be easily distinguished from one another by the part of speech they represent (participles always function as adjectives). Since a gerund or gerund phrase always functions as a noun, it can be used as the subject of a sentence, the predicate nominative, or the object of a verb or preposition.

Examples:

We want to be known for *teaching the poor*. (Object of preposition)

*Coaching this team* is the best job of my life. (Subject)

We like *practicing our songs* in the basement. (Object of verb)

## INFINITIVES

An **infinitive** is a type of verbal that can function as a noun, an adjective, or an adverb. An infinitive is made of the word *to* + the basic form of the verb. As with all other types of verbal phrases, an infinitive phrase includes the verbal itself and all of its complements or modifiers.

Examples:

*To join the team* is my goal in life. (Noun)

The animals have enough food *to eat for the night*. (Adjective)

People lift weights *to exercise their muscles*. (Adverb)

> **Review Video: Gerunds, Participles, and Infinitives**
> Visit mometrix.com/academy and enter code: 634263

## APPOSITIVE PHRASES

An **appositive** is a word or phrase that is used to explain or rename nouns or pronouns. Noun phrases, gerund phrases, and infinitive phrases can all be used as appositives.

Examples:

Terriers, *hunters at heart*, have been dressed up to look like lap dogs.

(The noun phrase *hunters at heart* renames the noun *terriers*.)

His plan, *to save and invest his money*, was proven as a safe approach.

(The infinitive phrase explains what the plan is.)

Appositive phrases can be **essential** or **nonessential**. An appositive phrase is essential if the person, place, or thing being described or renamed is too general for its meaning to be understood without the appositive.

Examples:

> **Essential**: Two Founding Fathers George Washington and Thomas Jefferson served as presidents.

> **Nonessential**: George Washington and Thomas Jefferson, two Founding Fathers, served as presidents.

### ABSOLUTE PHRASES

An absolute phrase is a phrase that consists of **a noun followed by a participle**. An absolute phrase provides **context** to what is being described in the sentence, but it does not modify or explain any particular word; it is essentially independent.

Examples:

> *The alarm ringing*, he pushed the snooze button.

> *The music paused*, she continued to dance through the crowd.

Note: Absolute phrases can be confusing, so don't be discouraged if you have a difficult time with them.

### PARALLELISM

When multiple items or ideas are presented in a sentence in series, such as in a list, the items or ideas must be stated in grammatically equivalent ways. In other words, if one idea is stated in gerund form, the second cannot be stated in infinitive form. For example, to write, *I enjoy reading and to study* would be incorrect. An infinitive and a gerund are not equivalent. Instead, you should write *I enjoy reading and studying*. In lists of more than two, it can be harder to keep straight, but all items in a list must be parallel.

Example:

> **Incorrect**: He stopped at the office, grocery store, and the pharmacy before heading home.

> The first and third items in the list of places include the article *the*, so the second item needs it as well.

> **Correct**: He stopped at the office, *the* grocery store, and the pharmacy before heading home.

Example:

> **Incorrect**: While vacationing in Europe, she went biking, skiing, and climbed mountains.

> The first and second items in the list are gerunds, so the third item must be as well.

> **Correct**: While vacationing in Europe, she went biking, skiing, and *mountain climbing*.

> **Review Video: Parallel Construction**
> Visit mometrix.com/academy and enter code: 831988

## SENTENCE PURPOSE

There are four types of sentences: declarative, imperative, interrogative, and exclamatory.

A **declarative** sentence states a fact and ends with a period.

> Example: *The football game starts at seven o'clock.*

An **imperative** sentence tells someone to do something and generally ends with a period. (An urgent command might end with an exclamation point instead.)

> Example: *Don't forget to buy your ticket.*

An **interrogative** sentence asks a question and ends with a question mark.

> Example: *Are you going to the game on Friday?*

An **exclamatory** sentence shows strong emotion and ends with an exclamation point.

> Example: *I can't believe we won the game!*

## SENTENCE STRUCTURE

Sentences are classified by structure based on the type and number of clauses present. The four classifications of sentence structure are the following:

**Simple:** A simple sentence has one independent clause with no dependent clauses. A simple sentence may have **compound elements** (i.e., compound subject or verb).

Examples:

> <u>Judy</u> *watered* the lawn. (single <u>subject</u>, single *verb*)
>
> <u>Judy and Alan</u> *watered* the lawn. (compound <u>subject</u>, single *verb*)
>
> <u>Judy</u> *watered* the lawn and *pulled* weeds. (single <u>subject</u>, compound *verb*)
>
> <u>Judy and Alan</u> *watered* the lawn and *pulled* weeds. (compound <u>subject</u>, compound *verb*)

**Compound:** A compound sentence has two or more <u>independent clauses</u> with no dependent clauses. Usually, the independent clauses are joined with a comma and a coordinating conjunction or with a semicolon.

Examples:

> <u>The time has come</u>, and <u>we are ready</u>.
>
> <u>I woke up at dawn</u>; <u>the sun was just coming up</u>.

**Complex:** A complex sentence has one <u>independent clause</u> and at least one *dependent clause*.

Examples:

> *Although he had the flu*, <u>Harry went to work</u>.
>
> <u>Marcia got married</u> *after she finished college.*

**Compound-Complex:** A compound-complex sentence has at least two <u>independent clauses</u> and at least one *dependent clause*.

Examples:

<u>John is my friend</u> *who went to India*, and <u>he brought back souvenirs</u>.

<u>You may not realize this</u>, but <u>we heard the music</u> *that you played last night*.

> **Review Video: Sentence Structure**
> Visit mometrix.com/academy and enter code: 700478

## SENTENCE FRAGMENTS

Usually when the term *sentence fragment* comes up, it is because you have to decide whether or not a group of words is a complete sentence, and if it's not a complete sentence, you're about to have to fix it. Recall that a group of words must contain at least one **independent clause** in order to be considered a sentence. If it doesn't contain even one independent clause, it would be called a **sentence fragment**. (If it contains two or more independent clauses that are not joined correctly, it would be called a run-on sentence.)

The process to use for **repairing** a sentence fragment depends on what type of fragment it is. If the fragment is a dependent clause, it can sometimes be as simple as removing a subordinating word (e.g., when, because, if) from the beginning of the fragment. Alternatively, a dependent clause can be incorporated into a closely related neighboring sentence. If the fragment is missing some required part, like a subject or a verb, the fix might be as simple as adding it in.

Examples:

**Fragment**: Because he wanted to sail the Mediterranean.

**Removed subordinating word**: He wanted to sail the Mediterranean.

**Combined with another sentence**: Because he wanted to sail the Mediterranean, he booked a Greek island cruise.

## RUN-ON SENTENCES

Run-on sentences consist of multiple independent clauses that have not been joined together properly. Run-on sentences can be corrected in several different ways:

**Join clauses properly**: This can be done with a comma and coordinating conjunction, with a semicolon, or with a colon or dash if the second clause is explaining something in the first.

Example:

**Incorrect**: I went on the trip, we visited lots of castles.

**Corrected**: I went on the trip, and we visited lots of castles.

**Split into separate sentences**: This correction is most effective when the independent clauses are very long or when they are not closely related.

Example:

> **Incorrect**: The drive to New York takes ten hours, my uncle lives in Boston.
>
> **Corrected**: The drive to New York takes ten hours. My uncle lives in Boston.

**Make one clause dependent**: This is the easiest way to make the sentence correct and more interesting at the same time. It's often as simple as adding a subordinating word between the two clauses.

Example:

> **Incorrect**: I finally made it to the store and I bought some eggs.
>
> **Corrected**: When I finally made it to the store, I bought some eggs.

**Reduce to one clause with a compound verb**: If both clauses have the same subject, remove the subject from the second clause, and you now have just one clause with a compound verb.

Example:

> **Incorrect**: The drive to New York takes ten hours, it makes me very tired.
>
> **Corrected**: The drive to New York takes ten hours and makes me very tired.

Note: While these are the simplest ways to correct a run-on sentence, often the best way is to completely reorganize the thoughts in the sentence and rewrite it.

> **Review Video: <u>Fragments and Run-on Sentences</u>**
> Visit mometrix.com/academy and enter code: 541989

## DANGLING AND MISPLACED MODIFIERS
### *DANGLING MODIFIERS*
A dangling modifier is a dependent clause or verbal phrase that does not have a **clear logical connection** to a word in the sentence.

Example:

> **Dangling**: *Reading each magazine article*, the stories caught my attention.
>
> The word *stories* cannot be modified by *Reading each magazine article*. People can read, but stories cannot read. Therefore, the subject of the sentence must be a person.
>
> **Corrected**: Reading each magazine article, *I* was entertained by the stories.

Example:

> **Dangling**: Ever since childhood, my grandparents have visited me for Christmas.
>
> The speaker in this sentence can't have been visited by her grandparents when *they* were children, since she wouldn't have been born yet. Either the modifier should be **clarified** or the sentence should be **rearranged** to specify whose childhood is being referenced.
>
> **Clarified**: Ever since I was a child, my grandparents have visited for Christmas.

**Rearranged**: Ever since childhood, I have enjoyed my grandparents visiting for Christmas.

## MISPLACED MODIFIERS

Because modifiers are grammatically versatile, they can be put in many different places within the structure of a sentence. The danger of this versatility is that a modifier can accidentally be placed where it is modifying the wrong word or where it is not clear which word it is modifying.

Example:

**Misplaced**: She read the book to a crowd *that was filled with beautiful pictures*.

The book was filled with beautiful pictures, not the crowd.

**Corrected**: She read the book *that was filled with beautiful pictures* to a crowd.

Example:

**Ambiguous**: Derek saw a bus nearly hit a man *on his way to work*.

Was Derek on his way to work? Or was the other man?

**Derek**: *On his way to work*, Derek saw a bus nearly hit a man.

**The other man**: Derek saw a bus nearly hit a man *who was on his way to work*.

## SPLIT INFINITIVES

A split infinitive occurs when a modifying word comes between the word *to* and the verb that pairs with *to*.

Example: To *clearly* explain vs. *To explain* clearly | To *softly* sing vs. *To sing* softly

Though considered improper by some, split infinitives may provide better clarity and simplicity in some cases than the alternatives. As such, avoiding them should not be considered a universal rule.

## DOUBLE NEGATIVES

Standard English allows **two negatives** only when a **positive** meaning is intended. For example, *The team was not displeased with their performance*. Double negatives to emphasize negation are not used in standard English.

**Negative modifiers** (e.g., never, no, and not) should not be paired with other negative modifiers or negative words (e.g., none, nobody, nothing, or neither). The modifiers *hardly, barely*, and *scarcely* are considered negatives in standard English, so they should not be used with other negatives.

# Knowledge of Language

## LEVEL OF FORMALITY

The relationship between writer and reader is important in choosing a **level of formality** as most writing requires some degree of formality. **Formal writing** is for addressing a superior in a school or work environment. Business letters, textbooks, and newspapers use a moderate to high level of formality. **Informal writing** is appropriate for *private letters, personal e-mails, and business correspondence between close associates.*

For your exam, you will want to be aware of informal and formal writing. One way that this can be accomplished is to watch for shifts in point of view in the essay. For example, unless writers are using a personal example, they will rarely refer to themselves (e.g., "*I* think that *my* point is very clear.") to avoid being informal when they need to be formal.

Also, be mindful of an author who addresses his or her audience **directly** in their writing (e.g., "Readers, *like you*, will understand this argument.") as this can be a sign of informal writing. Good writers understand the need to be consistent with their level of formality. Shifts in levels of formality or point of view can confuse readers and discount the message of an author's writing.

## CLICHÉS

Clichés are phrases that have been **overused** to the point that the phrase has no importance or has lost the original meaning. The phrases have no originality and add very little to a passage. Therefore, most writers will avoid the use of clichés. Another option is to make changes to a cliché so that it is not predictable and empty of meaning.

Examples:

> When life gives you lemons, make lemonade.
> Every cloud has a silver lining.

## JARGON

Jargon is a **specialized vocabulary** that is used among members of a trade or profession. Since jargon is understood by a small audience, writers tend to leave them to passages where certain readers will understand the vocabulary. Jargon includes exaggerated language that tries to impress rather than inform. Sentences filled with jargon are not precise and difficult to understand.

Examples:

> "He is going to *toenail* these frames for us." (toenailing refers to nailing at an angle)
> "They brought in a *kip* of material today." (a kip is a unit of measure equal to 1000 pounds)

## SLANG

Slang is an **informal** and sometimes private language that is understood by some individuals. Slang has some usefulness, but the language can have a small audience. So, most formal writing will not include this kind of language.

Examples:

> "Yes, the event was a *blast!*" (the speaker means that the event was a great experience)
> "That attempt was an *epic fail*." (the speaker means that the attempt was a spectacular failure.)

## COLLOQUIALISM

A colloquialism is a word or phrase that is found in informal writing. Unlike slang, **colloquial language** will be familiar to a greater range of people. Colloquial language can include some slang, but these are limited to contractions for the most part.

Examples:

> "Can *y'all* come back another time?" (y'all is a contraction of "you all")
> "Will you stop him from building this *castle in the air*?" (A "castle in the air" is an improbable or unlikely event.)

## POINT OF VIEW

Point of view is the **perspective** from which writing occurs. There are several possibilities:

- **First person** is written so that the *I* of the story is a participant or observer.
- **Second person** is written directly to the reader. It is a device to draw the reader in more closely. In second person, "you," the reader, are the one taking action in a the sentence.
- **Third person**, the most traditional form of point of view, is the omniscient narrator, in which the narrative voice, presumed to be the writer's, is presumed to know everything about the characters, plot, and action. Most writing uses this point of view.

> **Review Video: Point of View**
> Visit mometrix.com/academy and enter code: 383336

## PRACTICE MAKES PREPARED WRITERS

**Writing** is a skill that continues to need development throughout a person's life. For some people, writing seems to be a natural gift. They rarely struggle with writer's block. When you read their papers, you likely find their ideas persuasive. For others, writing is an intimidating task that they endure. As you prepare for the test, believe that you can improve your skills and be better prepared for reviewing several types of writing.

A traditional way to prepare for the English and Language Usage Section is to **read**. When you read newspapers, magazines, and books, you learn about new ideas. You can read newspapers and magazines to become informed about issues that affect many people. As you think about those issues and ideas, you can take a **position** and form **opinions**. Try to develop these ideas and your opinions by sharing them with friends. After you develop your opinions, try **writing** them down as if you were going to spread your ideas beyond your friends.

Remember that you are practicing for more than an exam. Two of the most valuable skills in life are the abilities to **read critically** and to **write clearly**. When you work on evaluating the arguments of a passage and explain your thoughts well, you are developing skills that you will use for a lifetime.

## BRAINSTORMING

Brainstorming is a technique that is used to find a creative approach to a subject. This can be accomplished by simple **free-association** with a topic. For example, with paper and pen, you write every thought that you have about the topic in a word or phrase. This is done without critical thinking. Everything that comes to your mind about the topic, you should put on your scratch paper. Then, you need to read the list over a few times. Next, you look for *patterns, repetitions, and clusters of ideas*. This allows a variety of fresh ideas to come as you think about the topic.

## FREE WRITING

Free writing is a more structured form of brainstorming. The method involves a limited amount of time (e.g., 2 to 3 minutes) and writing everything that comes to mind about the topic in complete sentences. When time expires, you need to review everything that has been written down. Many of your sentences may make little or no sense, but the insights and observations that can come from free writing make this method a valuable approach. Usually, free writing results in a fuller expression of ideas than brainstorming because thoughts and associations are written in complete sentences. However, both techniques can be used to complement each other.

## REVISIONS

A writer's choice of words is a signature of their **style**. Careful thought about the use of words can improve a piece of writing. A passage can be an exciting piece to read when attention is given to the use of specific nouns rather than general ones.

Example:

> **General**: His kindness will never be forgotten.
> **Specific**: His thoughtful gifts and bear hugs will never be forgotten.

**Revising** sentences is done to make writing more effective. **Editing** sentences is done to correct any errors. Sentences are the building blocks of writing, and they can be changed in regards to sentence length, sentence structure, and sentence openings. You should add **variety** to sentence length, structure, and openings so that the essay does not seem boring or repetitive. A careful analysis of a piece of writing will expose these stylistic problems, and they can be corrected before you finish your essay. Changing up your sentence structure and sentence length can make your essay more inviting and appealing to readers.

> **Review Video: Revising and Editing**
> Visit mometrix.com/academy and enter code: 674181

## RECURSIVE WRITING PROCESS

However you approach writing, you may find comfort in knowing that the revision process can occur in any order. The **recursive writing process** is not as difficult as the phrase may make it seem. Simply put, the recursive writing process means that you may need to revisit steps after completing other steps. Also implied in it is that there is no required order for the steps to take place. Indeed, you may find that **planning**, **drafting**, and **revising** (all a part of the writing process) can all take place at about the same time. The writing process involves moving back and forth between planning, drafting, and revising, followed by more planning, more drafting, and more revising until the writing is satisfactory.

> **Review Video: Recursive Writing Process**
> Visit mometrix.com/academy and enter code: 951611

## PARAGRAPHS

After the introduction of a passage, a series of **body paragraphs** will carry a message through to the conclusion. A paragraph should be unified around a **main point**. Normally, a good **topic sentence** summarizes the paragraph's main point. A topic sentence is a general sentence that introduces the paragraph.

The sentences that follow are a **support** to the topic sentence. However, the topic sentence can come as the final sentence to the paragraph if the earlier sentences give a clear explanation of the topic sentence. Overall, the paragraphs need to stay true to the main point. This means that any unnecessary sentences that do not advance the main point should be removed.

The **main point** of a paragraph requires adequate **development** (i.e., a substantial paragraph that covers the main point). A paragraph of only two or three sentences may not adequately cover a main point. An occasional short paragraph is fine as a **transitional device**. However, a well-developed argument will primarily consist of paragraphs with more than a few sentences.

> **Review Video: Drafting Body Paragraphs**
> Visit mometrix.com/academy and enter code: 724590

## METHODS OF DEVELOPING PARAGRAPHS

A common method of development with paragraphs can be done with **examples**. These examples are the supporting details to the main idea of a paragraph or a passage. When authors write about something that their audience may not understand, they can provide an example to show their point. When authors write about something that is not easily accepted, they can give examples to prove their point.

**Illustrations** are extended examples that require several sentences. Well-selected illustrations can be a great way for authors to develop a point that may not be familiar to their audience.

**Analogies** make comparisons between items that appear to have nothing in common. Analogies are employed by writers to provoke fresh thoughts about a subject. These comparisons may be used to explain the unfamiliar, to clarify an abstract point, or to argue a point. Although analogies are effective *literary devices*, they should be used carefully in arguments. Two things may be alike in some respects but completely different in others.

**Cause and effect** is an excellent device used when the cause and effect are accepted as true. One way that authors can use cause and effect is to state the effect in the topic sentence of a paragraph and add the causes in the body of the paragraph. With this method, an author's paragraphs can have structure which always strengthens writing.

## TYPES OF PARAGRAPHS

A **paragraph of narration** tells a story or a part of a story. Normally, the sentences are arranged in chronological order (i.e., the order that the events happened). However, flashbacks (i.e., beginning the story at an earlier time) can be included.

A **descriptive paragraph** makes a verbal portrait of a person, place, or thing. When specific details are used that appeal to one or more of the senses (i.e., sight, sound, smell, taste, and touch), authors give readers a sense of being present in the moment.

A **process paragraph** is related to time order (i.e., First, you open the bottle. Second, you pour the liquid, etc.). Usually, this describes a process or teaches readers how to perform a process.

**Comparing two things** draws attention to their similarities and indicates a number of differences. When authors **contrast**, they focus only on differences. Both comparisons and contrasts may be used point-by-point or in following paragraphs.

Reasons for starting a new paragraph include:

- To mark off the introduction and concluding paragraphs
- To signal a shift to a new idea or topic
- To indicate an important shift in time or place
- To explain a point in additional detail
- To highlight a comparison, contrast, or cause and effect relationship

## PARAGRAPH LENGTH

Most readers find that their comfort level for a paragraph is *between 100 and 200 words*. Shorter paragraphs cause too much starting and stopping, and give a choppy effect. Paragraphs that are too long often test the attention span of readers. Two notable exceptions to this rule exist. In scientific or scholarly papers, longer paragraphs suggest seriousness and depth. In journalistic writing, constraints are placed on paragraph size by the narrow columns in a newspaper format.

The first and last paragraphs of a text will usually be the **introduction** and **conclusion**. These special-purpose paragraphs are likely to be shorter than paragraphs in the body of the work. Paragraphs in the body of the essay follow the subject's **outline**; one paragraph per point in short essays and a group of paragraphs per point in longer works. Some ideas require more development than others, so it is good for a writer to remain flexible. A paragraph of excessive length may be divided, and shorter ones may be combined.

## COHERENT PARAGRAPHS

A smooth flow of sentences and paragraphs without gaps, shifts, or bumps will lead to paragraph **coherence**. Ties between old and new information can be smoothed by several methods:

- **Linking ideas clearly**, from the topic sentence to the body of the paragraph, is essential for a smooth transition. The topic sentence states the main point, and this should be followed by specific details, examples, and illustrations that support the topic sentence. The support may be direct or indirect. In **indirect support**, the illustrations and examples may support a sentence that in turn supports the topic directly.
- The **repetition of key words** adds coherence to a paragraph. To avoid dull language, variations of the key words may be used.
- **Parallel structures** are often used within sentences to emphasize the similarity of ideas and connect sentences giving similar information.
- Maintaining a **consistent verb tense** throughout the paragraph helps. Shifting tenses affects the smooth flow of words and can disrupt the coherence of the paragraph.

---

**Review Video: How to Write a Good Paragraph**
Visit mometrix.com/academy and enter code: 682127

---

# Vocabulary Acquisition

## CONTEXT CLUES

Learning new words is an important part of **comprehending** and **integrating** unfamiliar information. When a reader encounters a new word, he can stop and find it in the dictionary or the glossary of terms, but sometimes those reference tools aren't readily available or using them at the moment is impractical (e.g., during a test). Furthermore, most readers are usually not willing to take the time. Another way to determine the meaning of a word is by considering the **context** in which it is being used. These indirect learning hints are called **context clues**. They include definitions, descriptions, examples, and restatements. Because most words are learned by listening to conversations, people use this tool all the time even if they do it unconsciously. But to be effective in written text, context clues must be used judiciously because the unfamiliar word may have several subtle variations, and therefore the context clues could be misinterpreted.

Context refers to *how a word is used in a sentence*. Identifying context can help determine the definition of unknown words. There are different contextual clues such as definition, description, example, comparison, and contrast. The following are examples:

- **Definition**: the unknown word is clearly defined by the previous words. – "When he was painting, his instrument was a __." (paintbrush)
- **Description**: the unknown word is described by the previous words. – "I was hot, tired, and thirsty; I was __." (dehydrated)
- **Example**: the unknown word is part of a series of examples. – "Water, soda, and __ were the offered beverages." (coffee)
- **Comparison**: the unknown word is compared to another word. – "Barney is agreeable and happy like his __ parents." (positive)
- **Contrast**: the unknown word is contrasted with another word. – "I prefer cold weather to __ conditions." (hot)

> **Review Video: Context**
> Visit mometrix.com/academy and enter code: 613660

## SYNONYMS AND ANTONYMS

When you understand how words relate to each other, you will discover more in a passage. This is explained by understanding **synonyms** (e.g., words that mean the same thing) and **antonyms** (e.g., words that mean the opposite of one another). As an example, *dry* and *arid* are synonyms, and *dry* and *wet* are antonyms. There are many pairs of words in English that can be considered synonyms, despite having slightly different definitions. For instance, the words *friendly* and *collegial* can both be used to describe a warm interpersonal relationship, and one would be correct to call them **synonyms**. However, *collegial* (kin to *colleague*) is often used in reference to professional or academic relationships, and *friendly* has no such connotation. If the difference between two words is too great, then they should not be called synonyms. *Hot* and *warm* are not synonyms because their meanings are too distinct. A good way to determine whether two words are synonyms is to substitute one word for the other word and verify that the meaning of the sentence has not changed. Substituting *warm* for *hot* in a sentence would convey a different meaning. Although warm and hot may seem close in meaning, warm generally means that the temperature is moderate, and hot generally means that the temperature is excessively high.

**Antonyms** are words with opposite meanings. *Light* and *dark*, *up* and *down*, *right* and *left*, *good* and *bad*: these are all sets of antonyms. Be careful to distinguish between antonyms and pairs of words that are simply different. *Black* and *gray*, for instance, are not antonyms because gray is not the opposite of black. *Black* and *white*, on the other hand, are antonyms.

Not every word has an antonym. For instance, many nouns do not. What would be the antonym of *chair*? During your exam, the questions related to antonyms are more likely to concern adjectives. You will recall that adjectives are words that describe a noun. Some common adjectives include *purple, fast, skinny*, and *sweet*. From those four adjectives, *purple* is the item that lacks a group of obvious antonyms.

> **Review Video: <u>Synonyms and Antonyms</u>**
> Visit mometrix.com/academy and enter code: 105612

## DESCRIPTION

Occasionally, you will be able to define an unfamiliar word by looking at the **descriptive words** in the context. Consider the following sentence: *Fred dragged the recalcitrant boy kicking and screaming up the stairs.* The words *dragged, kicking*, and *screaming* all suggest that the boy does not want to go up the stairs. The reader may assume that *recalcitrant* means something like unwilling or protesting. In this example, an unfamiliar adjective was identified.

Additionally, using description to define an unfamiliar noun is a common practice compared to unfamiliar adjectives, as in this sentence: *Don's wrinkled frown and constantly shaking fist identified him as a curmudgeon of the first order.* Don is described as having a *wrinkled frown and constantly shaking fist* suggesting that a *curmudgeon* must be a grumpy person. **Contrasts** do not always provide detailed information about the unfamiliar word, but they at least give the reader some clues.

When a word has **more than one meaning**, readers can have difficulty with determining how the word is being used in a given sentence. For instance, the verb *cleave*, can mean either *join* or *separate*. When readers come upon this word, they will have to select the definition that makes the most sense. Consider the following sentence: *Hermione's knife cleaved the bread cleanly.* Since, a knife cannot join bread together, the word must indicate separation.

A slightly more difficult example would be the sentence: *The birds cleaved together as they flew from the oak tree.* Immediately, the presence of the word *together* should suggest that in this sentence *cleave* is being used to mean *join*. Discovering the intent of a word with multiple meanings requires the same tricks as defining an unknown word: *look for contextual clues and evaluate the substituted words*.

## STRUCTURAL ANALYSIS

An understanding of the basics of language is helpful, and often vital, to understanding what you read. The term **structural analysis** refers to looking at the parts of a word and breaking it down into its different **components** to determine the word's meaning. Parts of a word include prefixes, suffixes, and the root word. By learning the meanings of prefixes, suffixes, and other word fundamentals, you can decipher the meaning of words which may not yet be in your vocabulary.

**Prefixes** are common letter combinations at the beginning of words, while **suffixes** are common letter combinations at the end. The main part of the word is known as the **root**. Visually, it would look like this: prefix + root word + suffix. Look first at the individual meanings of the root word, prefix and/or suffix. Use knowledge of the meaning(s) of the prefix and/or suffix to see what information it adds to the root.

Even if the meaning of the root is unknown, one can use knowledge of the prefix's and/or suffix's meaning(s) to determine an *approximate meaning* of the word. For example, if one sees the word *uninspired* and does not know what it means, they can use the knowledge that *un-* means 'not' to know that the full word means "not inspired." Understanding the common prefixes and suffixes can illuminate at least part of the meaning of an unfamiliar word.

> **Review Video: Determining Word Meanings**
> Visit mometrix.com/academy and enter code: 894894

## AFFIXES

Affixes in the English language are **morphemes** that are added to words to create related but different words. **Derivational affixes** form new words based on and related to the original words. For example, the affix *–ness* added to the end of the adjective *happy* forms the noun *happiness.*

**Inflectional affixes** form different grammatical versions of words. For example, the plural affix *–s* changes the singular noun *book* to the plural noun *books*, and the past tense affix *–ed* changes the infinitive or present tense verb *look* to the past tense *looked.*

**Prefixes** are affixes placed in front of words. For example, *heat* means to make hot; *preheat*, using the prefix *pre-*, means to heat in advance. **Suffixes** are affixes placed at the ends of words. The *happiness* example above contains the suffix *–ness.* **Circumfixes** add parts both before and after words, such as how *light* becomes *enlighten* with the prefix *en-* and the suffix *–en.* **Interfixes** compound words via central affixes: *speed* and *meter* become *speedometer* via the interfix *–o–.*

> **Review Video: Affixes**
> Visit mometrix.com/academy and enter code: 782422

## PREFIXES
### AMOUNT

| Prefix | Definition | Examples |
|---|---|---|
| bi- | two | bisect, biennial |
| mono- | one, single | monogamy, monologue |
| poly- | many | polymorphous, polygamous |
| semi- | half, partly | semicircle, semicolon |
| uni- | one | uniform, unity |

### NEGATION

| Prefix | Definition | Examples |
|---|---|---|
| a- | without, lacking | atheist, agnostic |
| in- | not, opposing | incapable, ineligible |
| non- | not | nonentity, nonsense |
| un- | not, reverse of | unhappy, unlock |

### TIME AND SPACE

| Prefix | Definition | Examples |
|---|---|---|
| a- | in, on, of, up, to | abed, afoot |
| ab- | from, away, off | abdicate, abjure |
| ad- | to, toward | advance, adventure |
| ante- | before, previous | antecedent, antedate |
| anti- | against, opposing | antipathy, antidote |

| Prefix | Definition | Examples |
|--------|-----------|----------|
| cata- | down, away, thoroughly | catastrophe, cataclysm |
| circum- | around | circumspect, circumference |
| com- | with, together, very | commotion, complicate |
| contra- | against, opposing | contradict, contravene |
| de- | from | depart |
| dia- | through, across, apart | diameter, diagnose |
| dis- | away, off, down, not | dissent, disappear |
| epi- | upon | epilogue |
| ex- | out | extract, excerpt |
| hypo- | under, beneath | hypodermic, hypothesis |
| inter- | among, between | intercede, interrupt |
| intra- | within | intramural, intrastate |
| ob- | against, opposing | objection |
| per- | through | perceive, permit |
| peri- | around | periscope, perimeter |
| post- | after, following | postpone, postscript |
| pre- | before, previous | prevent, preclude |
| pro- | forward, in place of | propel, pronoun |
| retro- | back, backward | retrospect, retrograde |
| sub- | under, beneath | subjugate, substitute |
| super- | above, extra | supersede, supernumerary |
| trans- | across, beyond, over | transact, transport |
| ultra- | beyond, excessively | ultramodern, ultrasonic, ultraviolet |

*MISCELLANEOUS*

| Prefix | Definition | Examples |
|--------|-----------|----------|
| belli- | war, warlike | bellicose |
| bene- | well, good | benefit, benefactor |
| equi- | equal | equivalent, equilibrium |
| for- | away, off, from | forget, forswear |
| fore- | previous | foretell, forefathers |
| homo- | same, equal | homogenized, homonym |
| hyper- | excessive, over | hypercritical, hypertension |
| in- | in, into | intrude, invade |
| magn- | large | magnitude, magnify |
| mal- | bad, poorly, not | malfunction, malpractice |
| mis- | bad, poorly, not | misspell, misfire |
| mor- | death | mortality, mortuary |
| neo- | new | Neolithic, neoconservative |
| omni- | all, everywhere | omniscient, omnivore |
| ortho- | right, straight | orthogonal, orthodox |
| over- | above | overbearing, oversight |
| pan- | all, entire | panorama, pandemonium |
| para- | beside, beyond | parallel, paradox |
| phil- | love, like | philosophy, philanthropic |
| prim- | first, early | primitive, primary |
| re- | backward, again | revoke, recur |
| sym- | with, together | sympathy, symphony |
| vis- | to see | visage, visible |

## SUFFIXES

Suffixes are a group of letters, placed behind a root word, that carry a specific meaning. Suffixes can perform one of two possible functions. They can be used to create a new word, or they can shift the tense of a word without changing its original meaning. For example, the suffix -*ability* can be added to the end of the word *account* to form the new word *accountability*. *Account* means a written narrative or description of events, while *accountability* means the state of being liable. The suffix -*ed* can be added to *account* to form the word *accounted*, which simply shifts the word from present tense to past tense.

Sometimes adding a suffix can change the **spelling** of a root word. If the suffix begins with a vowel, the final consonant of the root word must be doubled. This rule applies only if the root word has one syllable or if the accent is on the last syllable. For example, when adding the suffix -*ery* to the root word *rob*, the final word becomes *robbery*. The letter *b* is doubled because *rob* has only one syllable. However, when adding the suffix -*able* to the root word *profit*, the final word becomes *profitable*. The letter *t* is not doubled because the root word *profit* has two syllables.

Spelling is not changed when the suffixes -*less, -ness, -ly*, or -*en* are used. The only exception to this rule occurs when the suffix -*ness* or -*ly* is added to a root word ending in *y*. In this case, the *y* changes to *i*. For example, *happy* becomes *happily*.

Certain suffixes require that the root word be **modified**. If the suffix begins with a vowel, e.g., -*ing*, and the root word ends in the letter *e*, the *e* must be dropped before adding the suffix. For example, the word *write* becomes *writing*. If the suffix begins with a consonant instead of a vowel, the letter *e* at the end of the root word does not need to be dropped. For example, *hope* becomes *hopeless*. The only exceptions to this rule are the words *judgment, acknowledgment,* and *argument.* If a root word ends in the letter *y* and is preceded by a consonant, the *y* is changed to *i* before adding the suffix. This is true for all suffixes except those that begin with *i.* For example, *plenty* becomes *plentiful.*

Here are some common suffixes, their meanings, and some examples of their use:

### ADJECTIVE SUFFIXES

| Suffix | Definition | Examples |
|---|---|---|
| -able (-ible) | capable of being | toler*able*, ed*ible* |
| -esque | in the style of, like | picturesque, grotesque |
| -ful | filled with, marked by | thankful, zestful |
| -ic | make, cause | terrific, beatific |
| -ish | suggesting, like | churlish, childish |
| -less | lacking, without | hopeless, countless |
| -ous | marked by, given to | religious, riotous |

### NOUN SUFFIXES

| Suffix | Definition | Examples |
|---|---|---|
| -acy | state, condition | accuracy, privacy |
| -ance | act, condition, fact | acceptance, vigilance |
| -ard | one that does excessively | drunkard, sluggard |
| -ation | action, state, result | occupation, starvation |
| -dom | state, rank, condition | serfdom, wisdom |
| -er (-or) | office, action | teach*er*, elevat*or*, hon*or* |
| -ess | feminine | waitress, duchess |
| -hood | state, condition | manhood, statehood |
| -ion | action, result, state | union, fusion |
| -ism | act, manner, doctrine | barbarism, socialism |
| -ist | worker, follower | monopolist, socialist |
| -ity (-ty) | state, quality, condition | acid*ity*, civil*ity*, royal*ty* |
| -ment | result, action | refreshment, disappointment |
| -ness | quality, state | greatness, tallness |
| -ship | position | internship, statesmanship |
| -sion (-tion) | state, result | revi*sion*, expedi*tion* |
| -th | act, state, quality | warmth, width |
| -tude | quality, state, result | magnitude, fortitude |

### VERB SUFFIXES

| Suffix | Definition | Examples |
|---|---|---|
| -ate | having, showing | separate, desolate |
| -en | cause to be, become | deepen, strengthen |
| -fy | make, cause to have | glorify, fortify |
| -ize | cause to be, treat with | sterilize, mechanize, criticize |

# Comprehensive Practice Tests

The table below shows the amount of time and number of questions that are on each practice test. It is recommended that you use a timer when taking the test to properly simulate the test taking conditions.

| Reading | Mathematics | Science | English and Language Usage | Total |
|---------|-------------|---------|----------------------------|-------|
| 53 items | 36 items | 53 items | 28 items | 170 items |
| 64 minutes | 54 minutes | 63 minutes | 28 minutes | 209 minutes |

**DIRECTIONS**: The questions you are about to take are multiple-choice with only one correct answer per question. Read each test item and mark your answer on the appropriate blank on the answer page that precedes each practice test.

When you have completed a practice test, you may check your answers with those on the answer key that follows each test.

Each practice test is followed by detailed answer explanations.

**Special feature**: In addition to the two full-length practice tests included in this section, you also have access to an **online interactive practice test!** Just follow the link below on your computer or mobile device to get started.

> **Online Interactive Practice Test**
> Visit mometrix.com/university/teas-bonus-practice-test

# TEAS Practice Test #1

|  | Reading |  | Mathematics | | Science |  | English and Language Usage |
|---|---|---|---|---|---|---|---|

| Reading | | Mathematics | Science | | English and Language Usage |
|---|---|---|---|---|---|

**Reading**

1. _____  46. _____
2. _____  47. _____
3. _____  48. _____
4. _____  49. _____
5. _____  50. _____
6. _____  51. _____
7. _____  52. _____
8. _____  53. _____
9. _____
10. _____
11. _____
12. _____
13. _____
14. _____
15. _____
16. _____
17. _____
18. _____
19. _____
20. _____
21. _____
22. _____
23. _____
24. _____
25. _____
26. _____
27. _____
28. _____
29. _____
30. _____
31. _____
32. _____
33. _____
34. _____
35. _____
36. _____
37. _____
38. _____
39. _____
40. _____
41. _____
42. _____
43. _____
44. _____
45. _____

**Mathematics**

1. _____
2. _____
3. _____
4. _____
5. _____
6. _____
7. _____
8. _____
9. _____
10. _____
11. _____
12. _____
13. _____
14. _____
15. _____
16. _____
17. _____
18. _____
19. _____
20. _____
21. _____
22. _____
23. _____
24. _____
25. _____
26. _____
27. _____
28. _____
29. _____
30. _____
31. _____
32. _____
33. _____
34. _____
35. _____
36. _____

**Science**

1. _____  46. _____
2. _____  47. _____
3. _____  48. _____
4. _____  49. _____
5. _____  50. _____
6. _____  51. _____
7. _____  52. _____
8. _____  53. _____
9. _____
10. _____
11. _____
12. _____
13. _____
14. _____
15. _____
16. _____
17. _____
18. _____
19. _____
20. _____
21. _____
22. _____
23. _____
24. _____
25. _____
26. _____
27. _____
28. _____
29. _____
30. _____
31. _____
32. _____
33. _____
34. _____
35. _____
36. _____
37. _____
38. _____
39. _____
40. _____
41. _____
42. _____
43. _____
44. _____
45. _____

**English and Language Usage**

1. _____
2. _____
3. _____
4. _____
5. _____
6. _____
7. _____
8. _____
9. _____
10. _____
11. _____
12. _____
13. _____
14. _____
15. _____
16. _____
17. _____
18. _____
19. _____
20. _____
21. _____
22. _____
23. _____
24. _____
25. _____
26. _____
27. _____
28. _____

| **Reading** | Number of Questions: **53** |
| --- | --- |
| | Time Limit: **64 Minutes** |

**1. Which of the answer choices gives the best definition for the underlined word in the following sentence?**

**Adelaide attempted to <u>assuage</u> her guilt over the piece of cheesecake by limiting herself to salads the following day.**

    a. increase
    b. support
    c. appease
    d. conceal – hide

**2. Which of the following would best support the argument that people cause global climate change?**

    a. The average global temperature has increased 1.5 degrees Fahrenheit since 1880.
    b. Common greenhouse gases include carbon dioxide and water vapor.
    c. Most of the greenhouse gases today come from burning things like coal and other fossil fuels for energy.
    d. The average person breathes out about 1.0 kg of carbon dioxide every day, while the average cow produces about 80 kg of methane.

*The next three questions are based on the following information.*

<u>The Dewey Decimal Classes</u>

000 Computer science, information, and general works
100 Philosophy and psychology
200 Religion
300 Social sciences
400 Languages
500 Science and mathematics
600 Technical and applied science
700 Arts and recreation
800 Literature
900 History, geography, and biography

**3. Lise is doing a research project on the various psychological theories that Sigmund Freud developed and on the modern response to those theories. She is not sure where to begin, so she consults the chart of Dewey Decimal Classes. To which section of the library should she go to begin looking for research material?**

    a. 100
    b. 200
    c. 300
    d. 900

4. During her research, Lise discovers that Freud's theory of the Oedipal complex was based on ancient Greek mythology that was made famous by Sophocles' play *Oedipus Rex*. To which section of the library should she go if she is interested in reading the play?

    a.  300
    b.  400
    c.  800
    d.  900

5. Also during her research, Lise learns about Freud's Jewish background, and she decides to compare Freud's theories to traditional Judaism. To which section of the library should she go for more information on this subject?

    a.  100
    b.  200
    c.  800
    d.  900

6. Which of the answer choices best describes the appropriateness of Mara's data sample in the following vignette?

Mara is conducting a study that will examine the ideas of middle school teachers, concerning the usage of iPhones in the classroom. She interviews all teachers who teach a computer software course.

    a.  The sample is biased because it only includes teachers who are immersed in the technology field
    b.  The sample is biased because the sample size is too small
    c.  The sample is biased because the sample size is too large
    d.  The sample is not biased and is appropriate for the study

7. Which of the answer choices gives the best definition for the underlined word in the following sentence?

Although his friends believed him to be enjoying a lavish lifestyle in the large family estate he had inherited, Enzo was in reality <u>impecunious</u>.

    a.  Penniless
    b.  Unfortunate
    c.  Emotional
    d.  Commanding

8. Follow the instructions below to transform the starting word into a different word.

- **Start with the word ESOTERIC**
- **Remove both instances of the letter E from the word**
- **Remove the letter I from the word**
- **Move the letter T from the middle of the word to the end of the word**
- **Remove the letter C from the word**

What new word has been spelled?

    a.  SECT
    b.  SORT
    c.  SORE
    d.  TORE

*The next two questions are based on the following chart, which reflects the enrollment and the income for a small community college.*

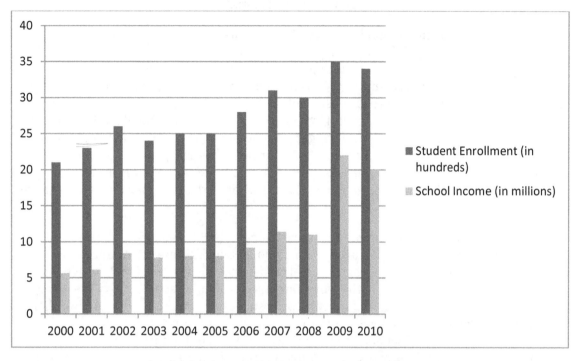

**9. Based on the chart, approximately how many students attended the community college in the year 2001?**

    a.  2100
    b.  2300
    c.  2500
    d.  2700

**10. In order to offset costs, the college administration decided to increase admission fees. Reviewing the chart above, during which year is it most likely that the college raised the price of admission?**

    a.  2002
    b.  2007
    c.  2009
    d.  2010

**11. If the statements listed below are true, which of the answer choices is a logical conclusion?**

**Literacy rates are lower today than they were fifteen years ago. Then, most people learned to read through the use of phonics. Today, whole language programs are favored by many educators.**

    a.  whole language is more effective at teaching people to read than phonics.
    b.  phonics is more effective at teaching people to read than whole language.
    c.  literacy rates will probably continue to decline over the next 15 years.
    d.  the definition of what it means to be literate is much stricter now.

*The next four questions are based on the following passage.*

## The Bermuda Triangle

The area known as the Bermuda Triangle has become such a part of popular culture that it can be difficult to separate fact from fiction. The interest first began when five Navy planes vanished in 1945, officially resulting from "causes or reasons unknown." The explanations about other accidents in the Triangle range from the scientific to the supernatural. Researchers have never been able to find anything truly mysterious about what happens in the Bermuda Triangle, if there even is a Bermuda Triangle. What is more, one of the biggest challenges in considering the phenomenon is deciding how much area actually represents the Bermuda Triangle. Most consider the Triangle to stretch from Miami out to Puerto Rico and to include the island of Bermuda. Others expand the area to include all of the Caribbean islands and to extend eastward as far as the Azores, which are closer to Europe than they are to North America.

The problem with having a larger Bermuda Triangle is that it increases the odds of accidents. There is near-constant travel, by ship and by plane, across the Atlantic, and accidents are expected to occur. In fact, the Bermuda Triangle happens to fall within one of the busiest navigational regions in the world, and the reality of greater activity creates the possibility for more to go wrong. Shipping records suggest that there is not a greater than average loss of vessels within the Bermuda Triangle, and many researchers have argued that the reputation of the Triangle makes any accident seem out of the ordinary. In fact, most accidents fall within the expected margin of error. The increase in ships from East Asia no doubt contributes to an increase in accidents. And as for the story of the Navy planes that disappeared within the Triangle, many researchers now conclude that it was the result of mistakes on the part of the pilots who were flying into storm clouds and simply got lost.

## 12. Which of the following describes this type of writing?
   a.  Narrative
   b.  Persuasive
   c.  Expository
   d.  Technical

## 13. Which of the following sentences is most representative of a summary sentence for this passage?
   a.  The problem with having a larger Bermuda Triangle is that it increases the odds of accidents.
   b.  The area that is called the Bermuda Triangle happens to fall within one of the busiest navigational regions in the world, and the reality of greater activity creates the possibility for more to go wrong.
   c.  One of the biggest challenges in considering the phenomenon is deciding how much area actually represents the Bermuda Triangle.
   d.  Researchers have never been able to find anything truly mysterious about what happens in the Bermuda Triangle, if there even is a Bermuda Triangle.

**14. With which of the following statements would the author most likely agree?**

    a. There is no real mystery about the Bermuda Triangle because most events have reasonable explanations.

    b. Researchers are wrong to expand the focus of the Triangle to the Azores, because this increases the likelihood of accidents.

    c. The official statement of "causes or reasons unknown" in the loss of the Navy planes was a deliberate concealment from the Navy.

    d. Reducing the legends about the mysteries of the Bermuda Triangle will help to reduce the number of reported accidents or shipping losses in that region.

**15. Which of the following represents an opinion statement on the part of the author?**

    a. The problem with having a larger Bermuda Triangle is that it increases the odds of accidents.

    b. The area known as the Bermuda Triangle has become such a part of popular culture that it can be difficult to sort through the myth and locate the truth.

    c. The increase in ships from East Asia no doubt contributes to an increase in accidents.

    d. Most consider the Triangle to stretch from Miami to Puerto Rico and include the island of Bermuda.

**16. Which of the following is a primary source?**

    a. A report of an original research experiment

    b. An academic textbook's citation of research

    c. A quotation of a researcher in a news article

    d. A website description of another's research

**17. The guide words at the top of a dictionary page are *intrauterine* and *invest*. Which of the following words is an entry on this page?**

    a. Intransigent

    b. Introspection

    c. Investiture

    d. Intone

*The next question is based on the following chart.*

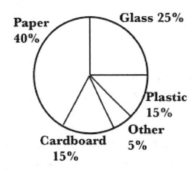

**18. A recycling company collects sorted materials from its clients. The materials are weighed and then processed for re-use. The chart shows the weights of various classes of materials that were collected by the company during a representative month. Which of the following statements is NOT supported by the data in the chart?**

  a.  Paper products, including cardboard, make up a majority of the collected materials.
  b.  One quarter of the materials collected are made of glass.
  c.  More plastic is collected than cardboard.
  d.  Plastic and cardboard together represent a larger portion of the collected materials than glass bottles.

**19. Ninette has celiac disease, which means that she cannot eat any product containing gluten. Gluten is a protein present in many grains such as wheat, rye, and barley. Because of her health condition, Ninette has to be careful about what she eats to avoid having an allergic reaction. She will be attending an all-day industry event, and she requested the menu in advance. Here is the menu:**

  • **Breakfast: Fresh coffee or tea, scrambled eggs, bacon or sausage**
  • **Lunch: Spinach salad (dressing available on the side), roasted chicken, steamed rice**
  • **Cocktail Hour: Various beverages, fruit and cheese plate**
  • **Dinner: Spaghetti and sauce, tossed salad, garlic bread**

**During which of these meals should Ninette be careful to bring her own food?**

  a.  Breakfast
  b.  Lunch
  c.  Cocktail Hour
  d.  Dinner

**20. Which of the following best provides detailed support for the claim that "seatbelts save lives"?**

  a.  A government website containing driving accident information
  b.  A blog developed by one of the largest car companies in the world
  c.  An encyclopedia entry on the seatbelt and its development
  d.  An instant message sent out by a famous race car driver

21. Which of the answer choices presents a valid inference based on the following scenario?

The latest movie by a certain director gets bad reviews before it opens in theatres. Consequently, very few people go to the movie and the director is given much less money to make his next movie, which is also unsuccessful.

a. This director makes terrible movies
b. The general public does not pay attention to movie reviews
c. The movie reviewers were right about the first movie
d. Movie reviewers exert influence on the movie quality

*The next three questions are based on the following table.*

| NAME | COMPOSITION (PER 100) | WORLD LITERATURE (PER 100) | TECHNICAL WRITING (PER 100) | LINGUISTICS (PER 100) |
|---|---|---|---|---|
| Textbook-Mania | $4500 | $5150 | $6000 | $6500 |
| Textbook Central | $4350 | $5200 | $6100 | $6550 |
| Bookstore Supply | $4675 | $5000 | $5950 | $6475 |
| University Textbooks | $4600 | $5000 | $6100 | $6650 |

*Note: Shipping is free for all schools that order 100 textbooks or more.*

22. A school needs to purchase 500 composition textbooks and 500 world literature textbooks. Which of the textbook suppliers can offer the lowest price?

a. Textbook Mania
b. Textbook Central
c. Bookstore Supply
d. University Textbooks

23. A school needs to purchase 1000 composition textbooks and 300 linguistics textbooks. Which of the textbook suppliers can offer the lowest price?

a. Textbook Mania
b. Textbook Central
c. Bookstore Supply
d. University Textbooks

24. A school needs to purchase 400 world literature textbooks and 200 technical writing textbooks. Which of the textbook suppliers can offer the lowest price?

a. Textbook Mania
b. Textbook Central
c. Bookstore Supply
d. University Textbooks

*The next four questions are based on the following graphic.*

**Table 1. Consumer Price Index for All Urban Consumers (CPI-U): U.S. city average, by expenditure category and commodity and service group**

(1982-84=100, unless otherwise noted)

| Item and group | Relative importance, December 2008 | Unadjusted indexes | | Unadjusted percent change to June 2009 from— | | Seasonally adjusted percent change from— | | |
|---|---|---|---|---|---|---|---|---|
| | | May 2009 | June 2009 | June 2008 | May 2009 | Mar. to Apr. | Apr. to May | May to June |
| **Expenditure category** | | | | | | | | |
| All items | 100.000 | 213.856 | 215.693 | -1.4 | 0.9 | 0.0 | 0.1 | 0.7 |
| All items (1967=100) | - | 640.616 | 646.121 | - | - | - | - | - |
| Food and beverages | 15.757 | 218.076 | 218.030 | 2.2 | .0 | -.2 | -.2 | .1 |
| Food | 14.629 | 217.826 | 217.740 | 2.1 | .0 | -.2 | -.2 | .0 |
| Food at home | 8.156 | 215.088 | 214.824 | .8 | -.1 | -.6 | -.5 | .0 |
| Cereals and bakery products | 1.150 | 252.714 | 253.008 | 3.0 | .1 | -.7 | -.2 | .0 |
| Meats, poultry, fish, and eggs | 1.898 | 203.789 | 204.031 | .6 | .1 | .0 | -.9 | -.2 |
| Dairy and related products [1] | .910 | 196.055 | 194.197 | -7.1 | -.9 | -1.3 | -.5 | -.9 |
| Fruits and vegetables | 1.194 | 274.006 | 272.608 | -1.9 | -.5 | .0 | -1.0 | 1.1 |
| Nonalcoholic beverages and beverage materials | .982 | 162.803 | 162.571 | 2.7 | -.1 | -1.0 | -.1 | .1 |
| Other food at home | 2.022 | 191.144 | 191.328 | 4.1 | .1 | -.8 | -.1 | .0 |
| Sugar and sweets | .300 | 196.403 | 197.009 | 6.2 | .3 | -.5 | .0 | .2 |
| Fats and oils | .241 | 200.679 | 201.127 | 2.5 | .2 | -1.4 | -.7 | .6 |
| Other foods | 1.481 | 205.587 | 205.654 | 3.9 | .0 | -.8 | .0 | -.2 |
| Other miscellaneous foods [1,2] | .433 | 122.838 | 122.224 | 3.2 | -.5 | .4 | .0 | -.5 |
| Food away from home [1] | 6.474 | 223.023 | 223.163 | 3.8 | .1 | .3 | .1 | .1 |
| Other food away from home [1,2] | .314 | 155.099 | 155.841 | 4.0 | .5 | .4 | .0 | .5 |
| Alcoholic beverages | 1.127 | 220.005 | 220.477 | 3.1 | .2 | -.1 | .3 | .2 |
| Housing | 43.421 | 216.971 | 218.071 | .1 | .5 | -.1 | -.1 | .0 |
| Shelter | 33.200 | 249.779 | 250.243 | 1.3 | .2 | .2 | .1 | .1 |
| Rent of primary residence [3] | 5.957 | 249.069 | 249.092 | 2.7 | .0 | .2 | .1 | .1 |
| Lodging away from home [2] | 2.478 | 135.680 | 138.318 | -6.9 | 1.9 | .5 | .1 | .3 |
| Owners' equivalent rent of primary residence [3,4] | 24.433 | 256.875 | 256.981 | 1.9 | .0 | .1 | .1 | .1 |
| Tenants' and household insurance [1,2] | .333 | 120.728 | 121.083 | 1.7 | .3 | -.1 | .0 | .3 |
| Fuels and utilities | 5.431 | 206.358 | 212.677 | -8.1 | 3.1 | -1.7 | -1.3 | -.8 |
| Household energy | 4.460 | 183.783 | 190.647 | -10.8 | 3.7 | -2.2 | -1.8 | -1.0 |
| Fuel oil and other fuels | .301 | 225.164 | 232.638 | -40.3 | 3.3 | -2.1 | -3.1 | 2.0 |
| Gas (piped) and electricity [3] | 4.159 | 189.619 | 196.754 | -7.8 | 3.8 | -2.2 | -1.7 | -1.2 |
| Water and sewer and trash collection services [2] | .971 | 159.517 | 159.831 | 6.2 | .2 | .6 | .6 | .4 |
| Household furnishings and operations | 4.790 | 129.644 | 129.623 | 1.6 | .0 | .0 | .0 | .0 |
| Household operations [1,2] | .781 | 149.468 | 149.995 | 1.3 | .4 | -.1 | -.9 | .4 |
| Apparel | 3.691 | 121.751 | 118.799 | 1.5 | -2.4 | -.2 | -.2 | .7 |
| Men's and boys' apparel | .923 | 117.146 | 112.849 | .7 | -3.7 | -1.7 | .4 | -.5 |
| Women's and girls' apparel | 1.541 | 109.460 | 106.455 | 2.1 | -2.7 | .2 | -.1 | 1.6 |
| Infants' and toddlers' apparel | .183 | 114.142 | 113.915 | 2.1 | -.2 | 1.3 | -1.6 | 2.2 |
| Footwear | .688 | 127.519 | 125.515 | 1.6 | -1.6 | .4 | .1 | .2 |
| Transportation | 15.314 | 175.997 | 183.735 | -13.2 | 4.4 | -.4 | .8 | 4.2 |
| Private transportation | 14.189 | 171.757 | 179.649 | -13.3 | 4.6 | -.3 | .9 | 4.5 |
| New and used motor vehicles [2] | 6.931 | 92.701 | 93.020 | -.6 | .3 | .4 | .5 | .4 |
| New vehicles | 4.480 | 135.162 | 135.719 | .9 | .4 | .4 | .5 | .7 |
| Used cars and trucks | 1.628 | 122.650 | 124.323 | -8.6 | 1.4 | -.1 | 1.0 | .9 |
| Motor fuel | 3.164 | 193.609 | 225.021 | -35.2 | 16.2 | -2.6 | 2.7 | 17.2 |
| Gasoline (all types) | 2.964 | 193.727 | 225.526 | -34.6 | 16.4 | -2.8 | 3.1 | 17.3 |
| Motor vehicle parts and equipment [1] | .382 | 134.347 | 134.270 | 5.0 | -.1 | .1 | -.2 | -.1 |
| Motor vehicle maintenance and repair [1] | 1.188 | 242.488 | 242.683 | 4.1 | .1 | .2 | -.1 | .1 |
| Public transportation | 1.125 | 228.878 | 232.540 | -12.1 | 1.6 | -.8 | -1.0 | -.5 |

**25. Which of the following expense categories decreased in the year prior to June 2009?**

   a.  Rent of primary residence
   b.  Boys' and men's apparel
   c.  Transportation
   d.  Meats, fish, and eggs

**26. On a seasonally adjusted basis, which of the following decreased by the greatest percentage between April and May of 2009?**

a. Gasoline
b. Fuel oil and other fuels
c. Infants' and toddlers' apparel
d. Fruits and vegetables

**27. According to the organization of the table, which of the following expense categories is not considered to be a component of the "Food at Home" category?**

a. Cereals and bakery products
b. Fats and oils
c. Other miscellaneous foods
d. Alcoholic beverages

**28. Which expenditure category was the most important in December of 2008?**

a. Housing
b. Food and Beverages
c. Apparel
d. Transportation

*The next question refers to the following image.*

**Starting Image**

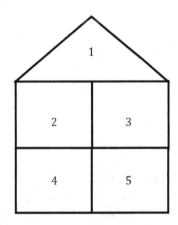

**Start with the shape pictured above. Follow the directions to alter its appearance.**

- **Rotate section 1 90° clockwise and move it to the right side, against sections 3 and 5.**
- **Remove section 4.**
- **Move section 2 immediately above section 3.**
- **Swap section 2 and section 5.**
- **Remove section 5.**
- **Draw a circle around the shape, enclosing it completely.**

**29. Which of the following does the shape now look like?**

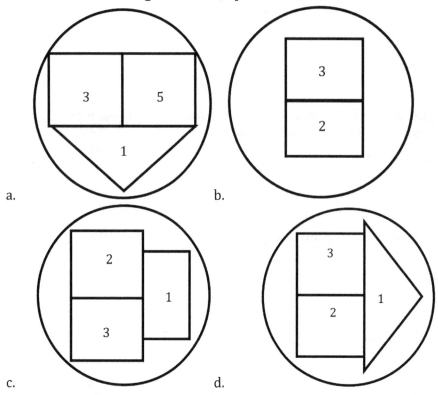

a.                                        b.

c.                                        d.

**30. Anna is planning a trip to Bretagne, or Brittany, in the northwestern part of France. Since she knows very little about it, she is hoping to find the most up-to-date information with the widest variety of details about hiking trails, beaches, restaurants, and accommodations. Which of the following guides will be the best for her to review?**

a. *The Top Ten Places to Visit in Brittany*, published by a non-profit organization in Bretagne looking to draw tourism to the region (2015)

b. *Getting to Know Nantes: Eating, Staying, and Sightseeing in Brittany's Largest City*, published by the French Ministry of Tourism (2014)

c. *Hiking Through Bretagne: The Best Trails for Discovering Northwestern France*, published by a company that specializes in travel for those wanting to experience the outdoors (2013)

d. *The Complete Guide to Brittany*, published by a travel book company that publishes guides for travel throughout Europe (2015)

*The next three questions are based on the following passage.*

An adult skeleton had 206 bones. The skeleton has two major divisions: the axial skeleton and the appendicular skeleton. Each bone belongs to either the axial skeleton or the appendicular skeleton. The axial skeleton, which consists of 80 bones including the skull, vertebrae, and rib, is located down the center of the body. The axial skeleton protects vital organs such as the brain and heart. The appendicular skeleton consists of 126 bones of the arms, legs, and the bones that attach these bones to the axial skeleton. The appendicular skeleton includes the scapulae (shoulder blades), clavicles (collarbones), and pelvic (hip) bones.

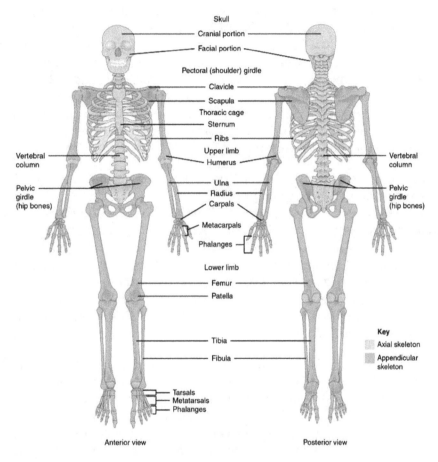

**31. Which of the following bones is not associated with the leg?**

   a.  Femur
   b.  Tibia
   c.  Patella
   d.  Radius

**32. Which of the following bones is not part of the appendicular skeleton?**

   a.  Skull
   b.  Clavicle
   c.  Scapula
   d.  Pelvic bone

**33. Which of the following bones are located in the hand?**

    a.  Fibula
    b.  Metacarpals
    c.  Metatarsals
    d.  Ulna

*The next three questions are based on the following passage.*

As little as three years before her birth, few would have thought that the child born Princess Alexandrina Victoria would eventually become Britain's longest reigning monarch, Queen Victoria. She was born in 1819, the only child of Edward, Duke of Kent, who was the fourth son of King George III. Ahead of Edward were three brothers, two of whom became king but none of whom produced a legitimate, surviving heir. King George's eldest son, who was eventually crowned King George IV, secretly married a Catholic commoner, Maria Fitzherbert, in 1783. The marriage was never officially recognized, and in 1795, George was persuaded to marry a distant cousin, Caroline of Brunswick. The marriage was bitter, and the two had only one daughter, Princess Charlotte Augusta. She was popular in England where her eventual reign was welcomed, but in a tragic event that shocked the nation, the princess and her stillborn son died in childbirth in 1817.

Realizing the precarious position of the British throne, the remaining sons of King George III were motivated to marry and produce an heir. The first in line was Prince Frederick, the Duke of York. Frederick married Princess Frederica Charlotte of Prussia, but the two had no children. After Prince Frederick was Prince William, the Duke of Clarence. William married Princess Adelaide of Saxe-Meiningen, and they had two sickly daughters, neither of whom survived infancy. Finally, Prince Edward, the Duke of Kent, threw his hat into the ring with his marriage to Princess Victoria of Saxe-Coburg-Saalfeld. The Duke of Kent died less than a year after his daughter's birth, but the surviving Duchess of Kent was not unaware of the future possibilities for her daughter. She took every precaution to ensure that the young Princess Victoria was healthy and safe throughout her childhood.

Princess Victoria's uncle, William, succeeded his brother George IV to become King William IV. The new king recognized his niece as his future heir, but he did not necessarily trust her mother. As a result, he was determined to survive until Victoria's eighteenth birthday to ensure that she could rule in her own right without the regency of the Duchess of Kent. The king's fervent prayers were answered: he died June 20, 1837, less than one month after Victoria turned eighteen. Though young and inexperienced, the young queen recognized the importance of her position and determined to rule fairly and wisely. The improbable princess who became queen ruled for more than sixty-three years, and her reign is considered to be one of the most important in British history.

**34. Which of the following is a logical conclusion that can be drawn from the information in the passage above?**

    a.   Victoria's long reign provided the opportunity for her to bring balance to England and right the wrongs that had occurred during the reigns of her uncles.

    b.   It was the death of Princess Charlotte Augusta that motivated the remaining princes to marry and start families.

    c.   The Duke of Kent had hoped for a son but was delighted with his good fortune in producing the surviving heir that his brothers had failed to produce.

    d.   King William IV was unreasonably suspicious of the Duchess of Kent's motivations, as she cared only for her daughter's well-being.

**35. What is the author's likely purpose in writing this passage about Queen Victoria?**

    a.   To persuade the reader to appreciate the accomplishments of Queen Victoria, especially when placed against the failures of her forebears.

    b.   To introduce the historical impact of the Victorian Era by introducing to readers the queen who gave that era its name.

    c.   To explain how small events in history placed an unlikely princess in line to become the queen of England.

    d.   To indicate the role that King George III's many sons played in changing the history of England.

**36. Based on the context of the passage, the reader can infer that this information is likely to appear in which of the following types of works?**

    a.   A scholarly paper

    b.   A mystery

    c.   A fictional story

    d.   A biography

*The next five questions are based on the following passage.*

In 1603, Queen Elizabeth I of England died. She had never married and had no heir, so the throne passed to a distant relative: James Stuart, the son of Elizabeth's cousin and one-time rival for the throne, Mary, Queen of Scots. James was crowned King James I of England. At the time, he was also King James VI of Scotland, and the combination of roles would create a spirit of conflict that haunted the two nations for generations to come.

The conflict developed as a result of rising tensions among the people within the nations, as well as between them. Scholars in the 21st century are far too hasty in dismissing the role of religion in political disputes, but religion undoubtedly played a role in the problems that faced England and Scotland. By the time of James Stuart's succession to the English throne, the English people had firmly embraced the teachings of Protestant theology. Similarly, the Scottish Lowlands was decisively Protestant. In the Scottish Highlands, however, the clans retained their Catholic faith. James acknowledged the Church of England and still sanctioned the largely Protestant translation of the Bible that still bears his name.

James's son King Charles I proved himself to be less committed to the Protestant Church of England. Charles married the Catholic Princess Henrietta Maria of France, and there were suspicions among the English and the Lowland Scots that Charles was quietly a Catholic. Charles's own political troubles extended beyond religion in this case, and he was beheaded in 1649. Eventually, his son King Charles II would be crowned, and this Charles is believed to have converted secretly to the Catholic Church. Charles II died without a legitimate heir, and his brother James ascended to the throne as King James II.

James was recognized to be a practicing Catholic, and his commitment to Catholicism would prove to be his downfall. James's wife Mary Beatrice lost a number of children during their infancy, and when she became pregnant again in 1687 the public became concerned. If James had a son, that son would undoubtedly be raised a Catholic, and the English people would not stand for this. Mary gave birth to a son, but the story quickly circulated that the royal child had died and the child named James's heir was a foundling smuggled in. James, his wife, and his infant son were forced to flee; and James's Protestant daughter Mary was crowned the queen.

In spite of a strong resemblance to the king, the young James was generally rejected among the English and the Lowland Scots, who referred to him as "the Pretender." But in the Highlands the Catholic princeling was welcomed. He inspired a group known as *Jacobites*, to reflect the Latin version of his name. His own son Charles, known affectionately as Bonnie Prince Charlie, would eventually raise an army and attempt to recapture what he believed to be his throne. The movement was soundly defeated at the Battle of Culloden in 1746, and England and Scotland have remained ostensibly Protestant ever since.

**37. Which of the following sentences contains an opinion on the part of the author?**

    a. James was recognized to be a practicing Catholic, and his commitment to Catholicism would prove to be his downfall.

    b. James' son King Charles I proved himself to be less committed to the Protestant Church of England.

    c. The movement was soundly defeated at the Battle of Culloden in 1746, and England and Scotland have remained ostensibly Protestant ever since.

    d. Scholars in the 21st century are far too hasty in dismissing the role of religion in political disputes, but religion undoubtedly played a role in the problems that faced England and Scotland.

**38. Which of the following is a logical conclusion based on the information that is provided within the passage?**

    a. Like Elizabeth I, Charles II never married and thus never had children.

    b. The English people were relieved each time that James II's wife Mary lost another child, as this prevented the chance of a Catholic monarch.

    c. Charles I's beheading had less to do with religion than with other political problems that England was facing.

    d. Unlike his son and grandsons, King James I had no Catholic leanings and was a faithful follower of the Protestant Church of England.

**39. Based on the information that is provided within the passage, which of the following can be inferred about King James II's son?**

 a. Considering his resemblance to King James II, the young James was very likely the legitimate child of the king and the queen.

 b. Given the queen's previous inability to produce a healthy child, the English and the Lowland Scots were right in suspecting the legitimacy of the prince.

 c. James "the Pretender" was not as popular among the Highland clans as his son Bonnie Prince Charlie.

 d. James was unable to acquire the resources needed to build the army and plan the invasion that his son succeeded in doing.

**40. Which of the following best describes the organization of the information in the passage?**

 a. Cause-effect

 b. Chronological sequence

 c. Problem-solution

 d. Comparison-contrast

**41. Which of the following best describes the author's intent in the passage?**

 a. To persuade

 b. To entertain

 c. To express feeling

 d. To inform

*The next two questions are based on the following statements.*

Lisa Grant: "Schools should make students wear uniforms. Everyone would look the same. Students would be able to respect each other based on their ideas and character because they would no longer be judged by their appearance."

Vivian Harris: "Students should not have to wear uniforms. Clothing is an important part of self-expression. Taking away that method of expression is suppressing that student's rights."

**42. What is one idea that the students above seem to agree on, based on their statements?**

 a. Students should be allowed to express themselves through apparel.

 b. Schools should give students a certain amount of respect.

 c. Students should focus more on school than on appearance.

 d. Schools would violate students' basic rights by enforcing a dress code.

**43. Which of the following statements could NOT provide support for BOTH arguments?**

 a. A number of local school districts have recently implemented dress codes.

 b. School administrators have been in talks with parents over the issue of uniforms.

 c. Students have reported that school uniforms are costly and typically ill-fitting.

 d. Several groups of students have been organized to discuss uniform dress codes.

*The next three questions are based on the following passage.*

NOTE: The instructor of a history class has just finished grading the essay exams from his students, and the results are not good. The essay exam was worth 70% of the final course score. The highest score in the class was a low B, and more than half of the class of 65 students failed the exam. In view of this, the instructor reconsiders his grading plan for the semester and sends out an email message to all students.

Dear Students:

The scores for the essay exam have been posted in the online course grade book. By now, many of you have probably seen your grade and are a little concerned. (And if you're not concerned, you should be—at least a bit!) At the beginning of the semester, I informed the class that I have a strict grading policy and that all scores will stand unquestioned. With each class comes a new challenge, however, and as any good instructor will tell you, sometimes the original plan has to change. As a result,

I propose the following options for students to make up their score:

1.  I will present the class with an extra credit project at the next course meeting. The extra credit project will be worth 150% of the point value of the essay exam that has just been completed. While I will not drop the essay exam score, I will give you more than enough of a chance to make up the difference and raise your overall score.
2.  I will allow each student to develop his or her own extra credit project. This project may reflect the tenor of option number 1 (above) but will allow the student to create a project more in his or her own line of interest. Bear in mind, however, that this is more of a risk. The scoring for option number 2 will be more subjective, depending on whether or not I feel that the project is a successful alternative to the essay exam. If it is, the student will be awarded up to 150% of the point value of the essay exam.
3.  I will provide the class with the option of developing a group project. Students may form groups of 3 to 4 and put together an extra credit project that reflects a stronger response to the questions in the essay exam. This extra credit project will also be worth 150% of the point value of the essay exam. Note that each student will receive an equal score for the project, so there is a risk in this as well. If you are part of a group in which you do most of the work, each member of the group will receive equal credit for it. The purpose of the group project is to allow students to work together and arrive at a stronger response than if each worked individually.

If you are interested in pursuing extra credit to make up for the essay exam, please choose one of the options above. No other extra credit opportunities will be provided for the course.

Good luck!

Dr. Edwards

**44. Which of the following describes this type of writing?**
   a.  Technical
   b.  Narrative
   c.  Persuasive
   d.  Expository

**45. Which of the following best describes the instructor's purpose in writing this email to his students?**

  a. To berate students for the poor scores that they made on the recent essay exam.
  b. To encourage students to continue working hard in spite of failure.
  c. To give students the opportunity to make up the bad score and avoid failing the course.
  d. To admit that the essay exam was likely too difficult for most students.

**46. Which of the following offers the best summary for the instructor's motive in sending the email to the students?**

  a. By now, many of you have probably seen your grade and are a little concerned. (And if you're not concerned, you should be—at least a bit!)
  b. With each class comes a new challenge, however, and as any good instructor will tell you, sometimes the original plan has to change.
  c. The purpose of the group project is to allow students to work together and arrive at a stronger response than if each worked individually.
  d. At the beginning of the semester, I informed the class that I have a strict grading policy and that all scores will stand unquestioned.

*The next seven questions are based on this passage.*

In the United States, where we have more land than people, it is not at all difficult for persons in good health to make money. In this comparatively new field there are so many avenues of success open, so many vocations which are not crowded, that any person of either sex who is willing, at least for the time being, to engage in any respectable occupation that offers, may find lucrative employment.

Those who really desire to attain an independence, have only to set their minds upon it, and adopt the proper means, as they do in regard to any other object which they wish to accomplish, and the thing is easily done. But however easy it may be found to make money, I have no doubt many of my hearers will agree it is the most difficult thing in the world to keep it. The road to wealth is, as Dr. Franklin truly says, "as plain as the road to the mill." It consists simply in expending less than we earn; that seems to be a very simple problem. Mr. Micawber, one of those happy creations of the genial Dickens, puts the case in a strong light when he says that to have annual income of twenty pounds per annum, and spend twenty pounds and sixpence, is to be the most miserable of men; whereas, to have an income of only twenty pounds, and spend but nineteen pounds and sixpence is to be the happiest of mortals.

Many of my readers may say, "we understand this: this is economy, and we know economy is wealth; we know we can't eat our cake and keep it also." Yet I beg to say that perhaps more cases of failure arise from mistakes on this point than almost any other. The fact is, many people think they understand economy when they really do not.

**47. Which of the following statements best expresses the main idea of the passage?**

  a. Getting a job is easier now than it ever has been before.
  b. Earning money is much less difficult than managing it properly.
  c. Dr. Franklin advocated getting a job in a mill.
  d. Spending money is the greatest temptation in the world.

**48. What would this author's attitude likely be to a person unable to find employment?**

    a.   descriptive

    b.   conciliatory

    c.   ingenuous

    d.   incredulous

**49. According to the author, what is more difficult than making money?**

    a.   managing money

    b.   traveling to a mill

    c.   reading Dickens

    d.   understanding the economy

**50. Who is the most likely audience for this passage?**

    a.   economists

    b.   general readers

    c.   teachers

    d.   philanthropists

**51. What is the best definition of *economy* as it is used in this passage?**

    a.   exchange of money, goods, and services

    b.   delegation of household affairs

    c.   efficient money management

    d.   less expensive

**52. Which word best describes the author's attitude towards those who believe they understand money?**

    a.   supportive

    b.   incriminating

    c.   excessive

    d.   patronizing

**53. This passage is most likely taken from a(n) _____.**

    a.   self-help manual

    b.   autobiography

    c.   epistle

    d.   novel

| **Mathematics** | Number of Questions: 36 |
|---|---|
| | Time Limit: 54 Minutes |

**1. Which of the following is the percentage equivalent of 0.0016?**

    a. 16%
    b. 160%
    c. 1.6%
    d. 0.16%

**2. Curtis is taking a road trip through Germany, where all distance signs are in metric. He passes a sign that states the city of Dusseldorf is 45 kilometers away. Approximately how far is this in miles?**

    a. 42 miles
    b. 37 miles
    c. 28 miles
    d. 16 miles

**3. On a floor plan drawn at a scale of 1:100, the area of a rectangular room is 30 cm$^2$. What is the actual area of the room?**

    a. 30,000 cm$^2$
    b. 300 m$^2$
    c. 3,000 m$^2$
    d. 30 m$^2$

**4. Mandy can buy 4 containers of yogurt and 3 boxes of crackers for $9.55. She can buy 2 containers of yogurt and 2 boxes of crackers for $5.90. How much does one box of crackers cost?**

    a. $1.75
    b. $2.00
    c. $2.25
    d. $2.50

*The next two questions are based on the following information:*

    Pernell's scores on her last five chemistry exams were 81, 92, 87, 89, and 94.

**5. What is the approximate average of her scores?**

    a. 81
    b. 84
    c. 89
    d. 91

**6. What is the *median* of Pernell's scores?**

    a. 87
    b. 89
    c. 92
    d. 94

7. Gordon purchased a television when his local electronics store had a sale. The television was offered at 30% off its original price of $472. What was the sale price that Gordon paid?

    a.  $141.60
    b.  $225.70
    c.  $305.30
    d.  $330.40

8. Simplify the following expression: $\frac{2}{3} \div \frac{4}{15} \times \frac{5}{8}$

    a.  $1\frac{9}{16}$
    b.  $1\frac{1}{4}$
    c.  $2\frac{1}{8}$
    d.  2

9. Simplify the following expression: $0.0178 \times 2.401$

    a.  2.0358414
    b.  0.0427378
    c.  0.2341695
    d.  0.3483240

10. Tom needs to buy ink cartridges and printer paper. Each ink cartridge costs $30. Each ream of paper costs $5. He has $100 to spend. Which of the following inequalities may be used to find the combinations of ink cartridges and printer paper that he may purchase?

    a.  $30c + 5p \leq 100$
    b.  $30c + 5p < 100$
    c.  $30c + 5p > 100$
    d.  $30c + 5p \geq 100$

11. Solve for $x$: $4(2x - 6) = 10x - 6$

    a.  $x = 5$
    b.  $x = -7$
    c.  $x = -9$
    d.  $x = 10$

12. Erma has her eye on two sweaters at her favorite clothing store, but she has been waiting for the store to offer a sale. This week, the store advertises that all clothing purchases, including sweaters, come with an incentive: 25% off a second item of equal or lesser value. One sweater is $50 and the other is $44. If Erma purchases the sweaters during the sale, what will she spend?

    a.  $79
    b.  $81
    c.  $83
    d.  $85

13. Simplify the following expression: $1.034 + 0.275 - 1.294$

    a.  0.015
    b.  0.15
    c.  1.5
    d.  −0.15

14. The graph below shows the weekly church attendance among residents in the town of Ellsford, with the town having five different denominations: Episcopal, Methodist, Baptist, Catholic, and Orthodox. Approximately what percentage of church-goers in Ellsford attends Catholic churches?

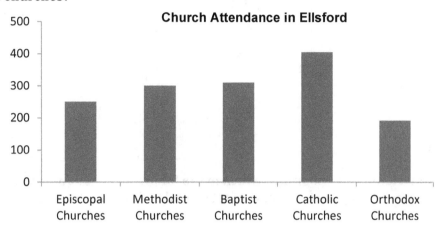

a. 23%
b. 28%
c. 36%
d. 42%

15. Jerry needs to load four pieces of equipment on to a factory elevator that has a weight limit of 800 pounds. Jerry weighs 200 pounds. What would the average weight of each item have to be so that the elevator's weight limit is not exceeded assuming Jerry accompanies the equipment?

a. 128 pounds
b. 150 pounds
c. 175 pounds
d. 180 pounds

16. Simplify the following expression: $4\frac{2}{3} \div 1\frac{1}{6}$

a. 2
b. $3\frac{1}{3}$
c. 4
d. $4\frac{1}{2}$

17. Solve for $x$: $2x + 4 = x - 6$

a. $x = -12$
b. $x = 10$
c. $x = -16$
d. $x = -10$

18. Solve for $x$: $2x - 7 = 3$

a. $x = 4$
b. $x = 3$
c. $x = -2$
d. $x = 5$

**19. What kind of association does the scatter plot show?**

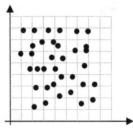

   a.   linear, positive
   b.   linear, negative
   c.   quadratic
   d.   no association

**20. If Stella's current weight is 56 kilograms, which of the following is her approximate weight in pounds? (Note: 1 kilogram is approximately equal to 2.2 pounds.)**

   a.   123 pounds
   b.   110 pounds
   c.   156 pounds
   d.   137 pounds

**21. Which of the following is listed in order from *least to greatest*?**

   a.   $-\frac{3}{4}, -7\frac{4}{5}, -8, 18\%, 0.25, 2.5$
   b.   $-8, -7\frac{4}{5}, -\frac{3}{4}, 0.25, 2.5, 18\%$
   c.   $18\%, 0.25, -\frac{3}{4}, 2.5, -7\frac{4}{5}, -8$
   d.   $-8, -7\frac{4}{5}, -\frac{3}{4}, 18\%, 0.25, 2.5$

**22. Between the years 2000 and 2010, the number of births in the town of Daneville increased from 1432 to 2219. Which of the following is the approximate percent of increase in the number of births during those ten years?**

   a.   55%
   b.   36%
   c.   64%
   d.   42%

**23. Simplify the following expression: $\frac{1}{4} \times \frac{3}{5} \div 1\frac{1}{8}$**

   a.   $\frac{8}{15}$
   b.   $\frac{27}{160}$
   c.   $\frac{2}{15}$
   d.   $\frac{27}{40}$

24. While at the local ice skating rink, Cora went around the rink 27 times total. She slipped and fell 20 of the 27 times she skated around the rink. What approximate percentage of the times around the rink did Cora *not* slip and fall?

    a.  37%

    b.  74%

    c.  26%

    d.  15%

25. A can has a radius of 1.5 inches and a height of 3 inches. Which of the following best represents the volume of the can?

    a.  $17.2 \text{ in}^3$

    b.  $19.4 \text{ in}^3$

    c.  $21.2 \text{ in}^3$

    d.  $23.4 \text{ in}^3$

26. Simplify the following expression: $3\frac{1}{6} - 1\frac{5}{6}$

    a.  $2\frac{1}{3}$

    b.  $1\frac{1}{3}$

    c.  $2\frac{1}{9}$

    d.  $\frac{5}{6}$

27. Four more than a number, $x$, is 2 less than $\frac{1}{3}$ of another number, $y$. Which of the following algebraic equations correctly represents this sentence?

    a.  $x + 4 = \frac{1}{3}y - 2$

    b.  $4x = 2 - \frac{1}{3}y$

    c.  $4 - x = 2 + \frac{1}{3}y$

    d.  $x + 4 = 2 - \frac{1}{3}y$

28. Margery is planning a vacation, and she has added up the cost. Her round-trip airfare will cost $572. Her hotel cost is $89 per night, and she will be staying at the hotel for five nights. She has allotted a total of $150 for sightseeing during her trip, and she expects to spend about $250 on meals. As she books the hotel, she is told that she will receive a discount of 10% per night off the price of $89 after the first night she stays there. Taking this discount into consideration, what is the amount that Margery expects to spend on her vacation?

    a.  $1328.35

    b.  $1373.50

    c.  $1381.40

    d.  $1417.60

**29. Given the double bar graph shown below, which of the following statements is true?**

## Number of Vehicles Owned

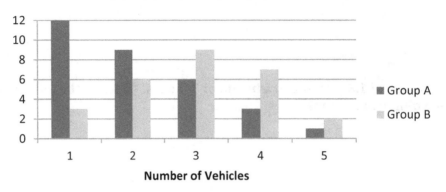

a. Group A is negatively skewed, while Group B is approximately normal.
b. Group A is positively skewed, while Group B is approximately normal.
c. Group A is approximately normal, while Group B is negatively skewed.
d. Group A is approximately normal, while Group B is positively skewed.

**30. A gift box has a length of 14 inches, a height of 8 inches, and a width of 6 inches. How many square inches of wrapping paper are needed to wrap the box?**

a. 56
b. 244
c. 488
d. 672

**31. After a hurricane struck a Pacific island, donations began flooding into a disaster relief organization. The organization provided the opportunity for donors to specify where they wanted the money to be used, and the organization provided four options. When the organization tallied the funds received, they allotted each to the designated need. Reviewing the chart below, what percentage of the funds was donated to support construction costs?**

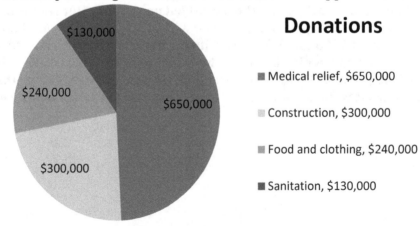

a. 49%
b. 23%
c. 18%
d. 10%

32. Arrange the following numbers above from least to greatest: $\frac{7}{3}, \frac{9}{2}, \frac{10}{9}, \frac{7}{8}$

   a. $\frac{10}{9}, \frac{7}{3}, \frac{9}{2}, \frac{7}{8}$

   b. $\frac{9}{2}, \frac{7}{3}, \frac{10}{9}, \frac{7}{8}$

   c. $\frac{7}{3}, \frac{9}{2}, \frac{10}{9}, \frac{7}{8}$

   d. $\frac{7}{8}, \frac{10}{9}, \frac{7}{3}, \frac{9}{2}$

33. Simplify the following expression: $\frac{2}{7} \div \frac{5}{6}$

   a. $\frac{2}{5}$

   b. $\frac{35}{12}$

   c. $\frac{5}{21}$

   d. $\frac{12}{35}$

34. Simplify the following expression: $7 + 16 - (5 + 6 \times 3) - 10 \times 2$

   a. $-42$

   b. $-20$

   c. 23

   d. 20

35. The table below shows the cost of renting a bicycle for 1, 2, or 3 hours. Which answer choice shows the equation that best represents the data? Let $C$ represent the cost of the rental and $h$ stand for the number of hours of rental time.

| Hours | 1 | 2 | 3 |
|-------|------|------|-------|
| Cost | $3.60 | $7.20 | $10.80 |

   a. $C = 3.60h$

   b. $C = h + 3.60$

   c. $C = 3.60h + 10.80$

   d. $C = \frac{10.80}{h}$

36. Chan receives a bonus from his job. He pays 30% in taxes, gives 30% to charity, and uses another 25% to pay off an old debt. He has $600 remaining from his bonus. What was the total amount of Chan's bonus?

   a. $3000

   b. $3200

   c. $3600

   d. $4000

| **Science** | Number of Questions: **53** |
|---|---|
| | Time Limit: **63 Minutes** |

### 1. Which of the following is NOT consistent with the scientific method?

a. Observe the data, noting potential outliers, and then analyze the results.
b. Develop a new hypothesis based on a conclusion from a previous experiment.
c. Conduct an experiment and then make a hypothesis that fits the results.
d. Communicate the results of an experiment that did not confirm the hypothesis.

### 2. Which of the following is FALSE regarding the use of qualitative and quantitative data in scientific research?

a. Quantitative data is collected through numerical measurements.
b. Quantitative data is more accurate than qualitative data.
c. Qualitative data is focused on perspectives and behavior.
d. Qualitative data is collected through observation and interviews.

*The next question refers to the following graphic.*

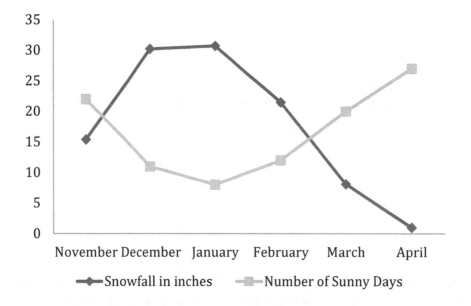

### 3. The chart above shows the average snowfall in inches for a town on Michigan's Upper Peninsula, during the months November through April. Which of the following can be concluded based on the information that is provided in the chart?

a. April is not a good month to go skiing in the Upper Peninsula.
b. Snowfall blocks the sunshine and reduces the number of sunny days.
c. The fewest sunny days occur in the months with the heaviest snowfall.
d. There is no connection between the amount of snowfall and the number of sunny days.

**4. Which of the following statements correctly describes the function of the corresponding physiologic structure?**

   a. The trachea connects the throat and the stomach, encouraging food to follow this path through contractions.

   b. The esophagus is the cylindrical portion of the respiratory tract that joins the larynx with the lungs.

   c. The diaphragm is a muscle that controls the height of the thoracic cavity, decreasing the height on contraction, and increasing the height on relaxation causing expiration.

   d. The epiglottis covers the trachea during swallowing, preventing food from entering the airway.

**5. Which of the following is an example of the location and function of cartilage in the body?**

   a. The dense connective tissue that comprises the better part of the structural skeleton.

   b. The supportive pads that provide cushion at joints, such as between the vertebrae of the spinal cord.

   c. The connective structure made of fibrous collagen that connects muscles and bones, such as the connection of the patella to the quadricep.

   d. The layer beneath the skin and on the outside of internal organs that provides cushioning and protection.

**6. Two criteria for classifying epithelial tissue are:**

   a. cell type and cell function.

   b. cell shape and cell type.

   c. cell layers and cell shape.

   d. cell function and cell layers.

**7. Where is the parathyroid gland located?**

   a. On the lateral lobes of the thyroid gland, on the posterior aspect.

   b. On the pyramidal lobe of the thyroid gland, on the posterior aspect.

   c. On the lateral lobes of the thyroid gland, on the anterior aspect.

   d. On the left lateral lobe of the thyroid gland, on the anterior aspect.

**8. How many organ systems are in the human body?**

   a. 12

   b. 15

   c. 9

   d. 11

**9. Which element or structure within the respiratory system is responsible for removing foreign matter from the lungs?**

   a. Bronchial tubes

   b. Cilia

   c. Trachea

   d. Alveoli

**10. Organized from highest to lowest, what is the hierarchy of the human body's structures is as follows: organism, organ systems, organs, tissues. Which of the following comes next?**

    a.   Organs, cells, tissues, molecules, atoms.
    b.   Organ system, organism, organ, cells, tissues, atoms, molecules.
    c.   Organism, organ systems, organs, tissues, cells, molecules, atoms.
    d.   Organism, organ, cells, tissues, molecules, atoms.

*The next two questions are based on the periodic table.*

| 1<br>IA | | | | | | | | | | | | | | | | | 18<br>VIIIA |
|---|---|---|---|---|---|---|---|---|---|---|---|---|---|---|---|---|---|
| 1<br>**H**<br>1.01 | 2<br>IIA | | | | | | | | | | | 13<br>IIIA | 14<br>IVA | 15<br>VA | 16<br>VIA | 17<br>VIIA | 2<br>**He**<br>4.00 |
| 3<br>**Li**<br>6.94 | 4<br>**Be**<br>9.01 | | | | | | | | | | | 5<br>**B**<br>10.81 | 6<br>**C**<br>12.01 | 7<br>**N**<br>14.01 | 8<br>**O**<br>16.00 | 9<br>**F**<br>19.00 | 10<br>**Ne**<br>20.18 |
| 11<br>**Na**<br>22.99 | 12<br>**Mg**<br>24.31 | 3<br>IIIB | 4<br>IVB | 5<br>VB | 6<br>VIB | 7<br>VIIB | 8 | 9<br>VIIIB | 10 | 11<br>IB | 12<br>IIB | 13<br>**Al**<br>26.98 | 14<br>**Si**<br>28.09 | 15<br>**P**<br>30.97 | 16<br>**S**<br>32.07 | 17<br>**Cl**<br>35.45 | 18<br>**Ar**<br>39.95 |
| 19<br>**K**<br>39.1 | 20<br>**Ca**<br>40.08 | 21<br>**Sc**<br>44.96 | 22<br>**Ti**<br>47.88 | 23<br>**V**<br>50.94 | 24<br>**Cr**<br>52.00 | 25<br>**Mn**<br>54.94 | 26<br>**Fe**<br>55.85 | 27<br>**Co**<br>58.93 | 28<br>**Ni**<br>58.69 | 29<br>**Cu**<br>63.55 | 30<br>**Zn**<br>65.39 | 31<br>**Ga**<br>69.72 | 32<br>**Ge**<br>72.61 | 33<br>**As**<br>74.92 | 34<br>**Se**<br>78.96 | 35<br>**Br**<br>79.90 | 36<br>**Kr**<br>83.80 |
| 37<br>**Rb**<br>85.47 | 38<br>**Sr**<br>87.62 | 39<br>**Y**<br>88.91 | 40<br>**Zr**<br>91.22 | 41<br>**Nb**<br>92.91 | 42<br>**Mo**<br>95.94 | 43<br>**Tc**<br>(98) | 44<br>**Ru**<br>101.07 | 45<br>**Rh**<br>102.91 | 46<br>**Pd**<br>106.42 | 47<br>**Ag**<br>107.87 | 48<br>**Cd**<br>112.41 | 49<br>**In**<br>114.82 | 50<br>**Sn**<br>118.71 | 51<br>**Sb**<br>121.76 | 52<br>**Te**<br>127.6 | 53<br>**I**<br>126.9 | 54<br>**Xe**<br>131.29 |
| 55<br>**Cs**<br>132.9 | 56<br>**Ba**<br>137.3 | 57<br>**La***<br>138.9 | 72<br>**Hf**<br>178.5 | 73<br>**Ta**<br>180.9 | 74<br>**W**<br>183.9 | 75<br>**Re**<br>186.2 | 76<br>**Os**<br>190.2 | 77<br>**Ir**<br>192.2 | 78<br>**Pt**<br>195.1 | 79<br>**Au**<br>197.0 | 80<br>**Hg**<br>200.6 | 81<br>**Tl**<br>204.4 | 82<br>**Pb**<br>207.2 | 83<br>**Bi**<br>209 | 84<br>**Po**<br>(209) | 85<br>**At**<br>(210) | 86<br>**Rn**<br>(222) |
| 87<br>**Fr**<br>(223) | 88<br>**Ra**<br>(226) | 89<br>**Ac^**<br>(227) | 104<br>**Rf**<br>(261) | 105<br>**Db**<br>(262) | 106<br>**Sg**<br>(263) | 107<br>**Bh**<br>(264) | 108<br>**Hs**<br>(265) | 109<br>**Mt**<br>(268) | 110<br>**Ds**<br>(271) | 111<br>**Rg**<br>(272) | | | | | | | |

| * | 58<br>**Ce**<br>140.1 | 59<br>**Pr**<br>140.9 | 60<br>**Nd**<br>144.2 | 61<br>**Pm**<br>(145) | 62<br>**Sm**<br>150.4 | 63<br>**Eu**<br>152.0 | 64<br>**Gd**<br>157.3 | 65<br>**Tb**<br>158.9 | 66<br>**Dy**<br>162.5 | 67<br>**Ho**<br>164.9 | 68<br>**Er**<br>167.3 | 69<br>**Tm**<br>168.9 | 70<br>**Yb**<br>173.0 | 71<br>**Lu**<br>175.0 |
|---|---|---|---|---|---|---|---|---|---|---|---|---|---|---|
| ^ | 90<br>**Th**<br>232.0 | 91<br>**Pa**<br>(231) | 92<br>**U**<br>238.0 | 93<br>**Np**<br>(237) | 94<br>**Pu**<br>(244) | 95<br>**Am**<br>(243) | 96<br>**Cm**<br>(247) | 97<br>**Bk**<br>(247) | 98<br>**Cf**<br>(251) | 99<br>**Es**<br>(252) | 100<br>**Fm**<br>(257) | 101<br>**Md**<br>(258) | 102<br>**No**<br>(259) | 103<br>**Lr**<br>(260) |

*Note: The row labeled with * is the <u>Lanthanide Series</u>, and the row labeled with ^ is the <u>Actinide Series</u>.*

**11. On average, how many neutrons does one atom of bromine (Br) have?**

    a.   35
    b.   44.90
    c.   45
    d.   79.90

*[handwritten: N = 79.9 − 35 = ; Mass# − Atomic# = Neutrons]*

**12. On average, how many protons does one atom of zinc (Zn) have?**

    a.   30
    b.   35
    c.   35.39
    d.   65.39

*[handwritten: electron = Protons]*

**13. Which statement below correctly describes the movement of molecules in the body and/or in relation to the external environment?**

    a.  Osmosis is the movement of a solution from and area of low solute concentration to an area of high solute concentration.

    b.  Diffusion is the process in the lungs by which oxygen is transported from the air to the blood.

    c.  Dissipation is the transport of molecules across a semipermeable membrane from an area of low concentration to high concentration, requiring energy.

    d.  Reverse osmosis is the movement of molecules in a solution from an area of high concentration to an area of lower concentration.

**14. Which gland is responsible for the regulation of calcium levels?**

    a.  The parathyroid glands

    b.  The pituitary gland

    c.  The adrenal glands

    d.  The pancreas

**15. Which statement matches the function to the organ of the digestive system?**   *1. duodenum*

    a.  The large intestine reabsorbs water into the body to form solid waste.   *2. jejunum*

    b.  The duodenum is the middle section of the small intestine in which acids, fat, and sugar are absorbed.

    c.  The jejunum is the first part of the small intestine that receives chyme from the stomach and further digests it prior to entering the large intestine.

    d.  The gallbladder produces insulin to assist in the transport of sugars from the blood to the organs.

**16. In your garden, you noticed that the tomato plants did better on the north side of your house than the west side and you decided to figure out why. They are both planted with the same soil that provides adequate nutrients to the plant, and they are watered at the same time during the week. Over the course of a week, you begin to measure the amount of sunlight that hits each side of the house and determine that the north side gets more light because the sunlight is blocked by the house's shadow on the west side. What is the name of the factor in your observations that affected the tomato plants growth?**

    a.  The control

    b.  The independent variable

    c.  The dependent variable

    d.  The conclusion

**17. Which of the following describes one responsibility of the integumentary system?**

    a.  Distributing vital substances (such as nutrients) throughout the body

    b.  Blocking pathogens that cause disease

    c.  Sending leaked fluids from cardiovascular system back to the blood vessels

    d.  Storing bodily hormones that influence gender traits

**18. When are the parasympathetic nerves active within the nervous system?**

    a.  When an individual experiences a strong emotion, such as fear or excitement.

    b.  When an individual feels pain or heat.

    c.  When an individual is either talking or walking.

    d.  When an individual is either resting or eating.

**19. Which of the following best describes the relationship between the circulatory system and the integumentary system?**

a. Removal of excess heat from body.
b. Hormonal influence on blood pressure.
c. Regulation of blood's pressure and volume.
d. Development of blood cells within marrow.

**20. Which of the following statements describes the path of blood entering into the heart?**

a. Blood enters the heart through the pulmonary vein, into the right atrium, through the tricuspid valve to the right ventricle.
b. Once the right ventricle is full, blood exits into the pulmonary artery and then empties into the left ventricle.
c. After traveling through the lungs, oxygenated blood enters into the left atrium, then through the mitral valve to the left ventricle.
d. Once the left ventricle is full, the left tricuspid valve shuts, the ventricle contracts, and blood exits through the aorta.

**21. The part of the human excretory system most responsible for maintaining normal body temperature is the:**

a. kidney.
b. bladder.
c. liver.
d. sweat glands.

**22. A part of which body system controls fluid loss, protects deep tissues, and synthesizes vitamin D?**

a. The skeletal system.
b. The muscular system.
c. The lymphatic system.
d. The integumentary system.

**23. There are three insects that are being compared under a microscope. As a scientist, you decide that measuring them would be an important part of recording their data. Which unit of measurement would best for this situation?**

a. Centimeters.
b. Meters.
c. Micrometers.
d. Kilometers.

**24. The respiratory system _____ oxygen for and _____ carbon dioxide from the circulatory system.**

a. creates; filters
b. provides; removes
c. ionizes; absorbs
d. eliminates; destroys

25. **Which statement below accurately describes the function of its element?**
    a. Collagen is a spongy fatty compound that creates a padding between bones and other structures.
    b. Hemoglobin is the amount of red blood cells that are present in blood, which can reflect disease states, hydration, and blood loss.
    c. Lymph is tissue that forms into nodes through which blood is filtered and cleaned.
    d. An antigen stimulates the production of antibodies.

26. **Which group of major parts and organs make up the immune system?**
    a. Lymphatic system, spleen, tonsils, thymus, and bone marrow.
    b. Brain, spinal cord, and nerve cells.
    c. Heart, veins, arteries, and capillaries.
    d. Nose, trachea, bronchial tubes, lungs, alveolus, and diaphragm.

*The next two questions are based on the following information.*

A student is conducting an experiment using a ball that is attached to the end of a string on a pendulum. The student pulls the ball back so that it is at an angle to its resting position. As the student releases the ball, it swings forward and backward. The student measures the time it takes the ball to make one complete period. A period is defined as the time it takes the ball to swing forward and back again to its starting position. This is repeated using different string lengths.

27. **The student formed the following hypothesis:**

**Lengthening the string of the pendulum increases the time it takes the ball to make one complete period.**

**What correction would you have the student make to the hypothesis?**
    a. Turn it into an "if/then" statement.
    b. Add the word "will" in the middle after the word "pendulum."
    c. Switch the order of the sentence so that the phrase about the period comes first, and the phrase about the string's length is last.
    d. No corrections are needed.

28. **What would be an appropriate control variable for this experiment?**
    a. The period
    b. The length of the string
    c. The mass of the ball
    d. The color of the ball

29. **Which of the following does not exist in RNA?**
    a. Uracil
    b. Thymine
    c. Cytosine
    d. Guanine

DNA: T A G C
RNA: U C G A

**30. In which of the following muscle types are the filaments arranged in a disorderly manner?**

    a. Cardiac.
    b. Smooth.
    c. Skeletal.
    d. Rough.

**31. Which of the following hormones is correctly matched with the gland/organ it is produced by?**

    a. Insulin; kidney.
    b. Testosterone; thyroid.
    c. Melatonin; pineal.⁻
    d. Epinephrine; gall bladder.

**32. Which of the following best describes a section that divides the body into equal right and left parts?**

    a. Midsagittal plane.
    b. Coronal plane.
    c. Oblique plane.
    d. Frontal plane.

**33. In the development of genetic traits, one gene must match to one _____ for the traits to develop correctly.**

    a. Codon
    b. Protein
    c. Amino acid
    d. Chromosome

**34. Which of the following is not composed of striated muscle?**

    a. Quadriceps.
    b. Uterus.
    c. Triceps.
    d. Gastrocnemius.

**35. Which of the following is NOT found in the dorsal cavity of the body?**

    a. Cerebellum
    b. Heart
    c. Brainstem
    d. Spine

**36. Which of the following best describes the careful ordering of molecules within solids that have a fixed shape?**

    a. Physical bonding
    b. Polar molecules
    c. Metalloid structure
    d. Crystalline order

**37. Which of the following statement properly describes how the structure moves during inspiration?**

a. The lungs contract on inspiration.
b. The diaphragm moves downward on inspiration.
c. The ribs remain fixed during inspiration.
d. The heart moves inward on inspiration.

**38. Which of the following describes the transport network that is responsible for the transference of proteins throughout a cell?**

a. Golgi apparatus
b. Endoplasmic reticulum
c. Mitochondria
d. Nucleolus

**39. What occurs during the *anaphase* of mitosis?**

a. Chromosomes, originally in pairs, separate from their daughters and move to the opposite ends (or poles) of the cell.
b. The mitotic spindle fibers begin to form.
c. The chromosomes align in the middle of the cell.
d. Two nuclei form, surrounded each by a nuclear membrane.

**40. Using the table below, what conclusions can be made about the students' scores?**

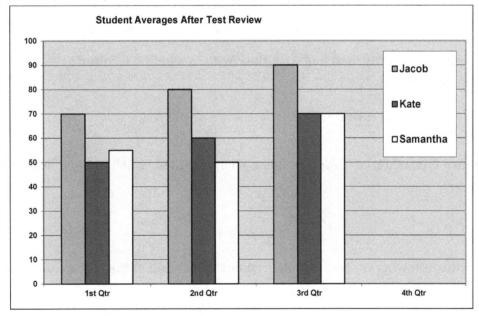

a. The scores increased as the year progressed.
b. The girls did better than the boys on the test each quarter.
c. The test was about math.
d. The scores were heavily impacted by the test reviews that were provided.

**41. Which of the following statements is correct about normal human lung anatomy?**

    a.  The right lung has three lobes; the left lung has two lobes.
    b.  The right lung has two lobes; the left lung has three lobes.
    c.  Both lungs have two lobes.
    d.  Both lungs have three lobes.

**42. All of the following are parts of the cardiac system EXCEPT the:**

    a.  ventricle.
    b.  alveoli.
    c.  atrium.
    d.  septum.

**43. If a biologist is describing the physical and visible expression of a genetic trait, which of the following is he referring to?**

    a.  Phenotype.
    b.  Allele.
    c.  Gamete.
    d.  Genotype.

**44. Which of the following does NOT produce hormones?**

    a.  Pituitary gland.
    b.  The Pons.
    c.  Pancreas.
    d.  Ovaries.

**45. Which organ is correctly matched with the cavity in which it is found?**

    a.  Spleen; pelvic cavity.
    b.  Brain; vertebral canal.
    c.  Bladder; abdominal cavity.
    d.  Heart; thoracic cavity.

**46. A substance is considered *acidic* if it has a pH of less than which of the following?**

    a.  12
    b.  9
    c.  7
    d.  4

**47. Which of the following choices best describes the location of the trachea in relation to the esophagus?**

    a.  Lateral
    b.  Anterior
    c.  Posterior
    d.  Dorsal

**48. A triple beam balance would show the units of measurement in which form?**

    a.  Liters
    b.  Grams
    c.  Meters
    d.  Gallons

**49. Which of the following best describes a section that divides the body into equal upper and lower portions?**

    a. Coronal
    b. Transverse
    c. Oblique
    d. Median

**50. Which of the following best describes one of the roles of RNA?**

    a. Manufacturing the proteins needed for DNA
    b. Creating the bonds between the elements that compose DNA
    c. Sending messages about the correct sequence of proteins in DNA
    d. Forming the identifiable "*double helix*" shape of DNA

**51. Which of the following do *catalysts* alter to control the rate of a chemical reaction?**

    a. Substrate energy
    b. Activation energy
    c. Inhibitor energy
    d. Promoter energy

**52. Which of the following components of the human integumentary system is the deepest?**

    a. Stratum basale.
    b. Epidermis.
    c. Hypodermis.
    d. Dermis.

**53. The Punnett square shown here indicates a cross between two parents, one with alleles BB and the other with alleles Bb. Select the correct entry for the upper right box in the Punnett square, which is indicated with the letter, *x*:**

|   | B | B |
|---|---|---|
| **B** |   | *x* |
| **b** |   |   |

    a. Bb
    b. bB
    c. BB
    d. bb

| **English and Language Usage** | Number of Questions: **28** |
| | Time Limit: **28 Minutes** |

**1. Which of the following nouns represents the correct plural form of the word *syllabus*?**

    a. Syllabus
    b. Syllaba
    c. Syllabi
    d. Syllabis

**2. Which of the following words functions as an adjective in the sentence below?**

**The Welsh kingdom of Gwynedd existed as an independent state from the early 5th century, when the Romans left Britain, until the late 13th century, when the king of England took control of Wales.**

    a. Independent
    b. Century
    c. King
    d. Control

**3. *Bi, re,* and *un* are:**

    a. Suffixes, appearing at the beginning of base words to change their meaning
    b. Suffixes, appearing at the end of base words to enhance their meaning
    c. Prefixes, appearing at the beginning of base words to emphasize their meaning
    d. Prefixes, appearing at the beginning of base words to change their meanings

**4. Which of the following sentences shows the correct use of quotation marks?**

    a. Grady asked Abe, 'Did you know that an earthquake and a tsunami hit Messina, Italy, in 1908?'
    b. Grady asked Abe, "Did you know that an earthquake and a tsunami hit Messina, Italy, in 1908"?
    c. Grady asked Abe, "Did you know that an earthquake and a tsunami hit Messina, Italy, in 1908?"
    d. Grady asked Abe, " 'Did you know that an earthquake and a tsunami hit Messina, Italy, in 1908'?"

**5. *Since, whether,* and *accordingly* are examples of which type of signal words?**

    a. Common, or basic, signal words
    b. Compare/contrast words
    c. Cause–effect words
    d. Temporal sequencing words

**6. Which of the answer choices identifies the misspelled word in the sentence below?**

**Donald considered the job offer carefully, but he ultimately decided that the low salary was not acceptable given his previous experience.**

    a. carefully
    b. decided
    c. salary
    d. acceptible

**7. Which of the answer choices best combines the following four sentences into two sentences?**

**I'm usually good about keeping track of my keys. I lost them. I spent hours looking for them. I found them in the freezer.**

  a. I lost my keys, even though I'm usually good about keeping track of them. I found them in the freezer and spent hours looking for them.
  b. I spent hours looking for my keys and found them in the freezer. I had lost them, even though I'm usually good about keeping track of them.
  c. I'm usually good about keeping track of my keys, but I lost them. After spending hours looking for them, I found them in the freezer.
  d. I'm usually good about keeping track of my keys, but I lost them in the freezer. I had to spend hours looking for them.

**8. Which of the answer choices gives the best definition of the underlined word in the following sentence?**

**The warning against smoking may have been <u>tacit</u>, but Beryl instinctively knew that her mother wanted her to avoid picking up the habit.**

  a. complicated
  b. empty
  c. wordy
  d. unstated

**9. Which of the answer choices shows the correct punctuation of the city and the state in the following sentence?**

**After living in Oak Ridge Missouri all her life, Cornelia was excited about her trip to Prague.**

  a. After living in Oak Ridge, Missouri, all her life, Cornelia was excited about her trip to Prague.
  b. After living in Oak Ridge, Missouri all her life, Cornelia was excited about her trip to Prague.
  c. After living in Oak, Ridge, Missouri all her life, Cornelia was excited about her trip to Prague.
  d. After living in Oak Ridge Missouri all her life, Cornelia was excited about her trip to Prague.

**10. What transition should be added to the beginning of sentence 2 below?**

**(1) I zoned out in class, turned work in late, talked out in class, and handed in assignments after the due date. (2) Mr. Shanbourne just nodded.**

  a. Surprisingly
  b. Actually
  c. Furthermore
  d. Instead

**11. The following words all end in the same suffix, -*ism*: polytheism, communism, nationalism. Considering the meaning of these three words, how does the suffix -*ism* apply to all of them?**

  a. Doctrine
  b. Condition
  c. Characteristic
  d. State of being

**12. What is the most effective way to rewrite the following sentence?**

**She is saying that some of the students are wearing to school is being distracting and inappropriate.**

  a. Some of the outfits students wear to school, she is saying, are distracting and not appropriate.
  b. The outfits are distracting and inappropriate, she says, that students wear to school.
  c. She says that some of the outfits that students wear to school are distracting and inappropriate.
  d. She says that it is distracting and inappropriate that students wear outfits to school.

**13. Which of the following is an example of a correctly punctuated sentence?**

  a. Beatrice is very intelligent, she just does not apply herself well enough in her classes to make good grades.
  b. Beatrice is very intelligent: she just does not apply herself well enough in her classes to make good grades.
  c. Beatrice is very intelligent she just does not apply herself well enough in her classes to make good grades
  d. Beatrice is very intelligent; she just does not apply herself well enough in her classes to make good grades.

**14. What is the most effective way to combine the two sentences below?**

**Some members of the Sons of Liberty constructed a paper obelisk. An obelisk is the same shape as the Washington Monument.**

  a. Some members of the Sons of Liberty constructed a paper obelisk, which is the same shape as the Washington Monument.
  b. Some members of the Sons of Liberty constructed a paper obelisk which is the same shape as the Washington Monument.
  c. Some members of the Sons of Liberty constructed a paper obelisk, that is the same shape as the Washington Monument.
  d. Some members of the Sons of Liberty constructed a paper obelisk; which is the same shape as the Washington Monument.

**15. Which of the following is a compound sentence?**

  a. Tabitha and Simon started the day at the zoo and then went to the art museum for the rest of the afternoon.
  b. Tabitha and Simon started the day at the zoo, and then they went to the art museum for the rest of the afternoon.
  c. After starting the day at the zoo, Tabitha and Simon then went to the art museum for the rest of the afternoon.
  d. Tabitha and Simon had a busy day, because they started at the zoo, and then they went to the art museum for the rest of the afternoon.

**16. Which of the following follows the rules of capitalization?**

  a. Dashiell visited his Cousin Elaine on Tuesday.
  b. Juniper sent a card to Uncle Archibald who has been unwell.
  c. Flicka and her Mother spent the day setting up the rummage sale.
  d. Lowell and his twin Sister look alike but have very different personalities.

**17. What is the most likely meaning of the underlined phrase in the sentence below?**

The Western perspective expects moral actions to be <u>quid pro quo</u>; to put it another way, a Westerner assumes that if he or she does something considered "good," then he or she should and will be rewarded.

    a. "something for nothing."
    b. "good merits money."
    c. "to each his own."
    d. "this for that."

**18. Which of the following sets of words correctly fill in the blanks in the sentence below?**

We cannot allow the budget cuts to _____ the plans to improve education; the futures of _____ children are at stake.

    a. effect; your
    b. affect; you're
    c. effect; you're
    d. affect; your

**19. Which of the answer choices gives the best definition of the underlined word in the following sentence?**

*The experience of being the survivor of a plane crash left an <u>indelible</u> impression on Johanna, and she suffered from nightmares for years afterwards.*

    a. candid
    b. permanent
    c. inexpressible
    d. indirect

**20. Which of the following sentences contains an incorrect use of capitalization?**

    a. For Christmas, we are driving to the South to visit my grandmother in Mississippi.
    b. Last year, we went to East Texas to go camping in Piney Woods.
    c. Next month, we will visit my Aunt Darla who lives just East of us.
    d. When my sister-in-law Susan has her baby, I will take the train north to see her.

**21. Which of the following sentences is grammatically correct?**

    a. Krista was not sure who to hold responsible for the broken window.
    b. Krista was not sure whom was responsible for the broken window.
    c. Krista was not sure whom to hold responsible for the broken window.
    d. Krista was not sure on who she should place responsibility for the broken window.

**22. The word *capacity* functions as which part of speech in the following sentence?**

    *Irish politician Constance Markiewicz was the first woman elected to the British House of Commons, but she never served in that capacity due to her activity in forming the Irish Republic.*

    a. Verb
    b. Noun
    c. Adverb
    d. Pronoun

**23. Which of the following sentences represents the best style and clarity of expression?**

    a.  Without adequate preparation, the test was likely to be a failure for Zara.

    b.  The test was likely to be a failure for Zara without adequate preparation.

    c.  Without adequate preparation, Zara expected to fail the test.

    d.  Zara expected to fail the test without adequate preparation.

**24. Which of the following sentences contains a correct example of subject-verb agreement?**

    a.  All of the board members are in agreement on the issue.

    b.  Each of the students were concerned about the test scores for the final exam.

    c.  Neither of the children are at home right now.

    d.  Any of the brownie recipes are perfect for the bake sale.

**25. Which of the answer choices gives the best definition of the underlined word in the following sentence?**

**Despite the important achievement of the election of our first African American president, the need for knowledge and education about African American history is still unmet to a <u>substantial</u> degree.**

    a.  base

    b.  considerable

    c.  minor

    d.  trivial

**26. Which of the following is a simple sentence?**

    a.  Phillippa walked the dog, and Primula gave the dog a bath.

    b.  Phillippa walked and bathed the dog, and Primula helped.

    c.  Phillippa walked the dog, while Primula gave the dog a bath.

    d.  Phillippa and Primula walked the dog and gave the dog a bath.

**27. Which of the following sentences is most correct in terms of style, clarity, and punctuation?**

    a.  The possible side effects of the medication that the doctor had prescribed for her was a concern for Lucinda, and she continued to take the medication.

    b.  The medication that the doctor prescribed had side effects concerning Lucinda who continued to take it.

    c.  Lucinda was concerned about side effects from the medication that her doctor had prescribed, so she continued to take it.

    d.  Although Lucinda was concerned about the possible side effects, she continued to take the medication that her doctor had prescribed for her.

**28. What does the prefix *poly-* mean in the word *polygon?***

    a.  few

    b.  several

    c.  none

    d.  many

# Answer Key and Explanations for Test #1

## Reading

**1. C:** To *assuage* is to lessen the effects of something, in this case Adelaide's guilt over eating the piece of cheesecake. The context of the sentence also suggests that she feels sorry for eating it and wants to compensate the following day.

**2. C:** This choice shows how greenhouse gases are released from burning coal and other fuels, which people need for power. The first, second, and third choices are facts, but don't show a relationship to the main idea.

**3. A:** To find information on Freud's psychological theories, Lise should go to class 100.

**4. C:** In this case, Lise needs to find a work of literature instead of a work of psychology, so she should consult the 800s.

**5. B:** To study Jewish traditions further, Lise should consult the 200s, which is devoted to books on religion.

**6. A:** The sample is biased because the study wishes to examine all middle school teachers' ideas, regarding usage of iPhones in the classroom, while the sample only represents ideas of those teachers teaching technology courses.

**7. A:** The sentence indicates a contrast between the appearance and the reality. Enzo's friends believe him to be wealthy, due to the large home that he inherited, but he is actually penniless.

**8. B:** The word SORT results from following all of the directions that are provided.

**9. B:** The enrollment in 2001 falls directly between 2000 and 2500, so 2300 is accurate. Note that the enrollment for 2000 falls much closer to 2000, so 2100 is a best estimate for that year.

**10. C:** The tuition appears to rise alongside the enrollment, until the year 2009 when it jumps significantly. Since the enrollment between 2008 and 2009 does not justify the immediate jump in income for the school, an increase in tuition costs makes sense.

**11. B:** It can be concluded that phonics is a more effective way to learn to read for two reasons. First, the passage states that literacy rates are lower now than they were 15 years ago, meaning that more people knew how to read 15 years ago. Then, the passage states that phonics was the main way people learned how to read then. Therefore, based on these two facts, it can be concluded that phonics is more effective.

**12. C:** The passage is *expository* in the sense that it looks more closely into the mysteries of the Bermuda Triangle and *exposes* information about what researchers have studied and now believe.

**13. D:** This sentence is the best summary statement for the entire passage, because it wraps up clearly what the author is saying about the results of studies on the Bermuda Triangle.

**14. A:** Of all the sentences provided, this is the one with which the author would most likely agree. The passage suggests that most of the "mysteries" of the Bermuda Triangle can be explained in a reasonable way. The passage mentions that some expand the Triangle to the Azores, but this is a point of fact, and the author makes no mention of whether or not this is in error. The author quotes the Navy's response to the disappearance of the planes, but there is no reason to believe the author questions this response. The author raises questions about the many myths surrounding the Triangle, but at no point does the author connect these myths with what are described as accidents that fall "within the expected margin of error."

**15. C:** The inclusion of the statement about the ships from East Asia is an opinion statement, as the author provides no support or explanation. The other statements within the answer choices offer supporting evidence and explanatory material, making them acceptable for an expository composition.

**16. A:** When a researcher has conducted an original experiment and reports the results, findings, and associated conclusions in a research report, that report is considered a primary source. Academic textbooks, journal articles, articles in other periodicals, and authoritative databases may all be primary sources. When an academic textbook cites research (B) by others, that citation is considered a secondary source as it refers to information originally presented by others. When a news article quotes a researcher's writing (C), that is also a secondary source. So is a description given on a website of another person's research (D).

**17. B:** Only the word *introspection* can fall between *intrauterine* and *invest*. The words *intransigent* and *intone* come before, and the word *investiture* follows.

**18. C:** The chart shows that plastic and cardboard materials both comprise 15% of the collected materials, and therefore it is incorrect to say that there is more plastic than cardboard. They are present in equal quantities.

**19. D:** The spaghetti and the garlic bread are definitely concerns for Ninette if she is unable to consume products with wheat in them. With all other meals, there appear to be gluten-free options that she can eat.

**20. A:** The government website would publish the most recent data on seatbelt information, like how many people wore seatbelts in the accident and how many survived. Choices B and C are more likely to be opinion-based. Choice D is tempting, but it would not give someone the most up-to-date information.

**21. D:** The negative reviews led to the poor quality of the second movie.

**22. B:** This question and the two that follow require simple multiplication and addition. Since the quantities needed are the same for both texts, one need only find the supplier with the lowest combined price (per 100) for the two texts. Textbook Central's combined price for 100 each of the two texts is $9,550. The closest competitor is University Textbook with a combined price of $9,600. The other two suppliers come in at $9,650 and $9,675. The total for the transaction with Textbook Central is $47,750.

**23. B:** Once again, Textbook Central prevails. In this case, it is not even necessary to do the calculations. The cost for composition textbooks is $4350 (per 100) and for linguistics textbooks is $6550 (per 100). The lower cost for the composition textbooks–$150 less per 100 than the closest company in cost–outweighs the slight difference in cost for the linguistics textbooks.

**24. C:** Bookstore Supply has the lowest cost of the four for the technical writing textbooks, and it has a comparable cost to University Textbook for the world literature textbooks. The slight difference for the technical writing textbooks will make the overall cost lower than University Textbook's and give Bookstore Supply the competitive edge in cost.

**25. C:** This should be read from the column labeled "Unadjusted percent change to June 2009 from June 2008", a period of one year. For transportation, the index is down 13.2%. This is the only negative change among the choices given.

**26. B:** Read this answer in the second column from the right. Fuel oil and other fuels decreased by 3.1% during this period. Gasoline increased by 3.1%. The other commodities decreased, but by lesser amounts.

**27. D:** In the table, components of each category are shown by indentation under the name of the category itself. There may be sub-categories within each category that are further indented. All of the Choices are indented under "Food at Home" except for "Alcoholic Beverages", which is a separate category.

**28. A:** Read this from the second column in the table, "Relative Importance December 2008". These numbers represent the average percentage of household budgets that are spent on the expenditure category. The greatest number, 43.421%, is on the row corresponding to housing.

**29. D:** Answer choice D is the only option that correctly follows the instructions in the question. Sections 4 and 5 are removed; section 1 is placed on the right sides along sections 3 and 2; and there is a circle drawn around the entire shape. Answer choice A places section 1 in the wrong location and fails to switch sections 2 and 5. Answer choice B incorrectly removes section 1 altogether. Answer choice C changes the shape of section 1 to a rectangle and reverses sections 2 and 3.

**30. D:** Anna is ultimately looking for a good all-around guidebook for the region. *The Top Ten Places to Visit in Brittany* might have some useful information, but it will not provide enough details about hiking trails, beaches, restaurants, and accommodations. *Getting to Know Nantes* limits the information to one city, and Anna's destination in Brittany is not identified. *Hiking Through Bretagne* limits the information to one activity. These three guidebooks might offer great supplemental information, but *The Complete Guide to Brittany* is the most likely to offer *all* of the information that Anna needs for her trip.

**31. D:** According to Figure 1, the radius is a bone in the lower arm. The femur, tibia, and patella are located in the leg. Therefore, choice D is correct.

**32. A:** According to the passage, the skull is part of the axial skeleton. Therefore, choice A is correct.

**33. B:** According to Figure 1, the metacarpals are located in the hand. The metatarsals are located in the foot. The fibula is in the leg, and the ulna is in the arm. Therefore, choice B is correct.

**34. B:** The passage does not state this outright, but the author indicates that the younger sons of King George III began considering the option of marrying and producing heirs *after* Princess Charlotte Augusta died. Since she was the heir-apparent, her death left the succession undetermined. The author mentions very little about any "wrongs" that Victoria's uncles committed, so this cannot be a logical conclusion. The passage says nothing about the Duke of Kent's preference for a male heir over a female. (In fact, it was likely that he was delighted to have any heir.) And the author does not provide enough detail about the relationship between the Duchess of Kent and King William IV to infer logically that his suspicions were "unreasonable" or that the duchess cared only for her daughter's well-being.

**35. C:** The author actually notes in the last paragraph that Victoria was an "improbable princess who became queen" and the rest of the passage demonstrates how it was a series of small events that changed the course of British succession. The passage is largely factual, so it makes little sense as a persuasive argument. The author mentions the Victorian Era, but the passage is more about Queen Victoria's family background than it is about the era to which she gave her name. And the passage is more about how the events affected Victoria (and through her, England) than it is about the direct effect that George III's sons had on English history.

**36. D:** This passage is most likely to belong in some kind of biographical reference about Queen Victoria. A scholarly paper would include more analysis instead of just fact. The information in the passage does not fit the genre of mystery at all. And since the passage recounts history, it is not an obvious candidate for a fictional story.

**37. D:** All other sentences in the passage offer some support or explanation. Only the sentence in answer choice D indicates an unsupported opinion on the part of the author.

**38. C:** The author actually says, "Charles's own political troubles extended beyond religion in this case, and he was beheaded in 1649." This would indicate that religion was less involved in this situation than in other situations. There is not enough information to infer that Charles II never married; the passage only notes that he had no legitimate children. (In fact, he had more than ten illegitimate children by his mistresses.) And while the chance of a Catholic king frightened many in England, it is reaching beyond logical inference to assume that people were relieved when the royal children died. Finally, the author does not provide enough detail for the reader to assume that James I had *no* Catholic leanings. The author only says that James recognized the importance of committing to the Church of England.

**39. A:** The author notes, "In spite of a strong resemblance to the king, the young James was generally rejected among the English and the Lowland Scots, who referred to him as "the Pretender." This indicates that there *was* a resemblance, and this increases the likelihood that the child was, in fact, that of James and Mary Beatrice. Answer choice B is too much of an opinion statement that does not have enough support in the passage. The passage essentially refutes answer choice C by pointing out that James "the Pretender" was welcomed in the Highlands. And there is little in the passage to suggest that James was unable to raise an army and mount an attack.

**40. B:** The passage is composed in a chronological sequence with each king introduced in order of reign.

**41. D:** The passage is largely informative in focus, and the author provides extensive detail about this period in English and Scottish history. There is little in the passage to suggest persuasion, and the tone of the passage has no indication of a desire to entertain. Additionally, the passage is historical, so the author avoids expressing feelings and instead focuses on factual information (with the exception of the one opinion statement).

**42. B:** Both of the speakers are arguing over the respect due to an individual, but they are going about it in different ways.

**43. C:** This detail would only really support the argument against wearing school uniforms, while the other three choices could all appear as details in support of either side of the argument.

**44. A:** Technical passages focus on presenting specific information and have a tone of formality. Narrative writing focuses on telling a story, and the passage offers no indication of this. Persuasive writing attempts to persuade the reader to agree with a certain position; the instructor offers the students information but leaves the decision up to each student. Expository passages reveal analytical information to the reader. The instructor is more focused on providing the students with information than with offering the students analytical details. (The analysis, it appears, will be up to the students if they choose to complete an extra credit project.)

**45. C:** Answer choice C fits the tone of the passage best. The instructor is simply offering students the chance to make up the exam score (which is worth 70% of their grade) and thus avoid failing the course. The instructor does not berate students at any point, nor does the instructor admit that the exam was too difficult. Additionally, the instructor offers encouragement to the students should they choose to complete an extra credit project, but that is not the primary purpose of this email.

**46. B:** This question asks for the best summary of the instructor's motive. In the opening paragraph, the instructor notes that his original grading plan has to change to reflect the exam scores. Because they were low, he now wants to give students a chance to make up for their low scores. Answer choice B thus summarizes his motive effectively. The instructor introduces his email with the notes about the scores being posted, but, given the information that is provided in the message, this is not the sole motive for his writing. Answer choice A limits the motive to the details about the group project, and the instructor provides three options. Answer choice D overlooks the instructor's further note about how the grading policy sometimes has to bend to reflect circumstances.

**47. B:** The author asserts both that earning money is increasingly easy and that managing money is difficult.

**48. D:** The author seems to believe that there are plenty of lucrative jobs for everyone.

**49. A:** The author insists that many people who have no trouble earning money waste it through lavish spending.

**50. B:** This passage is clearly intended for a non-expert adult readership.

**51. C:** Here, the author is speaking of money management on a personal or household level.

**52. D:** The author suggests that many people who believe they understand economy in fact do not.

**53. A:** It seems clear that the author is about to describe the correct means of personal economy for a self-help manual.

# Mathematics

**1. D:** To derive a percentage from a decimal, multiply by 100: $0.0016(100) = 0.16\%$.

**2. C:** One kilometer is about 0.62 miles, so $45(0.62)$ is 27.9, or approximately 28 miles.

**3. D:** Since there are 100 cm in a meter, on a 1:100 scale drawing, each centimeter represents one meter. Therefore, an area of one square centimeter on the drawing represents one square meter in actuality. Since the area of the room in the scale drawing is 30 cm$^2$, the room's actual area is 30 m$^2$.

Another way to determine the area of the room is to write and solve an equation, such as this one: $l/100 \times w/100 = 30$ cm$^2$, where $l$ and $w$ are the dimensions of the actual room

$$lw/1000 = 30 \text{ cm}^2$$

$$\text{Area} = 300,000 \text{ cm}^2$$

Since this is not one of the answer choices, convert cm² to m²:

$$300{,}000 \text{ cm}^2 \times \frac{1 \text{ m}}{100 \text{ cm}} \times \frac{1 \text{ m}}{100 \text{ cm}} = 30 \text{ m}^2.$$

**4. C:** The situation may be modeled by the system:

$$4x + 3y = 9.55$$
$$2x + 2y = 5.90$$

Multiplying the bottom equation by –2 gives:

$$4x + 3y = 9.55$$
$$-4x - 4y = -11.80$$

Addition of the two equations gives $-y = -2.25$ or $y = 2.25$. Thus, one box of crackers costs $2.25.

**5. C:** To find the average of Pernell's scores, add them up and then divide by the number of scores (5 in this case). In other words,

$$81 + 92 + 87 + 89 + 94 = 443$$

$$443/5 = 88.6, \text{ or approximately } 89$$

**6. B:** To find the median, list the series of numbers from least to greatest. The middle number represents the median—in this case 81, 87, 89, 92, 94. The number 89 is in the middle, so it is the median.

**7. D:** The television is 30% off its original price of $472. 30% of 472 is 141.60, and 141.60 subtracted from 472 is 330.40. Thus, Gordon paid $330.40 for the television.

**8. A:** To simplify, proceed in the order of the operations: $\frac{2}{3} \div \frac{4}{15}$ is $\frac{2}{3} \times \frac{15}{4}$, or $\frac{30}{12}$, which simplifies to $\frac{5}{2}$. Next, multiply $\frac{5}{2}$ by $\frac{5}{8}$. The result is $\frac{25}{16}$, or $1\frac{9}{16}$.

**9. B:** This is a simple matter of multiplication. The product is 0.0427378.

**10. A:** The inequality will be less than or equal to, since he may spend $100 or less on his purchase.

**11. C:** Multiplying the equation results in the following:

$$8x - 24 = 10x - 6$$
$$-18 = 2x$$
$$-\frac{18}{2} = x = -9$$

**12. C:** Erma's sale discount will be applied to the less expensive sweater, so she will receive the $44 sweater for 25% off. This amounts to a discount of $11, so the cost of the sweater will be $33. Added to the cost of the $50 sweater, which is not discounted, Erma's total is $83.

**13. A:** Start by adding the first two expressions, and then subtract 1.294 from the sum:

$$1.034 + 0.275 - 1.294 = 1.309 - 1.294 = 0.015$$

**14. B:** Adding up the number of church-goers in Ellsford results in about 1450 residents who attend a church in the town each week. There are approximately 400 people in Ellsford who attend a Catholic church each week. This number represents about 28% of the 1450 church-goers in the town.

**15. B:** To solve, first subtract Jerry's weight from the total permitted: $800 - 200 = 600$. Divide 600 by 4 (the four pieces of equipment) to get 150, the average weight.

**16. C:** Turn both expressions into fractions, and then multiply the first by the reverse of the second:

$$= \frac{14}{3} \div \frac{7}{6}$$
$$= \frac{14}{3} \times \frac{6}{7}$$

The result is the whole number 4.

**17. D:** Begin by subtracting 4 from both sides, then subtract $x$ from both sides:

$$2x + 4 - 4 = x - 6 - 4$$
$$2x = x - 10$$
$$2x - x = x - 10 - x$$
$$x = -10$$

**18. D:** To solve the equation for $x$, you can follow the steps below:

$$2x - 7 = 3$$
$$2x - 7 + 7 = 3 + 7$$
$$2x = 10$$
$$\frac{2x}{2} = \frac{10}{2}$$
$$x = 5$$

**19. D:** The points do not show any trend line or trend curve at all. So, there is no association in the scatter plot.

**20. A:** To find the correct answer, simply multiply 56 by 2.2. The result is 123.2, or approximately 123. This is Stella's weight in pounds.

**21. D:** The smallest negative integers are those that have the largest absolute value. Therefore, the negative integers, written in order from least to greatest, are $-8, -7\frac{4}{5}, -\frac{3}{4}$. The percentage, 18%, can be written as the decimal, 0.18; 0.18 is less than 0.25. The decimal, 2.5, is the greatest rational number given. Thus, the values, $-8, -7\frac{4}{5}, -\frac{3}{4}, 18\%, 0.25, 2.5$, are written in order from least to greatest.

**22. A:** Begin by subtracting 1432 from 2219. The result is 787. Then, divide 787 by 1432 to find the percent of increase: 0.549, or 54.9%. Rounded up, this is approximately a 55% increase in births between 2000 and 2010.

**23. C:** Solve the equation in the order of operations: $\frac{1}{4} \times \frac{3}{5}$, or $\frac{3}{20}$. Follow this up with division, which requires a reversal of the fraction: $\frac{3}{20} \div \frac{9}{8}$, or $\frac{3}{20} \times \frac{8}{9}$, which equals $\frac{24}{180}$. The result simplifies to $\frac{2}{15}$.

**24. C:** Cora did *not* fall 7 out of 27 times. To find the solution, simply divide 7 by 27 to arrive at 0.259, or 25.9%. Rounded up, this is approximately 26%.

**25. C:** The volume of a cylinder may be calculated using the formula $V = \pi r^2 h$, where $r$ represents the radius and $h$ represents the height. Substituting 1.5 for $r$ and 3 for $h$ gives $V = \pi(1.5)^2(3)$, which simplifies to $V \approx 21.2$.

**26. B:** Since the denominator is the same for both fractions, this is simple subtraction. Start by turning each expression into a fraction: $\frac{19}{6} - \frac{11}{6}$. The result is $\frac{8}{6}$, or $1\frac{2}{6} = 1\frac{1}{3}$.

**27. A:** The expression "Four more than a number, $x$" can be interpreted as $x + 4$. This is equal to "2 less than $\frac{1}{3}$ of another number, $y$," or $\frac{1}{3}y - 2$. Thus, the equation is $x + 4 = \frac{1}{3}y - 2$.

**28. C:** Start by adding up the costs of the trip, excluding the hotel cost: $572 + $150 + $250 = $972. Then, calculate what Margery will spend on the hotel. The first of her five nights at the hotel will cost her $89. For each of the other four nights, she will get a discount of 10% per night, or $8.90. This discount of $8.90 multiplied by the four nights is $35.60. The total she would have spent on the five nights without the discount is $445. With the discount, the amount goes down to $409.40. Add this amount to the $972 for a grand total of $1381.40.

**29. B:** Data is said to be positively skewed when there are a higher number of lower values, indicating data that is skewed right. An approximately normal distribution shows an increase in frequency, followed by a decrease in frequency, of approximately the same rate.

**30. C:** The surface area of a rectangular prism may be calculated using the formula

$$SA = 2lw + 2wh + 2hl$$

Substituting the dimensions of 14 inches, 6 inches, and 8 inches gives:

$$SA = 2(14)(6) + 2(6)(8) + 2(8)(14)$$

Thus, the surface area is 488 square inches.

**31. B:** Start by locating the section of the pie chart that represents construction. It looks close to a quarter of the pie chart, which means that it is probably 23%, but you can verify by adding up the numbers. The total amount of all donations is about $1.3 million and the amount given for construction is $0.3 million. $\frac{0.3}{1.3} = 0.227 \approx 23\%$.

**32. D:** Turn the fractions into mixed numbers to see the amounts more clearly. The result is that $\frac{7}{8}$ is smaller than $\frac{10}{9}$, or $1\frac{1}{9}$, which is smaller than $\frac{7}{3}$, or $2\frac{1}{3}$, which is smaller than $\frac{9}{2}$, or $4\frac{1}{2}$.

**33. D:** In order to divide the terms, they must first be rearranged as a multiplication by keeping the first fraction as is, changing the division sign to multiplication, and taking the reciprocal of the second fraction: $\frac{2}{7} \times \frac{6}{5}$. Then, multiply the new terms: $\frac{2}{7} \times \frac{6}{5} = \frac{12}{35}$. In Answer A, a common denominator was found, but the numerators were not also adjusted. Therefore, $\frac{2}{7}$ became $\frac{2}{42}$ and $\frac{5}{6}$ became $\frac{5}{42}$. Then, the fraction division process resulted in $\frac{2}{42} \div \frac{5}{42} = \frac{2}{42} \times \frac{42}{5} = \frac{2}{5}$. In Answer B, the reciprocal was taken of the first fraction instead of the second fraction before multiplying the terms. In Answer C, the fractions were incorrectly just multiplied as is.

**34. B:** Start by calculating the amount in parentheses, completing the multiplication first: $5 + 6 \times 3$, which is $5 + 18$ or $23$. Then calculate the product at the end: $10 \times 2$ which is $20$ and complete the equation:

$$= 7 + 16 - 23 - 20$$
$$= 23 - 23 - 20$$
$$= 0 - 20$$
$$= -20$$

**35. A:** This equation is a linear relationship that has a slope of 3.60 and passes through the origin. The table shows that for each hour of rental, the cost increases by $3.60. This matches with the slope of the equation. Of course, if the bicycle is not rented at all (0 hours), there will be no charge ($0). If plotted on the Cartesian plane, the line would have a y intercept of 0. Choice A is the only one that follows these requirements.

**36. D:** The correct answer is $4000. Chan has paid out a total of $30\% + 30\% + 25\% = 85\%$ of his bonus for the items in the question. So, the $600 is the remaining 15%. To find out his total bonus, solve $\frac{100}{15} \times 600 = \$4000$.

# Science

**1. C:** According to the principles of the scientific method, it is imperative that the hypothesis be established prior to the experiment as that is what the experiment should be testing. If the results do not support the hypothesis, that is acceptable, and often very informative. Once the experiment is complete, use the information gained to develop a new hypothesis to test.

**2. B:** The two types of measurement important in science are quantitative (when a numerical result is used) and qualitative (when descriptions or qualities are reported). Qualitative data is collected through observation and interviews, and focuses on the informant's behavior and perspectives. Both qualitative and quantitative data are equally important in scientific research, and when combined and analyzed together provide a full picture of the focus of the question at hand. Additionally, both qualitative and quantitative data can be accurate, or may be skewed by bias, therefore both should be thoroughly analyzed.

**3. C:** The chart shows two specific changes: snowfall levels from November to April and sunny days from November to April. Based on the chart alone, the only information that can be determined is that the fewest sunny days coincide with the months that have the heaviest snowfall. Anything further reaches beyond the immediate facts of the chart and moves into the territory of requiring other facts. As for answer choice D, it uses the word "relationship," which is not required in the question. The question only asks for what can be concluded.

**4. D:** The epiglottis covers the trachea during swallowing, thus preventing food from entering the airway. The trachea, also known as the windpipe, is a cylindrical portion of the respiratory tract that joins the larynx with the lungs. The esophagus connects the throat and the stomach. When a person swallows, the esophagus contracts to force the food down into the stomach. Like other structures in the respiratory system, the esophagus secretes mucus for lubrication. The diaphragm is a muscle that controls the height of the thoracic cavity, increasing the height on contraction (inspiration), and decreasing the height on relaxation (expiration).

**5. B:** The pads that support the vertebrae are made up of cartilage. Cartilage, a strong form of connective tissue, cushions and supports the joints. Cartilage also makes up the larynx and the outer ear. Bone is a form of connective tissue that comprises the better part of the skeleton. It includes both organic and inorganic substances. Tendons connect the muscles to other structures of the body, typically bones. Tendons can increase and decrease in length as the bones move. Fat is a combination of lipids; in humans, fat forms a layer beneath the skin and on the outside of the internal organs.

**6. C:** Cell layers and cell shape are the criteria for classifying epithelial tissue. Cell layers refers to the amount of cells that separate the basement membrane from the surface, such as a simple single layer, a stratified layer (2 or more), or a pseudostratified layer. Cell shapes refer to the shape of the outer cells and can be squamous, columnar or cuboidal.

**7. A:** The parathyroid gland is located on the lateral lobes of the thyroid gland in the neck, on the posterior aspect. It is part of the endocrine system. When the supply of calcium in blood diminishes to unhealthy levels, the parathyroid gland motivates the secretion of a hormone that encourages the bones to release calcium into the bloodstream. The parathyroid gland also regulates the amount of phosphate in the blood by stimulating the excretion of phosphates in the urine.

**8. D:** There are 11 organ systems in the human body: circulatory, digestive, endocrine, integumentary, lymphatic, muscular, nervous, reproductive, respiratory, skeletal, and urinary.

**9. B:** The cilia are the tiny hairs in the respiratory system that are responsible for removing foreign matter from the lungs. The cilia are located within the bronchial tubes, but it is the cilia that have the responsibility for removing inappropriate materials before they enter the lungs.

**10. C:** The order of hierarchy of human body structures is as follows: Organism, organ systems, organs, tissues, cells, molecules, and atoms. Muscles are types of tissues, so muscles do not have a separate place in the hierarchy but instead fall within the types of tissues.

**11. B:** To determine the average number of neutrons in one atom of an element, subtract the atomic number from the average atomic mass. For Bromine (Br), subtract its atomic number (35) from its average atomic mass (79.9) to acquire the average number of neutrons, 44.9.

**12. A:** The number of protons is the same for every atom of a given element and is the element's atomic number: in this case, 30 for Zinc (Zn).

**13. B:** In the lungs, oxygen is transported from the air to the blood through the process of *diffusion*, in which molecules passively move from an area of high concentration to low concentration. Specifically, the alveolar membranes withdraw the oxygen from the air in the lungs into the bloodstream. *Osmosis* is the passive movement of a water from an area of low solute concentration to an area of higher solute concentration through a permeable membrane. *Reverse osmosis* is the active transport of water opposite the concentration gradient from an area of low solute concentration to high solute concentration. *Dissipation* is a more general reference of the spread or loss of energy.

**14. A:** The parathyroid glands are four small glands that sit on top of the thyroid gland and regulate calcium levels by secreting parathyroid hormone. The hormone regulates the amount of calcium and magnesium that is excreted by the kidneys into the urine.

**15. A:** The large intestine's main function is the reabsorption of water into the body to form solid waste. It also allows for the absorption of vitamin K produced by microbes living inside the large intestine. The duodenum is the first section of the small intestine that receives partially digested food from the stomach, also called chyme, further digesting it with the help of enzymes released by the gall bladder, before it enters into the small intestine. The pancreas (not the gall bladder) releases insulin to assist in the removal and transport of sugar in the body. The jejunum is the second portion of the small intestine in which amino acids, fatty acids, and sugars are absorbed.

**16. B:** The conclusion was that the amount of sunlight received by the plants was affecting their growth. The independent variable was the amount of light that was given to the plants and could have been manipulated by the experimenter by moving the plants or adding equal parts of light. No control was used in this experiment.

**17. B:** The integumentary system includes skin, hair, and mucous membranes, all of which are responsible–in part, at least–for blocking disease-causing pathogens from entering the blood stream. The circulatory system distributes vital substances through the body. The lymphatic system sends leaked fluids from the cardiovascular system back to the blood vessels. The reproductive system stores bodily hormones that influence gender traits.

**18. D:** The parasympathetic nerves are active when an individual is either resting or eating. The sympathetic nerves are active when an individual experiences a strong emotion, such as fear or excitement. Feeling pain and heat fall under the responsibility of the sensory neurons. Talking and walking fall under the responsibility of the ganglia within the sensory-somatic nervous system.

**19. A:** The integumentary system (i.e., the skin, hair, mucous membranes, etc.) coordinates with the circulatory system to remove excess heat from the body. The superficial blood vessels (those nearest the surface of the skin) dilate to allow the heat to exit the body. The hormonal influence on blood pressure is the result of the relationship between the circulatory system and the endocrine system. The urinary system is responsible for assisting in the regulation of blood's pressure and volume. The skeletal system is responsible for assisting in the development of blood vessels within the marrow.

**20. C:** Blood returns to the heart from both the inferior and superior vena cava, entering into the right atrium, through the tricuspid valve, and into the right ventricle. Once the right ventricle is full, the tricuspid valve closes, and upon heart contraction, the blood is pumped through the pulmonary artery, becoming oxygenated in the lungs. The blood returns to the heart from the lungs through the pulmonary vein, into the left atrium, through the mitral valve, and into the left ventricle. When the left ventricle is full, the mitral valve closes, and the heart contracts and distributes the newly oxygenated blood throughout the body through the aortic valve and into the aorta.

**21. D:** Blood is cooled as it passes through capillaries surrounding the sweat glands. Heat is absorbed along with excess salt and water and transferred to the glands as sweat. Droplets of sweat then evaporate from the skin surface to dissipate heat and cool the body. The kidney, bladder, and liver are not involved in regulating body temperature.

**22. D:** The skin is a part of the integumentary system, along with the hair, nails, nerves, and glands. The skin controls fluid loss, protects deep tissues, and synthesizes vitamin D. The skeletal system gives the body its bony supporting structure, protects vital organs, collaborates with muscles in body movement, stores calcium, and produces red blood cells. The muscular system maintains posture, collaborates with the bones in body movement, uses energy, and generates heat. The lymphatic system retrieves fluids leaked from capillaries and contains white blood cells, and parts of it support parts of the immune system.

**23. C:** The best use of the International System of Units (SI) for this situation would be the use of the micrometer as it is the smallest unit of measurement provided and the scientist is using a microscope to view the insects.

**24. B:** The respiratory system inhales air, of which oxygen is one component. From that inhaled air, the respiratory system delivers oxygen to the circulatory system through gas exchange. It then removes carbon dioxide ($CO_2$) from the circulatory system as we exhale. The respiratory system does not create or destroy anything (A, D). It also does not ionize the oxygen (C).

**25. D:** The name for a substance that stimulates the production of antibodies is an *antigen*. An antigen is any substance perceived by the immune system as dangerous. When the body senses an antigen, it produces an antibody. *Collagen* is one of the components of bone, tendon, and cartilage. It is a spongy protein that can be turned into gelatin by boiling. *Hemoglobin* is the part of red blood cells that carries oxygen. In order for the blood to carry enough oxygen to the cells of the body, there has to be a sufficient amount of hemoglobin. *Lymph* is a near-transparent fluid that performs a number of functions in the body: It removes bacteria from tissues, replaces lymphocytes in the blood, and moves fat away from the small intestine. Lymph contains white blood cells. The lymph *node* is the tissue through which lymph travels in this filtering process.

**26. A:** The immune system consists of the lymphatic system, spleen, tonsils, thymus, and bone marrow. The nervous system consists of the brain, spinal cord, and nerve cells. The circulatory system consists of the heart, veins, arteries, and capillaries. The respiratory system consists of the nose, trachea, bronchial tubes, lungs, alveolus, and diaphragm.

**27. A:** Turn it into an "if/then" statement. A formalized hypothesis written in the form of an if/then statement can then be tested. A statement may make a prediction or imply a cause/effect relationship, but that does not necessarily make it a good hypothesis. In this example, the student could rewrite the statement in the form of an if/then statement such as, "If the length of the string of the pendulum is varied, then the time it takes the ball to make one complete period changes." This hypothesis is testable, and doesn't simply make a prediction or a conclusion. The validity of the hypothesis can then be supported or disproved by experimentation and observation.

**28. C:** The mass of the ball. The mass of the ball is appropriately called a control variable for the experiment. A control or controlled variable is a factor that could be varied, but for testing purposes should remain the same throughout all experiments, otherwise, it could affect the results. In this case, if the mass of the ball was changed, it could also affect the length of the period. The length of the string is meant to be an independent variable, one that is changed during experiments to observe the results upon the dependent variable, which is the variable (or variables) that are affected. In this case, the period would be the dependent variable.

**29. B:** The substance thymine does not exist in RNA. The bases of RNA include uracil, cytosine, guanine, and adenine.

**30. B:** Smooth muscle tissue is said to be arranged in a disorderly fashion because it is not striated like the other two types of muscle: cardiac and skeletal. Striations are lines that can only be seen with a microscope. *Smooth* muscle is typically found in the supporting tissues of hollow organs and blood vessels. *Cardiac* muscle is found exclusively in the heart; it is responsible for the contractions that pump blood throughout the body. *Skeletal* muscle, by far the most preponderant in the body, controls the movements of the skeleton. The contractions of skeletal muscle are responsible for all voluntary motion. There is no such thing as *rough* muscle.

**31. C:** *Melatonin* is produced by the pineal gland. One of the primary functions of melatonin is regulation of the circadian cycle, which is the rhythm of sleep and wakefulness. *Insulin* helps regulate the amount of glucose in the blood. Without insulin, the body is unable to convert blood sugar into energy. *Testosterone* is the main hormone produced by the testes; it is responsible for the development of adult male sex characteristics. *Epinephrine*, also known as adrenaline, performs a number of functions: It quickens and strengthens the heartbeat and dilates the bronchioles. Epinephrine is one of the hormones secreted when the body senses danger.

**32. A:** The midsagittal plane refers to a lengthwise cut that divides the body into equal right and left portions; it is also called the medial plane. The frontal or coronal plane refers to a cut that divides the body into anterior and posterior sections. The oblique plane is when a cylindrical organ is sectioned with an angular cut across the organ.

**33. B:** In the development of genetic traits, one gene must match to a protein for a genetic trait to develop correctly.

**34. B:** Skeletal or striated muscles are voluntary muscles that help support the skeletal structures. Examples of striated muscles are the biceps, triceps, quadriceps, gluteus, and gastrocnemius muscles to name a few. Smooth or involuntary muscles are muscles primarily found in the visceral organs such as the intestines, prostate, reproductive organs, bladder and trachea.

**35. B:** The vertebral cavity (containing the spine) can be found in the dorsal cavity along with the cranial cavity (containing the brain). The ventral body cavity is divided into several subsections: the thoracic and abdominopelvic cavities. The heart is in the thoracic cavity, the stomach is in the abdominal cavity, and the testes are in the pelvic cavity.

**36. D:** Solids with a fixed shape have a crystalline order that defines and maintains that shape.

**37. B:** The diaphragm moves downward or contracts to increase the space in the thoracic cavity. This downward motion inflates the lungs and contracts the ribs. The heart's position does not change during inspiration or expiration.

**38. B:** The endoplasmic reticulum is the cell's transport network that moves proteins from one part of the cell to another. The Golgi apparatus assists in the transport but is not the actual transport network. Mitochondria are organelles ("tiny organs") that help in the production of ATP, which the cells need to operate properly. The nucleolus participates in the production of ribosomes that are needed to generate proteins for the cell.

**39. A:** There are four phases of mitosis: the prophase, metaphase, anaphase, and telophase. During the prophase of mitosis, the mitotic spindle fibers begin to form. Next, during the metaphase, the chromosomes line up in the middle of the cell. Next, in the anaphase of mitosis, the chromosomes, originally in pairs, separate and move to the opposite ends of the cells. Then, during the telophase, two nuclei form around the separated chromosomes, each surrounded by a nuclear membrane.

**40. A:** The table reflects student scores for each quarter. The trend that can be seen in the graph is an increase in scores as the year progressed. The graph label mentions a test review, but there is not enough information about that to know if that is the reason for the scores changing.

**41. A:** The right lung has three segments: upper, medial and lower. The left lung has two lobes: upper and lower. The lobes are further divided into segments. The right lung comprises ten segments: three in the right upper, two in the right medial lobe, and five in the right lower lobe. The left lung comprises eight segments: four in the left upper lobe and four in the left lower lobe.

**42. B:** Alveoli are air sacs found within the lung parenchyma and are not part of the cardiac system. The septum is dividing wall between the right and left sides of the heart. The heart has four chambers: the upper two chambers are the right and left atrium and the lower two chambers are the right and left ventricles.

**43. A:** The physical expression—such as hair color—is the result of the phenotype. The genotype is the basic genetic code. Allele are two or more alternative gene forms that generally arises via mutation, and are located in the same part of a chromosome. A gamete is a germ cell (female or male) that can unite with the opposite sex germ cell in the process of zygote formation of sexual reproduction.

**44. B:** The endocrine system is made up of the pituitary gland, thyroid gland, parathyroid glands, adrenal glands, pancreas, ovaries, and testicles. They secrete hormones which help regulate mood, growth and development, tissue function, metabolism, and sexual function and reproductive processes. The Pons is located in the brain stem and relays nerve signals that coordinate messages between the brain and the body.

**45. D:** The heart is located in the thoracic cavity. The thoracic cavity extends from the neck to the diaphragm, which divides the abdominal cavity from the thoracic cavity. Some of the major structures contained in the thoracic cavity are the ribs, heart, lungs, mediastinum, trachea, and the esophagus. The spleen is located in the abdominal cavity. The brain is located in the cranial cavity. The bladder is located in the pelvic cavity.

**46. C:** The number of 7 is the "breaking point" between basic and acidic. Above 7 solutions are considered basic; below 7 solutions are considered acidic. For instance, milk, with a pH of 6.5, is actually considered acidic. Bleach, with a pH of 12.5, is considered basic.

**47. B:** The trachea is anterior or ventral to the esophagus. The trachea is separated from the esophagus by the epiglottis, which is a flap of cartilage that covers one while the other is in use. The trachea's proximal portion is connected to the larynx and the distal portion splits off into the right and left bronchi.

**48. B:** All of the answers use the System of International Units (SI) of measurement with the exception of gallons. A liter is the measurement of a liquid. Grams are a unit of measurement for the weight of an object, which would be measured on the triple beam balance. Meters measure length.

**49. B:** The transverse plane separates the body into equal upper and lower portions. The oblique plane is when a cylindrical organ is sectioned with an angular cut across the organ. The midsagittal or medial plane refers to a lengthwise cut that divides the body into equal right and left portions. The frontal or coronal plane refers to a cut that divides the body into anterior and posterior sections.

**50. C:** RNA has several roles, one of which is to act as the messenger and deliver information about the correct sequence of proteins in DNA. The ribosomes do the actual manufacturing of the proteins. Hydrogen, oxygen, and nitrogen work to create the bonds within DNA. And far from having a double helix shape, RNA has what would be considered a more two-dimensional shape.

**51. B:** Catalysts alter the activation energy during a chemical reaction and therefore control the rate of the reaction. The substrate is the actual surface that enzymes use during a chemical reaction (and there is no such term as *substrate energy*). Inhibitors and promoters participate in the chemical reaction, but it is the activation energy that catalysts alter to control the overall rate as the reaction occurs.

**52. C:** The stratum basale is the lowest level of the epidermis, which is the surface level. The dermis is a layer of connective tissue immediately beneath the epidermis. The hypodermis, while not a layer of skin, is part of the integumentary system and it is just below the dermis.

**53. C:** Crossing the corresponding alleles from each parent will yield a result of BB in the upper right box of this Punnett square.

# English and Language Usage

**1. C:** The word *syllabi* is the correct plural form of *syllabus*. The other answer choices reflect incorrect plural forms. Specifically, *syllabus* does not change the form at all, and the Latin root of *syllabus* would require some change. At the same time, *syllaba*—while an accurate plural for some words with Latin roots—is incorrect in this case. And *syllabis* is a double form of the plural, so it cannot be correct.

**2. A:** The word *independent* is an adjective that modifies the word *state*, describing what kind of state the kingdom of Gwynedd was. The words *century*, *king*, and *control* are all nouns in this context.

**3. D:** Prefixes, appearing at the beginning of base words to change their meanings. Suffixes appear at the end of words. Prefixes are attached to the beginning of words to change their meanings. *Un+happy, bi+monthly,* and *re+examine* are prefixes that, by definition, change the meanings of the words to which they are attached.

**4. C:** Answer choice C is correct, because the quotation is a standard quotation (requiring double quotes) as well as a question. Additionally, the question mark belongs inside the quotation marks. Answer choice A correctly places the question mark inside the quotation marks, but the use of single quotes is incorrect for standard quotations. Answer choice B is incorrect, because it places the question mark outside the quotation marks. Answer choice D uses the layered quotes, which are unnecessary in this case, since the sentence presents only one quotation instead of more than one.

**5. C:** Cause–effect words. Signal words give the reader hints about the purpose of a particular passage. Some signal words are concerned with comparing/contrasting, some with cause and effect, some with temporal sequencing, some with physical location, and some with a problem and its solution. The words *since, whether,* and *accordingly* are words used when describing an outcome. Outcomes have causes.

**6. D:** *Acceptable* is the correct spelling of the word.

**7. C:** Answer choice C offers the most effective combination of the sentences with the use of the conjunction *but* and the dependent clause starting with *after*. All other answer choices result in choppy or unclear combinations of the four sentences.

**8. D:** If Beryl knew something instinctively, it is safe to say that her mother's warning was not stated outright. Therefore, answer choice D is the best option. Answer choice A makes little sense. Answer choice B makes sense only if Beryl suspects her mother does not care whether or not she smokes. Answer choice C has a meaning that is the opposite of the one implied in the sentence.

**9. A:** Correct punctuation requires a comma after both city and state when both fall within the sentence, even when the city and state fall within an opening dependent clause that has a comma after it. All answer choices that do not have a comma after the state as well as the city are incorrect.

Answer choice C is incorrect because it adds a comma after *Oak* for no clear reason as the name of the city in full is clearly *Oak Ridge*.

**10. A:** The transition "surprisingly" indicates that the reaction was unexpected, or even contradictory to the circumstance of the speaker not turning his work in on time and talking-out in class. The other answer choices do not make as much sense to coordinate these two sentences.

**11. A:** The suffix *-ism* here suggests a doctrine that is followed, whether that be the doctrine of polytheism (a religious doctrine), communism (a social doctrine), or nationalism (a political doctrine).

**12. C:** This version begins with a subject and verb and is followed by a clause. Choice A is incorrect because the words are out of order and don't logically follow the previous sentence. The sentence should begin with 'She says' because it is the school principal's opinion being expressed. This choice is also incorrect because it uses the words *not appropriate* instead of *inappropriate*. Choice B is incorrect because the clause "that students wear to schools" should come after the word *outfits*. Choice D is incorrect because the word order changes the meaning of the sentence by stating that any outfits are distracting and inappropriate.

**13. D:** The semicolon correctly joins the two sentences. Answer choice A is incorrect, because it uses a comma splice to join two independent clauses. (To join two independent clauses, a comma needs to be accompanied by a coordinating conjunction.) The colon in answer choice B is incorrect because the information in the second clause does not clearly define or explain the previous clause. Answer choice C is incorrect because it offers no punctuation to separate the two independent clauses and thus creates more confusion than clarity.

**14. A:** A comma should be used to separate the independent clause beginning with *some members* from the non-essential phrase beginning with *which is*. Choice B is incorrect because it is missing the comma. Choice C is incorrect because it incorrectly uses *that* instead of *which*. Choice D is incorrect because it uses a semicolon instead of a comma.

**15. B:** Answer choice B contains two independent clauses that are joined with a comma and the coordinating conjunction *and*. Answer choice A, though it contains a compound subject and a compound verb, is still a simple sentence. Answer choice C opens with a dependent clause, so it is a complex sentence. Answer choice D is a compound-complex sentence because it includes a dependent clause as well as two independent clauses.

**16. B:** Answer choice B correctly capitalizes *Uncle Archibald*, where *Uncle Archibald* is used as one whole to a specific name, which makes it a proper noun. If the sentence said "her uncle Archibald," then *uncle* would remain lower case. In answer choice A, the word *cousin* needs no capitalization, because it is used to describe Elaine but is not used as part of her name. (The only distinctions are when the word is used within a direct address or opens a sentence.) Similarly, *mother* and *sister* do not need to be capitalized unless they are the first word of the sentence or are used to directly address someone.

**17. D:** Within the context of the sentence, it seems as if "*quid pro quo*" means something like "if I do something, then I will be rewarded with something good." Choice A is not a good choice because it says "if I don't do anything, I will get something good." Choice B is inappropriate because money is not mentioned. While choice C might seem like a good choice, the phrase is not put in another way to talk about what people deserve as much as it talks about what people should do or how they should behave. Choice D is the best choice because "something for something" implies the sort of exchange described in the passage.

**18. D:** The word *affect* is a verb in this context and is the correct usage within the sentence. The possessive pronoun *your* also correctly modifies *children*, so answer choice D is correct. All other answer choices incorrectly apply the words to the sentence.

**19. B:** The context of the sentence suggests that the trauma of surviving the plane crash left long-term memories that haunted Johanna for many years. As a result, *permanent* is the best meaning of *indelible*. The other meanings make little sense in the context of the sentence. The only possible option is *indirect*, but there is nothing about the sentence to suggest that the nightmares are indirect impressions of a traumatic experience.

**20. C:** The word *east* in answer choice C is simply a directional indication and does not need to be capitalized in the context of the sentence. All other uses of capitalization are correct in the context of the sentences. The word *South* should be capitalized when it refers to a region of the United States (as indicated by the mention of Mississippi). The word *East* should be capitalized when it refers to the region of Texas. And the word *north* does not need to be capitalized when it is simply a directional indication (as in answer choice D).

**21. C:** The word *whom* correctly indicates the objective case—as in "to hold him/her responsible"—so answer choice C is correct. The word *who* in answer choice A incorrectly indicates the subjective case. Similarly, answer choice B is incorrect because it incorrectly applies the objective whom instead of the subjective who. Answer choice D is incorrect because the word who is the subjective case (instead of the objective case) here.

**22. B:** The word *capacity* is a noun in this context, so answer choice B is correct. Because the word functions as the object of the preposition, the options of verb and adverb cannot be correct. Answer choice D is incorrect because the word *capacity* is not a pronoun in any context.

**23. C:** Answer choice C summarizes the ideas within the sentence simply and clearly. Answer choice A moves the ideas around to make them awkward instead of effective. Answer choice B creates a dangling modifier with the phrase without adequate preparation, so it cannot be correct. Similarly, answer choice D makes this phrase a dangling modifier that makes the flow of thought awkward instead of clear.

**24. A:** The pronoun *all* is plural, so it requires the plural verb *are*. The pronouns *each* and *neither* are singular and require singular verbs (not provided in answer choices B and C). The pronoun *any* can be either singular or plural depending on the context of the sentence. In this case, *any* suggests a singular usage, so answer choice D is incorrect with the plural verb.

**25. B:** The use of substantial in this sentence has a meaning that is closest to "considerable." The other choices are antonyms of substantial.

**26. D:** While answer choice D is arguably the longest of the four sentences, it is actually a simple sentence. It contains a compound subject and a compound verb, but because it represents only one independent clause it still functions as a simple sentence. Answer choices A and B contain two independent clauses and are thus compound sentences. Answer choice C contains a dependent clause, so it is a complex sentence.

**27. D:** Answer choice D correctly arranges the ideas to reflect the most effective meaning of the sentence. All other answer choices place the ideas in such a way as to create confusion or incorrect punctuation instead of clarity.

**28. D:** The prefix poly- means "many." A is incorrect because the prefix *poly-* does not mean "few." B is incorrect because the prefix poly- does not mean "several." C is incorrect because the prefix poly- does not mean "none."

# TEAS Practice Test #2

| Reading | | Mathematics | Science | | English and Language Usage |
|---------|---------|-------------|---------|---------|---------|
| 1. ____ | 46. ____ | 1. ____ | 1. ____ | 46. ____ | 1. ____ |
| 2. ____ | 47. ____ | 2. ____ | 2. ____ | 47. ____ | 2. ____ |
| 3. ____ | 48. ____ | 3. ____ | 3. ____ | 48. ____ | 3. ____ |
| 4. ____ | 49. ____ | 4. ____ | 4. ____ | 49. ____ | 4. ____ |
| 5. ____ | 50. ____ | 5. ____ | 5. ____ | 50. ____ | 5. ____ |
| 6. ____ | 51. ____ | 6. ____ | 6. ____ | 51. ____ | 6. ____ |
| 7. ____ | 52. ____ | 7. ____ | 7. ____ | 52. ____ | 7. ____ |
| 8. ____ | 53. ____ | 8. ____ | 8. ____ | 53. ____ | 8. ____ |
| 9. ____ | | 9. ____ | 9. ____ | | 9. ____ |
| 10. ____ | | 10. ____ | 10. ____ | | 10. ____ |
| 11. ____ | | 11. ____ | 11. ____ | | 11. ____ |
| 12. ____ | | 12. ____ | 12. ____ | | 12. ____ |
| 13. ____ | | 13. ____ | 13. ____ | | 13. ____ |
| 14. ____ | | 14. ____ | 14. ____ | | 14. ____ |
| 15. ____ | | 15. ____ | 15. ____ | | 15. ____ |
| 16. ____ | | 16. ____ | 16. ____ | | 16. ____ |
| 17. ____ | | 17. ____ | 17. ____ | | 17. ____ |
| 18. ____ | | 18. ____ | 18. ____ | | 18. ____ |
| 19. ____ | | 19. ____ | 19. ____ | | 19. ____ |
| 20. ____ | | 20. ____ | 20. ____ | | 20. ____ |
| 21. ____ | | 21. ____ | 21. ____ | | 21. ____ |
| 22. ____ | | 22. ____ | 22. ____ | | 22. ____ |
| 23. ____ | | 23. ____ | 23. ____ | | 23. ____ |
| 24. ____ | | 24. ____ | 24. ____ | | 24. ____ |
| 25. ____ | | 25. ____ | 25. ____ | | 25. ____ |
| 26. ____ | | 26. ____ | 26. ____ | | 26. ____ |
| 27. ____ | | 27. ____ | 27. ____ | | 27. ____ |
| 28. ____ | | 28. ____ | 28. ____ | | 28. ____ |
| 29. ____ | | 29. ____ | 29. ____ | | |
| 30. ____ | | 30. ____ | 30. ____ | | |
| 31. ____ | | 31. ____ | 31. ____ | | |
| 32. ____ | | 32. ____ | 32. ____ | | |
| 33. ____ | | 33. ____ | 33. ____ | | |
| 34. ____ | | 34. ____ | 34. ____ | | |
| 35. ____ | | 35. ____ | 35. ____ | | |
| 36. ____ | | 36. ____ | 36. ____ | | |
| 37. ____ | | | 37. ____ | | |
| 38. ____ | | | 38. ____ | | |
| 39. ____ | | | 39. ____ | | |
| 40. ____ | | | 40. ____ | | |
| 41. ____ | | | 41. ____ | | |
| 42. ____ | | | 42. ____ | | |
| 43. ____ | | | 43. ____ | | |
| 44. ____ | | | 44. ____ | | |
| 45. ____ | | | 45. ____ | | |

| **Reading** | Number of Questions: **53** |
|---|---|
| | Time Limit: **64 Minutes** |

*At first, the woman's contractions were only <u>intermittent</u>, so the nurse had trouble determining how far her labor had progressed.*

**1. Which of the following is the definition for the underlined word?**

   a.  frequent
   b.  irregular
   c.  painful
   d.  dependable

**2. Which of the following would be the best source to begin developing a position about civil rights for an oral debate?**

   a.  A blog created by a proponent of civil rights.
   b.  An interview with someone who took part in a civil rights march.
   c.  A history textbook detailing civil rights.
   d.  A speech by a famous civil rights leader.

*The heavy spring rain resulted in a <u>plethora</u> of zucchini in Kit's garden, and left her desperately giving the vegetables to anyone who was interested.*

**3. Which of the following is the definition for the underlined word in the sentence?**

   a.  irritation
   b.  quantity
   c.  abundance
   d.  waste

**4. The guide words at the top of a dictionary page are *needs* and *negotiate*. Which of the following words is an entry on this page?**

   a.  needle
   b.  neigh
   c.  neglect
   d.  nectar

*The next question is based on the following information.*

   <u>Chapter 4: The Fictional Writings of Dorothy L. Sayers</u>

   Plays
   Novels
   Short Stories
   Letters
   Mysteries

**5. Analyze the headings above. Which of the following does not belong?**

   a.  Novels
   b.  Plays
   c.  Mysteries
   d.  Letters

*The next three questions are based on the following passage.*

Among the first females awarded a degree from Oxford University, Dorothy L. Sayers proved to be one of the most versatile writers in post-war England. Sayers was born in 1893, the only child of an Anglican chaplain, and she received an unexpectedly good education at home. For instance, her study of Latin commenced when she was only six years old. She entered Oxford in 1912, at a time when the university was not granting degrees to women. By 1920, this policy had changed, and Sayers received her degree in medieval literature and modern languages after finishing university. That same year, she also received a master of arts degree.

Sayers's first foray into published writing was a collection of poetry released in 1916. Within a few years, she began work on the detective novels and short stories that would make her famous, due to the creation of the foppish, mystery-solving aristocrat Lord Peter Wimsey. Sayers is also credited with the short story mysteries about the character Montague Egg. In spite of her success as a mystery writer, Sayers continued to balance popular fiction with academic work; her translation of Dante's *Inferno* gained her respect for her ability to convey the poetry in English while still remaining true to the Italian *terza rima*. She also composed a series of twelve plays about the life of Christ, and wrote several essays about education and feminism. In her middle age, Dorothy L. Sayers published several works of Christian apologetics, one of which was so well-received that the archbishop of Canterbury attempted to present her with a doctorate of divinity. Sayers, for reasons known only to her, declined.

**6. Which of the following describes the type of writing used to create the passage?**
   a. narrative
   b. persuasive
   c. expository
   d. technical

**7. Which of the following sentences is the best summary of the passage?**
   a. Among the first females awarded a degree from Oxford University, Dorothy L. Sayers proved to be one of the most versatile writers in post-war England.
   b. Sayers was born in 1893, the only child of an Anglican chaplain, and she received an unexpectedly good education at home.
   c. Within a few years, she began work on the detective novels and short stories that would make her famous, due to the creation of the foppish, mystery-solving aristocrat Lord Peter Wimsey.
   d. In her middle age, Dorothy L. Sayers published several works of Christian apologetics, one of which was so well-received that the archbishop of Canterbury attempted to present her with a doctorate of divinity.

**8. Which of the following sentences contains an opinion statement by the author?**
   a. Among the first females awarded a degree from Oxford University, Dorothy L. Sayers proved to be one of the most versatile writers in post-war England.
   b. Sayers was born in 1893, the only child of an Anglican chaplain, and she received an unexpectedly good education at home.
   c. Her translation of Dante's Inferno gained her respect for her ability to convey the poetry in English while still remaining true to the Italian terza rima.
   d. Sayers, for reasons known only to her, declined.

*The next four questions are based on the following information.*

The Dewey Decimal Classes

> 000 Computer science, information, and general works
> 100 Philosophy and psychology
> 200 Religion
> 300 Social sciences
> 400 Languages
> 500 Science and mathematics
> 600 Technical and applied science
> 700 Arts and recreation
> 800 Literature
> 900 History, geography, and biography

**9. Jorgen is doing a project on the ancient Greek mathematician and poet Eratosthenes. In his initial review, Jorgen learns that Eratosthenes is considered the first person to calculate the circumference of the earth, and that he is considered the first to describe geography as it is studied today. To which section of the library should Jorgen go to find one of the early maps created by Eratosthenes?**

    a. 100
    b. 300
    c. 600
    d. 900

**10. Due to his many interests and pursuits, Eratosthenes dabbled in a variety of fields, and he is credited with a theory known as the sieve of Eratosthenes. This is an early algorithm used to determine prime numbers. To which section of the library should Jorgen go to find out more about the current applications of the sieve of Eratosthenes?**

    a. 000
    b. 100
    c. 400
    d. 500

**11. One ancient work claims that Eratosthenes received the nickname "beta" from those who knew him. This is a word that represents the second letter of the Greek alphabet, and it represented Eratosthenes's accomplishments in every area that he studied. To which section of the library should Jorgen go to learn more about the letters of the Greek alphabet and the meaning of the word "beta"?**

    a. 200
    b. 400
    c. 700
    d. 900

12. Finally, Jorgen learns that Eratosthenes was fascinated by the story of the Trojan War, and that he attempted to determine the exact dates when this event occurred. Jorgen is unfamiliar with the story of the Fall of Troy, so he decides to look into writings such as *The Iliad* and *The Odyssey*, by Homer. To which section of the library should Jorgen go to locate these works?

    a.  100
    b.  200
    c.  700
    d.  800

13. Which of the answer choices gives the best definition for the underlined word in the following sentence?

With all of the planning that preceded her daughter's wedding, Marci decided that picking out a new paint color for her own living room was largely <u>peripheral</u>.

    a.  meaningless
    b.  contrived
    c.  unimportant
    d.  disappointing

*The next two questions are based on the following chart.*

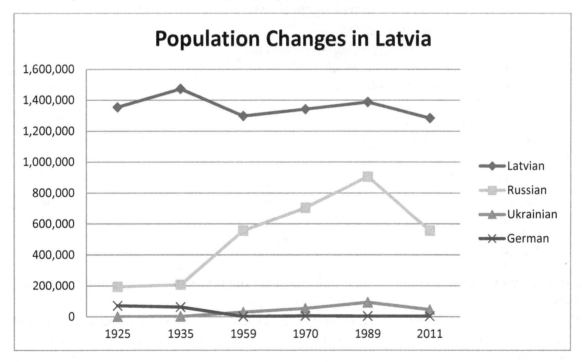

14. Between 1925 and 1991, Latvia was part of the Soviet Union. Since 1991, the population of which ethnic group in Latvia appears to have decreased the most?

    a.  Latvian
    b.  Russian
    c.  Ukrainian
    d.  German

15. After World War II ended in 1945, large numbers of non-Latvian workers entered the country, primarily to work at construction jobs. Among these non-Latvian ethnic groups, the increase in workers represented a population percentage shift of less than one percent before 1945 to more than three percent by the time of the Soviet Union's collapse. Which ethnic group shown on the chart best represents this shift?

    a. Latvian
    b. Russian
    c. Ukrainian
    d. German

16. Which answer choice represents the most useful resource for Hilaire in the following vignette?

Hilaire's professor instructed him to improve the word choice in his papers. As the professor noted, Hilaire's ideas are good, but he relies too heavily on simple expressions when a more complex word would be appropriate.

    a. Roget's Thesaurus
    b. Webster's Dictionary
    c. Encyclopedia Britannica
    d. University of Oxford Style Guide

17. Follow the instructions below to transform the starting word into a different word.

- **Start with the word CORPOREAL.**
- **Remove the C from the beginning of the word.**
- **Remove the O from the beginning of the word.**
- **Remove the O from the middle of the word.**
- **Move the E to follow the first R.**
- **Move the L to follow the P.**
- **Remove the second R.**
- **Add the letter Y to the end of the word.**

What is the new word?

    a. REALLY
    b. PRETTY
    c. REPLAY
    d. POWER

18. Which answer choice gives the best definition for the underlined word in the following sentence?

Although not considered the smartest student in her class, Klara was willing to work hard for her grades, and her <u>sedulous</u> commitment to her studies earned her top scores at graduation.

    a. diligent
    b. silent
    c. moderate
    d. complicated

19. Flemming is on a new diet that requires him to avoid all dairy products, as well as dairy byproducts. This will be a big change for him, so his doctor gives him information about foods that he might not realize often contain dairy products. These include bread, granola, deli meat, dry breakfast cereal, and energy bars. Which of the following items from Flemming's standard diet will still be safe to eat?

    a. puffed rice cereal
    b. breaded chicken parmesan
    c. sliced turkey sandwich
    d. yogurt made from coconut milk

*The next two questions are based on the following information.*

    Car Owner's Manual: Table of Contents:

    Chapter I: Vehicle Instruments
    Chapter II: Safety Options
    Chapter III: Audio, Climate, and Voice Controls
    Chapter IV: Pre-Driving and Driving
    Chapter V: Routine Maintenance
    Chapter VI: Emergencies
    Chapter VII: Consumer Resources

20. To which chapter should Regina turn if she needs to locate information about adjusting the air conditioning in the vehicle?

    a. I
    b. II
    c. III
    d. IV

21. To which chapter should Regina turn if she needs to find out what to do if the car begins overheating?

    a. II
    b. III
    c. IV
    d. VI

22. Of the resource options listed in the answer choices, which would not be considered a reliable, scholarly source for Nora in the following vignette?

Nora is preparing a large research project for the end of the term, and the instructor has required that all students make sure they are using reliable, scholarly resources in their papers.

    a. Encyclopedia Britannica
    b. Wikipedia
    c. Science.gov
    d. LexisNexis

*The next five questions are based on the following passage.*

In the United States, the foreign language requirement for high school graduation is decided at the state level. This means the requirement varies, with some states deciding to forego a foreign language requirement altogether (www.ncssfl.org). It is necessary that these states reconsider their position and amend their requirements to reflect compulsory completion of a course of one or more foreign languages. Studying a foreign language has become increasingly important for the global economy. As technology continues to make international business relations increasingly easy, people need to keep up by increasing their communication capabilities. High school graduates with foreign language credits have been shown to have an increased college acceptance rate. In addition, students who have mastered more than one language typically find themselves in greater demand when they reach the job market. Students who did not study a foreign language often find themselves unable to obtain a job at all.

### 23. What is the main idea of this passage?
a. Studying a foreign language will help graduating students find jobs after high school.
b. Studying a foreign language should be a mandatory requirement for high school graduation.
c. Studying a foreign language helps students gain an understanding of other cultures.
d. Studying a foreign language is essential if a student hopes to get into college.

### 24. Which of the following statements represents the best summary of the claims made in this passage?
a. Studying a foreign language is important if you want to graduate from high school and get a job.
b. Studying a foreign language is important for the global economy because of the technological advances that have been made in international communications.
c. Studying a foreign language is important for the global economy, college acceptance rates, and becoming a sought-after candidate in the job market.
d. Studying a foreign language is important for college acceptance rates and obtaining a job after college.

### 25. Which of the following statements represents an EXAGGERATED claim in support of the argument presented in this passage?
a. In the United States, the foreign language requirement for high school graduation is decided at the state level.
b. Studying a foreign language has become increasingly important for the global economy.
c. High school graduates with foreign language credits have been shown to have an increased college acceptance rate.
d. Students who did not study a foreign language often find themselves unable to obtain a job at all.

**26. Which of the following would be a useful source of information to determine the validity of the argument presented in this passage?**

    a.   A survey of high school students' preferences with regard to foreign language requirements.

    b.   A comparison of the correlation between a second language introduced at home and subsequent college acceptance rates.

    c.   A survey that asks parents to select the foreign language they would like their children to study in high school.

    d.   A comparison of the correlation between high school students' study of a foreign language and subsequent college acceptance rates.

**27. Which of the following would be the best concluding statement for this passage?**

    a.   States should consider how important foreign languages are for the global economy when making their policies regarding foreign language requirements for graduation from high school.

    b.   Policies regarding a foreign language requirement for graduation from high school should take into account the importance of foreign languages for the global economy and the correlation between foreign languages and increased college acceptance rates and employment opportunities.

    c.   High school graduation requirements should include a foreign language class because of the influence knowledge of a second language has on college acceptance rates.

    d.   Policies regarding a foreign language requirement for graduation from high school should take into account how difficult it is to obtain a job in today's economy for those who do not have knowledge of more than one language.

*The next four questions are based on the following information.*

<u>The Big Book of Herbs and Herbal Medicine</u>

Part I: How to Grow Herbs
Chapter 1: Choosing Your Herbs
Chapter 2: Planting Your Herbs
Chapter 3: Caring for Your Herbs

Part II: How to Cook with Herbs
Chapter 4: Herbs in Food
Chapter 5: Herbs in Beverages
Chapter 6: Herbs in Oils and Vinegars

Part III: How to Heal with Herbs
Chapter 7: Herbs for Children's Needs
Chapter 8: Herbs for Adult Needs
      Section 8–A: Women's Needs
      Section 8–B: Men's Needs
Chapter 9: Herbs for Immunity
Chapter 10: Herbs for Respiratory Conditions
Chapter 11: Herbs for Digestive Conditions
Chapter 12: Herbs for Detox
      Section 12–A: Circulatory Conditions
      Section 12–B: Musculoskeletal Conditions
      Section 12–C: Endocrine Conditions
      Section 12–D: Topical Conditions

Part IV: Alphabetical Herb Listing
Chapter 13: Herbs, A–I
Chapter 14: Herbs, J–O
Chapter 15: Herbs, P–Z

**28. Clothilde is looking for an herbal remedy to combat a recent outbreak of eczema. In which chapter should she look for more information?**

    a.   Chapter 8
    b.   Chapter 10
    c.   Chapter 11
    d.   Chapter 12

**29. Clothilde's sister has asked her to recommend an herbal therapy for her five-year-old daughter's chronic cough. In which chapter should Clothilde look for more information?**

    a.   Chapter 7
    b.   Chapter 9
    c.   Chapter 10
    d.   Chapter 12

**30. Clothilde's elderberry plant is nearly overgrown, and she is hoping to trim it back and use the elderflower to prepare a blend of tea, as well as a homemade wine. In which chapter should she look for more information about how to do this?**

    a. Chapter 3
    b. Chapter 4
    c. Chapter 5
    d. Chapter 13

**31. Clothilde realizes that she failed to maintain her elderberry plant as she should have, and she needs tips about how to keep the plant in good condition to avoid another overgrowth. In which chapter should she look for more information?**

    a. Chapter 2
    b. Chapter 3
    c. Chapter 13
    d. Chapter 14

*The next question is based on the following information.*

> LOOKING FOR ROOMMATE – CLEAN HOUSE / QUIET AREA / CLOSE TO UNIVERSITY
> Need one more female roommate for 3-bd house w/in walking distance of univ. Current occupants quiet, house clean/smoke-free. No pets. Long-term applicants preferred. Rent: $800/mo. Utilities/Internet included. Avail: Aug 15. Call Florence at 985-5687, or send an email to f.carpenter@email.com.

**32. Florence receives a number of calls about the roommate advertisement. Of the individuals described below, who seems like the best applicant?**

    a. Frances is a research assistant in the science department; she has a Yorkshire terrier.
    b. Adelaide works in the humanities department; she is looking for a three-month rental.
    c. Cosette is allergic to cigarette smoke; she needs a quiet place to study.
    d. Felix is a graduate student in the history department; he doesn't have a car.

**33. Which answer choice gives the best definition for the underlined word in the following sentence?**

**Based on the student's <u>florid</u> complexion, Vivienne knew that his nerves were getting the better of him before the debate.**

    a. rambling
    b. flushed
    c. unclear
    d. weak

*The next two questions are based on the following table.*

| COMPANY | ENGLISH BREAKFAST | EARL GREY | DARJEELING | OOLONG | GREEN |
|---|---|---|---|---|---|
| **Tea Heaven** | $25 | $27 | $26 | $32 | $30 |
| **Wholesale Tea** | $24 | $24 | $24 | $26 | $27 |
| **Tea by the Pound** | $22 | $25 | $30 | $28 | $29 |
| **Tea Express** | $25 | $28 | $26 | $29 | $30 |

Note: Prices per 16 oz. (1 pound)

**34. Noella runs a small tea shop and needs to restock. She is running very low on English Breakfast and Darjeeling tea, and she needs two pounds of each. Which company can offer her the best price on the two blends?**

    a. Tea Heaven
    b. Wholesale Tea
    c. Tea by the Pound
    d. Tea Express

**35. After reviewing her inventory, Noella realizes that she also needs one pound of Earl Grey and two pounds of green tea. Which company can offer her the best price on these two blends?**

    a. Tea Heaven
    b. Wholesale Tea
    c. Tea by the Pound
    d. Tea Express

*The next question is based on the following passage.*

When people are conducting research, particularly historical research, they usually rely on primary and secondary sources. Primary sources are the more direct type of information. They are accounts of an event that are produced by individuals who were actually present. Some examples of primary sources include a person's diary entry about an event, an interview with an eyewitness, a newspaper article, or a transcribed conversation. Secondary sources are pieces of information that are constructed through the use of other, primary sources. Often, the person who creates the secondary source was not actually present at the event. Secondary sources could include books, research papers, and magazine articles.

**36. From the passage it can be assumed that**

    a. primary sources are easier to find than secondary sources.
    b. primary sources provide more accurate information than secondary sources.
    c. secondary sources give more accurate information than primary sources.
    d. secondary sources are always used when books or articles are being written.

*The next question refers to the following graphic.*

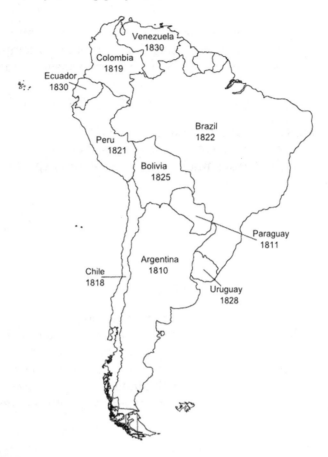

**37. The year listed with each country is when the nation gained independence. Which of the following conclusions is true?**

    a. The nations of North America were also fighting for independence at the same time as nations in South America.
    b. France lost most of its control in the New World because of these revolutions.
    c. Nations on the west coast gained independence first.
    d. South America had many revolutions in the first three decades of the 19th century.

*The next two questions are based on the following information.*

Dear library patrons:

    To ensure that all visitors have the opportunity to use our limited number of computers, we ask that each person restrict himself or herself to 30 minutes on a computer. For those needing to use a computer beyond this time frame, there will be a $3 charge for each 15-minute period.

We thank you in advance for your cooperation.

Pineville Library

**38. Which of the following is a logical conclusion that can be derived from the announcement above?**

    a. The library is planning to purchase more computers, but cannot afford them yet.

    b. The library is facing budget cuts, and is using the Internet fee to compensate for them.

    c. The library has added the fee to discourage patrons from spending too long on the computers.

    d. The library is offsetting its own Internet service costs by passing on the fee to patrons.

**39. Raoul has an upcoming school project, and his own computer is not working. He needs to use the library computer, and he has estimated that he will need to be on the computer for approximately an hour and a half. How much of a fee can Raoul expect to pay for his computer use at the library?**

    a. $6

    b. $9

    c. $12

    d. $15

*The next question is based on the following passage.*

    Victims of Marah's disease, a virtually unknown neurological condition, appear pain-free and content. Often, they also have a desire to engage in vigorous physical activities such as contact sports. Beneath it all, they are in great physical pain but have an inability to express it or act to reduce it, making diagnosis difficult. As a result, they are inaccurately diagnosed as very low on the pain scale, their discomfort level much lower than victims of severe sprains, despite the fact that sprains, although more painful, are temporary and comparatively easy to manage nature.

**40. This passage makes the argument that**

    a. the pain scale is not an accurate or adequate way to measure the physical discomfort of certain people, such as those suffering from Marah's disease

    b. sprain victims have more intense pain than Marah's sufferers, but they can manage their pain more easily

    c. the pain scale seems to put more emphasis on intensity of pain than duration

    d. victims of Marah's syndrome are often unable to deal effectively with their discomfort

*The next question is based on the following passage.*

    There is a clear formula that many students are taught when it comes to writing essays. The first is to develop an introduction, which outlines what will be discussed in the work. It also includes the thesis statement. Next come the supporting paragraphs. Each paragraph contains a topic sentence, supporting evidence, and finally a type of mini-conclusion that restates the point of the paragraph. Finally, the conclusion sums up the purpose of the paper and emphasizes that the thesis statement was proven.

**41. After the topic sentence,**

    a. a thesis statement is included.

    b. supporting evidence is presented.

    c. the conclusion is stated.

    d. the author outlines what will be discussed.

*The next question is based on the following passage.*

At one time, the use of leeches to treat medical problems was quite common. If a person suffered from a snake bite or a bee sting, leeches were believed to be capable of removing the poison from the body if they were placed on top of the wound. They have also been used for bloodletting and to stop hemorrhages, although neither of these leech treatments would be considered acceptable by present-day physicians. Today, leeches are still used on a limited basis. Most often, leeches are used to drain blood from clogged veins. This results in little pain for the patient and also ensures the patient's blood will not clot while it is being drained.

**42. The main purpose of the passage is**
   a. to discuss the benefits of using leeches to treat blocked veins.
   b. to give an overview of how leeches have been used throughout history.
   c. to compare which uses of leeches are effective and which are not.
   d. to explain how leeches can be used to remove poison from the body.

*The next two questions are based on the following passage.*

For lunch, she likes ham and cheese (torn into bites), yogurt, raisins, applesauce, peanut butter sandwiches in the fridge drawer, or any combo of these. She's not a huge eater. Help yourself too. Bread is on counter if you want to make a sandwich.

It's fine if you want to go somewhere, leave us a note of where you are. Make sure she's buckled and drive carefully! Certain fast food places are fun if they have playgrounds and are indoors. It's probably too hot for playground, but whatever you want to do is fine. Take a sippy cup of water and a diaper wherever you go. There's some money here for you in case you decide to go out for lunch with her.

As for nap, try after lunch. She may not sleep, but try anyway. Read her a couple of books first, put cream on her mosquito bites (it's in the den on the buffet), then maybe rock in her chair. Give her a bottle of milk, and refill as needed, but don't let her drink more than $2\frac{1}{2}$ bottles of milk or she'll throw up. Turn on music in her room, leave her in crib with a dry diaper and bottle to try to sleep. She likes a stuffed animal too. Try for 30–45 minutes. You may have to start the tape again. If she won't sleep, that's fine. We just call it "rest time" on those days that naps won't happen.

**43. To whom is this passage probably being written?**
   a. a mother
   b. a father
   c. a babysitter
   d. a nurse

**44. You can assume the writer of the passage is:**
   a. a mom
   b. a dad
   c. a teacher
   d. a parent

*The next two questions are based on the following passage.*

Volleyball is easy to learn and fun to play in a physical education class. With just one net and one ball, an entire class can participate. The object of the game is to get the ball over the net and onto the ground on the other side. At the same time, all players should be in the ready position to keep the ball from hitting the ground on their own side. After the ball has been served, the opposing team may have three hits to get the ball over the net to the other side. Only the serving team may score. If the receiving team wins the volley, the referee calls, "side out" and the receiving team wins the serve. Players should rotate positions so that everyone gets a chance to serve. A game is played to 15 points, but the winning team must win by two points. That means if the score is 14 to 15, the play continues until one team wins by two. A volleyball match consists of three games. The winner of the match is the team that wins two of the three games.

**45. Who can score in a volleyball game?**
    a.   the receiving team
    b.   the serving team
    c.   either team
    d.   there is no score

**46. How many people can participate in a volleyball game?**
    a.   14
    b.   15
    c.   half of a class
    d.   an entire class

*The next five questions are based on the following passage.*

Global warming and the depletion of natural resources are constant threats to the future of our planet. All people have a responsibility to be proactive participants in the fight to save Earth by working now to conserve resources for later. Participation begins with our everyday choices. From what you buy to what you do to how much you use, your decisions affect the planet and everyone around you. Now is the time to take action.

When choosing what to buy, look for sustainable products made from renewable or recycled resources. The packaging of the products you buy is just as important as the products themselves. Is the item minimally packaged in a recycled container? How did the product reach the store? Locally grown food and other products manufactured within your community are the best choices. The fewer miles a product traveled to reach you, the fewer resources it required.

You can continue to make a difference for the planet in how you use what you bought and the resources you have available. Remember the locally grown food you purchased? Don't pile it on your plate at dinner. Food that remains on your plate is a wasted resource, and you can always go back for seconds. You should try to be aware of your consumption of water and energy. Turn off the water when you brush your teeth, and limit your showers to five minutes. Turn off the lights, and don't leave appliances or chargers plugged in when not in use.

Together, we can use less, waste less, recycle more, and make the right choices. It may be the only chance we have.

**47. What is the author's tone?**

   a.  The author's tone is optimistic.

   b.  The author's tone is pessimistic.

   c.  The author's tone is matter-of-fact.

   d.  The author's tone is angry.

**48. Why does the author say it is important to buy locally grown food?**

   a.  Buying locally grown food supports people in your community.

   b.  Locally grown food travels the least distance to reach you, and therefore uses fewer resources.

   c.  Locally grown food uses less packaging.

   d.  Locally grown food is healthier for you because it has been exposed to fewer pesticides.

**49. What does the author imply will happen if people do not follow his suggestions?**

   a.  The author implies we will run out of resources in the next 10 years.

   b.  The author implies water and energy prices will rise sharply in the near future.

   c.  The author implies global warming and the depletion of natural resources will continue.

   d.  The author implies local farmers will lose their farms.

**50. "You should try to be aware of your consumption of water and energy."**

What does the word "consumption" mean in the context of this selection?

   a.  Using the greatest amount

   b.  Illness of the lungs

   c.  Using the least amount

   d.  Depletion of goods

**51. The author makes a general suggestion to the reader: "You should try to be aware of your consumption of water and energy." Which of the following is one way the author specifies that this suggestion be carried out?**

   a.  Food that remains on your plate is a wasted resource, and you can always go back for a second helping.

   b.  Locally grown food and other products manufactured within your community are the best choices.

   c.  Turn off the lights, and don't leave appliances or chargers plugged in when not in use.

   d.  Participation begins with our everyday choices.

*The next question is based on the following passage.*

The butterfly effect is a somewhat poorly understood mathematical concept, primarily because it is interpreted and presented incorrectly by the popular media. It refers to systems, and how initial conditions can influence the ultimate outcome of an event. The best way to understand the concept is through an example. You have two rubber balls. There are two inches between them, and you release them. Where will they end up? Well, that depends. If they're in a sloped, sealed container, they will end up two inches away from each other at the end of the slope. If it's the top of a mountain, however, they may end up miles away from each other. They could bounce off rocks; one could get stuck in a snow bank while the other continues down the slope; one could enter a river and get swept away. The fact that even a tiny initial difference can have a significant overall impact is known as the butterfly effect.

**52. The purpose of this passage is:**
   a.  To discuss what could happen to two rubber balls released on top of a mountain.
   b.  To show why you can predict what will happen to two objects in a sloped, sealed container.
   c.  To discuss the primary reason why the butterfly effect is a poorly understood concept.
   d.  To give an example of how small changes at the beginning of an event can have large effects.

*The next question refers to the following graphic.*

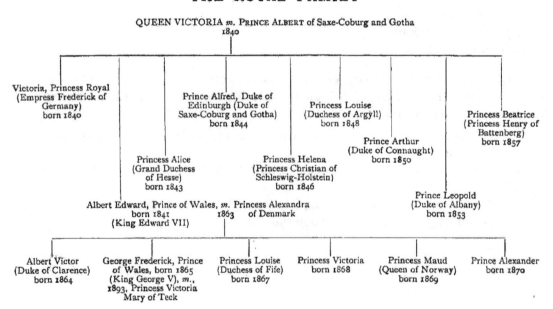

**53. In what way is the family tree organized?**
   a.  The oldest generation at the bottom, and the youngest generation at the top.
   b.  The youngest children on right and the oldest children on the left.
   c.  The youngest children on the left and the oldest children on the right.
   d.  The grandparents (Queen Victoria and Prince Albert) are on the top, followed by their children, grandchildren, and great-grandchildren on the bottom layers.

| **Mathematics** | Number of Questions: **36** |
| --- | --- |
| | Time Limit: **54 Minutes** |

1. Within a certain nursing program, 25% of the class wanted to work with infants, 60% of the class wanted to work with the elderly, 10% of the class wanted to assist general practitioners in private practices, and the rest were undecided. What fraction of the class wanted to work with the elderly?

    a. $\frac{1}{4}$

    b. $\frac{1}{10}$

    c. $\frac{3}{5}$

    d. $\frac{1}{20}$

2. Veronica has to create the holiday schedule for the neonatal unit at her hospital. She knows that 35% of the staff members will not be available because they are taking vacation days during the holiday. Of the remaining staff members who will be available, only 20% are certified to work in the neonatal unit. What percentage of the TOTAL staff is certified and available to work in the neonatal unit during the holiday?

    a. 7%
    b. 13%
    c. 65%
    d. 80%

3. A patient requires a 30% decrease in the dosage of his medication. His current dosage is 340 mg. What will his dosage be after the decrease?

    a. 70 mg
    b. 238 mg
    c. 270 mg
    d. 340 mg

4. A study about anorexia was conducted on 100 patients. Within that patient population 70% were women, and 10% of the men were overweight as children. How many male patients in the study were NOT overweight as children?

    a. 3
    b. 10
    c. 27
    d. 30

5. University Q has an extremely competitive nursing program. Historically, $\frac{3}{4}$ of the students in each incoming class major in nursing but only $\frac{1}{5}$ of those who major in nursing actually complete the program. If this year's incoming class has 100 students, how many students will complete the nursing program?

    a. 75
    b. 20
    c. 15
    d. 5

*The next two questions are based on the following information.*

> Four nurse midwives open a joint practice together. They use a portion of the income to pay for various expenses for the practice. Each nurse midwife contributes $2000 per month.

**6. The first midwife uses $\frac{2}{5}$ of her monthly contribution to pay the rent and utilities for the office space. She saves half of the remainder for incidental expenditures, and uses the rest of the money to purchase medical supplies. How much money does she spend on medical supplies each month?**

    a.  $600
    b.  $800
    c.  $1000
    d.  $1200

**7. The second midwife allocates $\frac{1}{2}$ of her funds to pay an office administrator, plus another $\frac{1}{10}$ for office supplies. What is the total fraction of the second midwife's budget that is spent on the office administrator and office supplies?**

    a.  $\frac{3}{5}$
    b.  $\frac{2}{12}$
    c.  $\frac{2}{20}$
    d.  $\frac{1}{20}$

**8. A mathematics test has a 4:2 ratio of data analysis problems to algebra problems. If the test has 18 algebra problems, how many data analysis problems are on the test?**

    a.  24
    b.  28
    c.  36
    d.  38

**9. Jonathan pays a $65 monthly flat rate for his cell phone. He is charged $0.12 per minute for each minute used, in a roaming area. Which of the following expressions represents his monthly cell phone bill for *x* roaming minutes?**

    a.  $65 + 0.12x$
    b.  $65x + 0.12$
    c.  $65.12x$
    d.  $65.12 + 0.12x$

**10. Robert is planning to drive 1,800 miles on a cross-country trip. If his car gets 30 miles to the gallon, and his tank holds 12 gallons of gas, how many tanks of gas will he need to complete the trip?**

    a.  3 tanks of gas
    b.  5 tanks of gas
    c.  30 tanks of gas
    d.  60 tanks of gas

11. A patient was taking 310 mg of antidepressant each day. However, the doctor determined that this dosage was too high and reduced the dosage by a fifth. Further observation revealed the dose was still too high, so he reduced it again by 20 mg. What is the final dosage of the patient's antidepressant?

    a.  20 mg
    b.  42 mg
    c.  228 mg
    d.  248 mg

12. A lab technician took 100 hairs from a patient to conduct several tests. The technician used $\frac{1}{7}$ of the hairs for a drug test. How many hairs were used for the drug test? Round your answer to the nearest hundredth.

    a.  14.00
    b.  14.20
    c.  14.29
    d.  14.30

13. What kind of association does the scatter plot show?

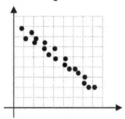

    a.  Positive, Linear Association
    b.  Negative, Linear Association
    c.  Non-linear Association
    d.  No association can be determined

14. Joshua has to earn more than 92 points on the state test in order to qualify for an academic scholarship. Each question is worth 4 points, and the test has a total of 30 questions. Let $x$ represent the number of test questions. Which of the following inequalities can be solved to determine the number of questions Joshua must answer correctly?

    a.  $4x < 30$
    b.  $4x < 92$
    c.  $4x > 30$
    d.  $4x > 92$

15. Susan decided to celebrate getting her first nursing job by purchasing a new outfit. She bought a dress for $69.99 and a pair of shoes for $39.99. She also bought accessories for $34.67. What was the total cost of Susan's outfit, including accessories?

    a.  $69.99
    b.  $75.31
    c.  $109.98
    d.  $144.65

**16. Given the histograms shown below, which of the following statements is true?**

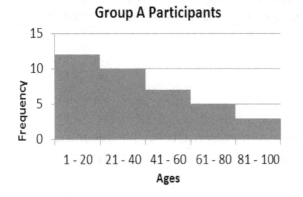

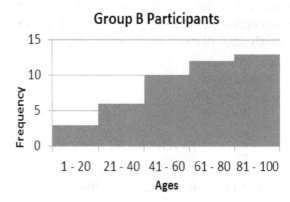

a. Group A is negatively skewed and has a mean that is less than the mean of Group B.
b. Group A is positively skewed and has a mean that is more than the mean of Group B.
c. Group B is negatively skewed and has a mean that is more than the mean of Group A.
d. Group B is positively skewed and has a mean that is less than the mean of Group A.

**17. Complete the following equation:**

$$2 + (2)(2) - 2 \div 2 = ?$$

a. 5
b. 3
c. 2
d. 1

**18. Which of the following is listed in order from *least to greatest*?**

a. $-2, -\frac{3}{4}, -0.45, 3\%, 0.36$
b. $-\frac{3}{4}, -0.45, -2, 0.36, 3\%$
c. $-0.45, -2, -\frac{3}{4}, 3\%, 0.36$
d. $-2, -\frac{3}{4}, -0.45, 0.36, 3\%$

**19. As part of a study, a set of patients will be divided into three groups: $\frac{4}{15}$ of the patients will be in Group Alpha, $\frac{2}{5}$ of the patients will be in Group Beta, and $\frac{1}{3}$ of the patients will be in Group Gamma. Order the groups from smallest to largest, according to the number of patients in each group.**

a. Group Alpha, Group Beta, Group Gamma
b. Group Alpha, Group Gamma, Group Beta
c. Group Gamma, Group Alpha, Group Beta
d. Group Gamma, Group Beta, Group Alpha

20. Solve for $x$:

$$2x + 6 = 14$$

   a. $x = 4$
   b. $x = 8$
   c. $x = 10$
   d. $x = 13$

21. In the 2008 Olympic Games, the semifinal heat for the Women's 200m event had the following results:

| Time (in seconds) |
|---|
| 22.33 |
| 22.50 |
| 22.50 |
| 22.61 |
| 22.71 |
| 22.72 |
| 22.83 |
| 23.22 |

What was the mean time for the women who ran this 200m event?

   a. 22.50 sec
   b. 22.66 sec
   c. 22.68 sec
   d. 22.77 sec

22. During week 1, Nurse Cameron worked 5 shifts. During week 2, she worked twice as many shifts as she did during week 1. During week 3, she added 4 shifts to the number of shifts she worked during week 2. Which equation below describes the number of shifts Nurse Cameron worked during week 3?

   a. shifts $= (2)(5) + 4$
   b. shifts $= (4)(5) + 2$
   c. shifts $= 5 + 2 + 4$
   d. shifts $= (5)(2)(4)$

23. Simplify the following expression:

$$(3)(-4) + (3)(4) - 1$$

   a. $-1$
   b. 1
   c. 23
   d. 24

24. **How many cubic inches of water could this aquarium hold if it were filled completely?**

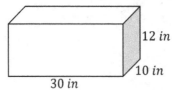

12 *in*

10 *in*

30 *in*

   a. 3600 cubic inches
   b. 52 cubic inches
   c. 312 cubic inches
   d. 1144 cubic inches

25. **What statement best describes the rate of change?**

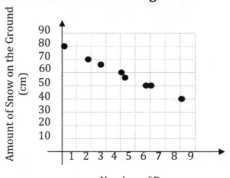

   a. Every day, the snow melts 10 centimeters.
   b. Every day, the snow melts 5 centimeters.
   c. Every day, the snow increases by 10 centimeters.
   d. Every day, the snow increases by 5 centimeters.

26. What are the dependent and independent variables in the graph below?

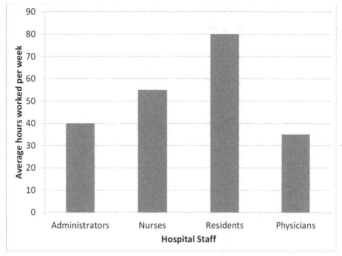

a. The dependent variable is Nurses. The independent variable is Physicians.
b. The dependent variable is Physicians. The independent variable is Nurses.
c. The dependent variable is Hospital Staff. The independent variable is Average hours worked per week.
d. The dependent variable is Average hours worked per week. The independent variable is Hospital Staff.

27. How many milligrams are in 5 grams?

a. 0.005 mg
b. 50 mg
c. 500 mg
d. 5000 mg

28. 9.5% of the people in a town voted for a certain proposition in a municipal election. If the town's population is 51,623, about how many people in the town voted for the proposition?

a. 3,000
b. 5,000
c. 7,000
d. 10,000

29. A charter bus driver drove at an average speed of 65 mph for 305 miles. If he stops at a gas station for 15 minutes, then drives another 162 miles at an average speed of 80 mph, how long, will it have been since he began the trip?

a. 0.96 hours
b. 6.44 hours
c. 6.69 hours
d. 6.97 hours

30. A box in the form of a rectangular solid has a square base of 5 feet in length, a width of 5 feet, and a height of $h$ feet. If the volume of the rectangular solid is 200 cubic feet, which of the following equations may be used to find $h$?

  a.  $5h = 200$
  b.  $5h^2 = 200$
  c.  $25h = 200$
  d.  $h = 200 \div 5$

31. Two even integers and one odd integer are multiplied together. Which of the following could be their product?

  a.  3.75
  b.  9
  c.  16.2
  d.  24

32. There are $\frac{80\ mg}{0.8\ ml}$ in Acetaminophen Concentrated Infant Drops. If the proper dosage for a four-year-old child is 240 mg, how many milliliters should the child receive?

  a.  0.8 mL
  b.  1.6 mL
  c.  2.4 mL
  d.  3.2 mL

33. Using the chart below, which equation describes the relationship between $x$ and $y$?

| $x$ | $y$ |
|---|---|
| 2 | 6 |
| 3 | 9 |
| 4 | 12 |
| 5 | 15 |

  a.  $x = 3y$
  b.  $y = 3x$
  c.  $y = \frac{1}{3}x$
  d.  $\frac{x}{y} = 3$

34. On a highway map, the scale indicates that 1 inch represents 45 miles. If the distance on the map is 3.2 inches, how far is the actual distance?

  a.  45 miles
  b.  54 miles
  c.  112 miles
  d.  144 miles

35. Andy has already saved $15. He plans to save $28 per month. Which of the following equations represents the amount of money he will have saved?

  a.  $y = 15 + 28x$
  b.  $y = 43x + 15$
  c.  $y = 43x$
  d.  $y = 28 + 15x$

36. Given the double bar graph shown below, which of the following statements is true?

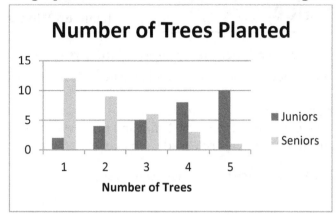

a. The number of trees planted by the Juniors is positively skewed, while the number of trees planted by the Seniors is approximately normal.
b. The number of trees planted by the Juniors is negatively skewed, while the number of trees planted by the Seniors is positively skewed.
c. The number of trees planted by the Juniors is positively skewed, while the number of trees planted by the Seniors is negatively skewed.
d. The number of trees planted by the Juniors is approximately normal, while the number of trees planted by the Juniors is positively skewed.

| | Number of Questions: **53** |
| :---: | :--- |
| **Science** | Time Limit: **63 Minutes** |

**1. Which of the following is NOT a function of the circulatory system?**

    a. Pumping blood throughout the body to provide tissues and organs with nutrients and oxygen.

    b. Removing toxins and waste from the blood

    c. Transmitting nerve impulses between the brain and the rest of the body.

    d. Transporting important hormones released from glands to their sites of action.

**2. Which item below is NOT a disease of the digestive system?**

    a. Crohn's disease.

    b. Diabetes.

    c. Ulcerative colitis.

    d. Diverticulosis.

**3. Which item below best describes the primary function of the nervous system?**

    a. The nervous system is the center of communication in the body.

    b. The nervous system is primarily responsible for helping the body breathe.

    c. The nervous system transports blood throughout the body.

    d. The nervous system helps the body break down food.

**4. Which of the following is NOT an element of the respiratory system?**

    a. Ribs.

    b. Trachea.

    c. Diaphragm.

    d. Alveoli.

**5. Which of the following cells is NOT part of the immune system?**

    a. Neurons.

    b. Dendritic cells.

    c. Macrophages.

    d. Mast cells.

**6. Which of the following is NOT one of the major types of bones in the human body?**

    a. Dense bone.

    b. Long bone.

    c. Short bone.

    d. Irregular bone.

**7. Which of the following bone types is embedded in tendons?**

    a. Long bones.

    b. Sesamoid bones.

    c. Flat bones.

    d. Vertical bones.

**8. Two nursing students will be completing a scientific experiment measuring the mass of chewed gum after one-minute chewing increments. Which lab equipment will the students most likely use?**

    a.  Triple beam balance.
    b.  Anemometer.
    c.  Hot plate.
    d.  Microscope.

**9. Which of the following is not a product of respiration?**

    a.  Carbon dioxide.
    b.  Water.
    c.  Oxygen.
    d.  ATP.

**10. Of the following, the blood vessel containing the least-oxygenated blood is:**

    a.  the aorta.
    b.  the vena cava.
    c.  the pulmonary artery.
    d.  the capillaries.

**11. Which layer of the heart contains striated muscle fibers for contraction of the heart?**

    a.  Pericardium.
    b.  Epicardium.
    c.  Endocardium.
    d.  Myocardium.

**12. Which blood vessel carries oxygenated blood back to the heart?**

    a.  Pulmonary vein.
    b.  Pulmonary artery.
    c.  Aorta.
    d.  Superior vena cava.

**13. Mrs. Jones's class conducted an experiment on the effects of sugar and artificial sweetener on the cookie recipe's overall color when baked. What would be the independent variable in the cookie experiment?**

    a.  The students should use the same ingredients in both recipes, but bake the cookies with sugar at 450 degrees and those with artificial sweetener at 475 degrees. They should increase the baking time on the artificial sweetener cookies, since the package instructs them to do so.
    b.  The students should use the same ingredients in both recipes, but increase the baking time on the artificial sweetener cookies, since the package instructs them to do so.
    c.  The students should use the same ingredients, same baking temperatures, and same baking times for both recipes.
    d.  The students should use the same ingredients and baking times in both recipes, but bake the cookies with sugar at 450 degrees and the artificial sweetener cookies at 475 degrees.

**14. Which part of the cell is often called the cell "power house" because it provides energy for cellular functions?**

    a.  Nucleus.

    b.  Cell membrane.

    c.  Mitochondria.

    d.  Cytoplasm.

**15. What function do ribosomes serve within the cell?**

    a.  Ribosomes are responsible for cell movement.

    b.  Ribosomes aid in protein synthesis.

    c.  Ribosomes help protect the cell from its environment.

    d.  Ribosomes have enzymes that help with digestion.

**16. What is the most likely reason that cells differentiate?**

    a.  Cells differentiate to avoid looking like all the cells around them.

    b.  Cells differentiate so that simple, non-specialized cells can become highly specialized cells.

    c.  Cells differentiate so that multicellular organisms will remain the same size.

    d.  Cells differentiate for no apparent reason.

**17. How is meiosis similar to mitosis?**

    a.  Both produce daughter cells that are genetically identical.

    b.  Both produce daughter cells that are genetically different.

    c.  Both occur in humans, animals, and plants.

    d.  Both occur asexually.

**18. In the suburban neighborhood of Northwoods, there have been large populations of deer, and residents have complained about them eating flowers and garden plants. What would be a logical explanation, based on observations, for the large increase in the deer population over the last two seasons?**

    a.  Increased quantity of food sources in surrounding areas.

    b.  Decreased population of a natural predator in Northwoods.

    c.  Deer migration from surrounding areas.

    d.  Increase in hunting licenses sold.

**19. How do DNA and RNA function together as part of the human genome?**

    a.  DNA carries genetic information from RNA to the cell cytoplasm.

    b.  RNA carries genetic information from DNA to the cell cytoplasm.

    c.  DNA and RNA carry genetic information from the cell nucleus to the cytoplasm.

    d.  DNA and RNA do not interact within the cell.

**20. The majority of nutrient absorption occurs in the:**

    a.  mouth.

    b.  stomach.

    c.  small intestine.

    d.  large intestine.

**21. What process should the DNA within a cell undergo before cell replication?**

    a. The DNA should quadruple so that daughter cells have more than enough DNA material after cell division.

    b. The DNA should triple so that daughter cells have three times the amount of DNA material after cell division.

    c. The DNA should replicate so that daughter cells have the same amount of DNA material after cell division.

    d. The DNA should split so that daughter cells have half the amount of DNA material after cell division.

**22. What basic molecular unit enables hereditary information to be transmitted from parent to offspring?**

    a. Genes.

    b. Blood.

    c. Traits.

    d. Cell.

**23. Which statement most accurately compares and contrasts the structures of DNA and RNA?**

    a. Both DNA and RNA have 4 nucleotide bases. Three of the bases are the same but the fourth base is thymine in DNA and uracil in RNA.

    b. Both DNA and RNA have the same 4 nucleotide bases. However, the nucleotides bond differently in the DNA when compared to RNA.

    c. Both DNA and RNA have 6 nucleotide bases. However, the shape of DNA is a triple helix and the shape of RNA is a double helix.

    d. Both DNA and RNA have a double helix structure. However, DNA contains 6 nucleotide bases and RNA contains 4 nucleotide bases.

**24. Which of the following characteristics is part of a person's genotype?**

    a. Brown eyes that appear hazel in the sunlight.

    b. CFTR genes that causes cystic fibrosis.

    c. Black hair that grows rapidly.

    d. Being a fast runner.

*The next two questions are based on the following information.*

Let $B$ represent the dominant gene for a full head of hair, and let $b$ represent the recessive gene for male pattern baldness. The following Punnett square represents the offspring of two people with recessive genes for baldness.

|   | **B** | **b** |
|---|---|---|
| **B** | Possibility 1 | Possibility 2 |
| **b** | Possibility 3 | Possibility 4 |

**25. According to the Punnett square, which selection includes all outcomes that would produce an offspring with male pattern baldness?**

    a. Possibility 1.

    b. Possibility 4.

    c. Possibilities 1, 2, and 3.

    d. Possibilities 2, 3, and 4.

**26. According to the Punnett square, which selection includes all outcomes that would produce an offspring with a full head of hair?**

    a. Possibility 1.

    b. Possibility 4.

    c. Possibilities 1, 2, and 3.

    d. Possibilities 2, 3, and 4.

**27. Where is the interstitial fluid found?**

    a. In the blood and lymphatic vessels.

    b. In the tissues around cells.

    c. In the cells.

    d. In the ventricles of the brain.

**28. Which type of cell secretes antibodies?**

    a. Bacterial cell.

    b. Viral cell.

    c. Lymph cell.

    d. Plasma cells.

**29. Chemical C is a catalyst in the reaction between chemical A and chemical B. What is the effect of chemical C?**

    a. Chemical C increases the rate of the reaction between A and B.

    b. Chemical C decreases the rate of the reaction between A and B.

    c. Chemical C initiates the reaction between A and B.

    d. Chemical C converts A from a base to an acid.

**30. What type of molecules are enzymes?**

    a. Water molecules.

    b. Protein molecules.

    c. Tripolar molecules.

    d. Inorganic molecules.

**31. Which structure controls the hormones secreted by the pituitary gland?**

    a. Hypothalamus.

    b. Adrenal gland.

    c. Testes.

    d. Pancreas.

**32. Where does gas exchange occur in the human body?**

    a. Alveoli.

    b. Bronchi.

    c. Larynx.

    d. Pharynx.

**33. All of the following are parts of the respiratory system EXCEPT the:**

    a. trachea.

    b. bronchi.

    c. esophagus.

    d. larynx.

**34. What lab equipment would most likely be used to measure a liquid solution?**

   a. Flask.
   b. Triple beam balance.
   c. Graduated cylinder.
   d. Test tube.

**35. An atom has 5 protons, 5 neutrons, and 6 electrons. What is the electric charge of this atom?**

   a. Neutral.
   b. Positive.
   c. Negative.
   d. Undetermined.

**36. All of the following are components of the genitourinary system EXCEPT:**

   a. the kidneys.
   b. the urethra.
   c. the rectum.
   d. the bladder.

**37. Which of the following best describes the structures found underneath each rib in descending order?**

   a. Vein, nerve, artery.
   b. Artery, vein, nerve.
   c. Vein, artery, nerve.
   d. Nerve, vein, artery.

*The table below contains information from the periodic table of elements.*

| Element | Atomic number | Approximate atomic weight |
| --- | --- | --- |
| H | 1 | 1 |
| He | 2 | 4 |
| Li | 3 | 7 |
| Be | 4 | 9 |

**38. Which pattern below best describes the elements listed in the table?**

   a. The elements are arranged in order by weight with H being the heaviest atom and Be being the lightest atom.
   b. The elements are arranged in order by electron charge with H having the most electrons and Be having the fewest electrons.
   c. The elements are arranged in order by protons with H having the most protons and Be having the fewest protons.
   d. The elements are arranged in order by protons with H having the fewest protons and Be having the most protons.

**39. Which of the following is true regarding the primary function of the spleen?**

   a. It produces bile to emulsify fats.
   b. It filters microorganisms and other foreign substances from the blood.
   c. It helps control blood glucose levels and regulates blood pressure.
   d. It regulates blood clotting factors.

**40. The process of changing from a liquid to a gas is called _____.**

    a. freezing
    b. condensation
    c. vaporization
    d. sublimation

**41. A nurse wants to investigate how different environmental factors affect her patients' body temperatures. Which tool would be the most helpful when the nurse conducts her investigation?**

    a. Scale.
    b. Yard stick.
    c. Thermometer.
    d. Blood pressure monitor.

**42. A scientific study has over 2000 data points. Which of the following methods is most likely to help the researcher gain usable information from the data?**

    a. Use statistical analysis to understand trends in the data.
    b. Look at each individual data point, and try to create a trend.
    c. Eliminate 90% of the data so that the sample size is more manageable.
    d. Stare at the data until a pattern pops out.

*The next question is based on the following information.*

> Many years ago, people believed that flies were created from spoiled food because spoiled food that was left out in the open often contained fly larvae. So a scientist placed fresh food in a sealed container for an extended period of time. The food spoiled, but no fly larvae were found in the food that was sealed.

**43. Based on this evidence, what is the most likely reason that spoiled food left out in the open often contained fly larvae?**

    a. The spoiled food evolved into fly larvae.
    b. Since the food was left out in the open, flies would lay eggs in the food.
    c. Fly larvae were spontaneously generated by the spoiled food.
    d. People only imagined they saw fly larvae in the spoiled food.

**44. The average life expectancy in the 21st century is about 75 years. The average life expectancy in the 19th century was about 40 years. What is a possible explanation for the longer life expectancy in the present age?**

    a. Advances in medical technology enable people to live longer.
    b. Knowledge about how basic cleanliness can help avoid illness has enabled people to live longer.
    c. The creation of various vaccines has enabled people to live longer.
    d. All of the statements above offer reasonable explanations for longer life expectancy.

**45. A doctor needs to convince his boss to approve a test for a patient. Which statement below best communicates a scientific argument that justifies the need for the test?**

    a.  The patient looks like he needs this test.

    b.  The doctor feels that the patient needs this test.

    c.  The patient's symptoms and health history suggest that this test will enable the correct diagnosis to help the patient.

    d.  The patient has excellent insurance that will pay for several tests, and the doctor would like to run as many tests as possible.

**46. Which of the following is a protein that interferes with virus production?**

    a.  Lysozyme.

    b.  Prion.

    c.  Interferon.

    d.  Keratin.

**47. Which of the following does not contain blood vessels?**

    a.  Hyperdermis.

    b.  Hypodermis.

    c.  Dermis.

    d.  Epidermis.

**48. What structure is responsible for the release of hormones that stimulate the gonads during puberty?**

    a.  Hypothalamus.

    b.  Midbrain.

    c.  Basal ganglia.

    d.  Hippocampus.

**49. Which of the following structures has the lowest blood pressure?**

    a.  Arteries.

    b.  Arteriole.

    c.  Venule.

    d.  Vein.

**50. Which of the heart chambers is the most muscular?**

    a.  Left atrium.

    b.  Right atrium.

    c.  Left ventricle.

    d.  Right ventricle.

**51. Which part of the brain interprets sensory information?**

    a.  Cerebrum.

    b.  Hindbrain.

    c.  Cerebellum.

    d.  Medulla oblongata.

**52. A vaccination is a way of acquiring which type of immunity?**

    a.   Passive natural immunity.
    b.   Active natural immunity.
    c.   Active artificial immunity.
    d.   Passive artificial immunity.

**53. Which component of the nervous system is responsible for lowering the heart rate?**

    a.   Central nervous system.
    b.   Sympathetic nervous system.
    c.   Parasympathetic nervous system.
    d.   Distal nervous system.

| **English and Language Usage** | Number of Questions: 28 |
|---|---|
| | Time Limit: 28 Minutes |

**1. Which of the following sentences shows the correct way to separate the items in the series?**

a.   These are actual cities in the United States: Unalaska, Alaska; Yreka, California; Two Egg, Florida; and Boring, Maryland.

b.   These are actual cities in the United States: Unalaska; Alaska, Yreka; California, Two Egg; Florid, and Boring; Maryland.

c.   These are actual cities in the United States: Unalaska, Alaska, Yreka, California, Two Egg, Florida, and Boring, Maryland.

d.   These are actual cities in the United States: Unalaska Alaska, Yreka California, Two Egg Florida, and Boring Maryland.

**2. Choose the sentence that most effectively follows the conventions of Standard Written English:**

a.   Wilbur and Orville Wright were two brothers, and they tested their prototype airplane on a beach in Kitty Hawk, North Carolina.

b.   The two brothers, Wilbur and Orville Wright, tested their prototype airplane on a beach in Kitty Hawk, North Carolina.

c.   Testing their prototype airplane on a beach in Kitty Hawk, North Carolina, were the two brothers, Wilbur and Orville Wright.

d.   The beach in Kitty Hawk, North Carolina was where the two brothers, Wilbur and Orville Wright, came and tested their prototype airplane.

**3. Which of the following types of language are not appropriate in a research paper?**

a.   colloquialisms

b.   contractions

c.   relative pronouns

d.   both A and B

**4. Which of the following sentences demonstrates the correct use of an apostrophe?**

a.   Lyle works for the courthouse, and among his responsibilities is getting the jurors meal's.

b.   Lyle works for the courthouse, and among his responsibilities is getting the juror's meals.

c.   Lyle works for the courthouse, and among his responsibilities is getting the jurors' meals.

d.   Lyle works for the courthouse, and among his responsibilities is getting the jurors meals'.

**5. Which of the following is a complex sentence?**

a.   Milton's favorite meal is spaghetti and meatballs, along with a side salad and garlic toast.

b.   Before Ernestine purchases a book, she always checks to see if the library has it.

c.   Desiree prefers warm, sunny weather, but her twin sister Destiny likes a crisp, cold day.

d.   Ethel, Ben, and Alice are working together on a school project about deteriorating dams.

**6. Which of the answer choices gives the best definition of the underlined word in the following sentence?**

Finlay flatly refused to take part in the piano recital, so his parents had to <u>cajole</u> him with the promise of a trip to his favorite toy store.

    a. prevent
    b. threaten
    c. insist
    d. coax

**7. Which of the following nouns is the correct plural form of the word *tempo*?**

    a. tempo
    b. tempae
    c. tempi
    d. tempos

**8. Which of the following sentences follows the rules of capitalization?**

    a. Kristia knows that her aunt Jo will be visiting, but she is not sure if her uncle will be there as well.
    b. During a visit to the monastery, Jess interviewed brother Mark about the daily prayer schedule.
    c. Leah spoke to her Cousin Martha about her summer plans to drive from Colorado to Arizona.
    d. Justinia will be staying with family in Chicago during the early Fall.

**9. Which of the answer choices gives the best definition of the underlined word in the following sentence?**

The discussion over the new park had begun well, but it soon descended into an <u>acrimonious</u> debate over misuse of tax revenues.

    a. shocking
    b. childish
    c. rancorous
    d. revealing

**10. Which of the following sentences does NOT use correct punctuation to separate independent clauses?**

    a. Anne likes to add salsa to her scrambled eggs; Gordon unaccountably likes his with peanut butter.
    b. Anne likes to add salsa to her scrambled eggs, however Gordon unaccountably likes his with peanut butter.
    c. Anne likes to add salsa to her scrambled eggs. Gordon unaccountably likes his with peanut butter.
    d. Anne likes to add salsa to her scrambled eggs, but Gordon unaccountably likes his with peanut butter.

**11. Considering both style and clarity, which of the answer choices best combines the following sentences?**

**Fenella wanted to attend the concert. She also wanted to attend the reception at the art gallery. She tried to find a way to do both in one evening. She failed.**

    a. Although Fenella wanted to attend the concert, she also wanted to attend the reception at the art gallery, so she tried to find a way to do both in one evening. She failed.

    b. Fenella wanted to attend both the concert and the reception at the art gallery, but she failed to find a way to do both in one evening.

    c. Fenella failed to find a way to attend both the concert and the reception at the art gallery.

    d. Because Fenella wanted to attend both the concert and the reception at the art gallery, she tried to find a way to do both in one evening. Unfortunately, she failed.

**12. Which of the answer choices gives the best definition of the underlined word in the following sentence?**

**Mara enjoyed great <u>felicity</u> when her missing dog found his way home.**

    a. Discomfort

    b. Anxiety

    c. Disbelief

    d. Happiness

**13. Based on the definition of the word *permeate* "to penetrate or pervade," which of the following is the most likely meaning of the prefix *per-*?**

    a. across

    b. by

    c. with

    d. through

**14. The following words share a common Greek-based suffix: *anthropology*, *cosmetology*, *etymology*, and *genealogy*. What is the most likely meaning of the suffix *-logy*?**

    a. record

    b. study

    c. affinity

    d. fear

**15. Which of the following words functions as an adverb in the sentence below?**

**Jacob had been worried about the speech, but in the end he did well.**

    a. worried

    b. about

    c. but

    d. well

**16. Which of the following would belong in a formal speech?**

    a. We all need to work together to make this school better. First, we need to organize a list of our issues. Then we need to form small groups to discuss them and find solutions. Finally, we need to implement those solutions.

    b. Our purpose is to work together to improve the quality of education at this school. Ideally, we need to organize a list of our issues. Secondly, we need to form small groups to discuss them and find solutions. Then, we need to implement some solutions.

    c. We all got to work together to make this school much better than before. First, we need to say what is on our mind. We got to form small groups to discuss them and find solutions. And, we need to talk about those solutions.

    d. It is possible for us to talk about the problems in school and solve them. Of course, we need to organize a list of our issues. For example, we should form small groups to discuss them and find solutions. Finally, we need to implement those solutions.

**17. Which of the following sentences contains a correct example of subject-verb agreement?**

    a. Neither Jeanne nor Pauline like the dinner options on the menu.

    b. All of the council likes the compromise that they have reached about property taxes.

    c. The faculty of the math department were unable to agree on the curriculum changes.

    d. Both Clara and Don feels that they need to be more proactive in checking on the contractors.

**18. Which of the answer choices gives the best definition of the underlined word in the following sentence?**

**The guest speaker was undoubtedly an <u>erudite</u> scholar, but his comments on nomological determinism seemed to go over the heads of the students in the audience.**

    a. authentic

    b. arrogant

    c. faulty

    d. knowledgeable

**19. What is the correct spelling of the word that completes the following sentence?**

**Wearing white to a funeral is considered by many to be ____.**

    a. sacrelegious

    b. sacriligious

    c. sacrilegious

    d. sacreligious

**20. What is the most effective way to combine the two sentences below?**

**German cuisine is known for its hearty, meat and potato dishes. Families often enjoy a rich Sunday dinner of roast meat, potatoes, and cabbage.**

    a. German cuisine is known for its hearty, meat and potato dishes but families often enjoy a rich Sunday dinner of roast meat, potatoes, and cabbage.

    b. German cuisine is known for its hearty, meat and potato dishes, but families often enjoy a rich Sunday dinner of roast meat, potatoes, and cabbage.

    c. German cuisine is known for its hearty, meat and potato dishes, and families often enjoy a rich Sunday dinner of roast meat, potatoes and cabbage.

    d. German cuisine is known for its hearty, meat and potato dishes, and families often enjoy a rich Sunday dinner of roast meat, potatoes, and cabbage.

**21. Which of the following is a simple sentence?**

   a.  Ben likes baseball, but Joseph likes basketball.

   b.  It looks like rain; be sure to bring an umbrella.

   c.  Although he was tired, Edgar still attended the recital.

   d.  Marjorie and Thomas planned an exciting trip to Maui.

**22. Which of the following words functions as a pronoun in the sentence below?**

**Anne-Charlotte and I will be driving together to the picnic this weekend.**

   a.  be

   b.  this

   c.  together

   d.  I

**23. Which of the following sentences is the best in terms of style, clarity, and conciseness?**

   a.  Ava has a leap year birthday; she is really twenty, and her friends like to joke that she is only five years old.

   b.  Because Ava has a leap year birthday, her friends like to joke that she is only five years old when she is really twenty.

   c.  Ava is twenty years old, her friends like to joke that she is five because she has a leap year birthday.

   d.  Although Ava has a leap year birthday, she is twenty years old, but her friends like to joke that she is five.

**24. Which of the answer choices gives the best definition of the underlined word in the following sentence?**

**The housekeeper Mrs. Vanderbroek had a fixed daily routine for running the manor and was not particularly <u>amenable</u> to any suggested changes.**

   a.  capable

   b.  agreeable

   c.  obstinate

   d.  critical

**25. Which of the following words does not function as an adjective in the sentence below?**

**A quick review of all available housing options indicated that Casper had little choice but to rent for now and wait for a better time to buy.**

   a.  quick

   b.  available

   c.  little

   d.  rent

**26. What is the most effective way to combine the two sentences below?**

**A lot of teens express themselves through fashion. Since many teens start earning their own money, they can buy their own clothes and choose the fashions that they want.**

  a. A lot of teens express themselves through fashion, and since many teens start earning their own money, they can buy their own clothes and choose the fashions that they want.
  b. A lot of teens express themselves through fashion and since many teens start earning their own money, they can buy their own clothes and choose the fashions that they want.
  c. A lot of teens express themselves through fashion, but since many teens start earning their own money, they can buy their own clothes and choose the fashions that they want.
  d. A lot of teens express themselves through fashion but since many teens start earning their own money, they can buy their own clothes and choose the fashions that they want.

**27. Use of formal language would be LEAST essential when addressing which of the following audiences?**

  a. a board of directors
  b. a grammar school class
  c. a gathering of college professors
  d. none of the above

**28. Which of the following words correctly fills in the blank in the sentence below?**

**The Bill of Rights protects the right to ____ arms, but one common mistake is to spell this as though the Founding Fathers were ensuring the right to go sleeveless.**

  a. bear
  b. bare
  c. barre
  d. baire

# Answer Key and Explanations for Test #2

## Reading

**1. B:** The word *intermittent* suggests that something occurs at imprecise intervals, so answer choice B is the best synonym. Answer choices A and D suggest the exact opposite of the meaning indicated in the sentence. Answer choice C likely reflects another element of the woman's labor, but it has nothing to do with the meaning of the word *intermittent*.

**2. C:** All of these are good sources to use while developing a position on Civil Rights; nonetheless, first you must first familiarize yourself with an overview of the issue. A history textbook probably would be the most comprehensive and the least affected by personal opinion. Speeches, interviews, and blogs are great next steps in the research process, but these choices may prove too subjective to provide a necessary overview of the issue.

**3. C:** The correct answer is *abundance.* The sentence suggests that Kit has more zucchini than she needs, and is therefore trying to offload zucchini on anyone who might want some. The *plethora* might lead to a mild *irritation*, but the words are definitely not synonyms. (In some cases, a *plethora* is certainly not an irritation.) The word *plethora* is related to a *quantity*, but it is a specific type of quantity: an excess. Because the word *quantity* can also describe a lack of something, these words are not synonyms. Kit is obviously trying to avoid *waste*, but the words *plethora* and *waste* are not synonyms. *Waste* would also not be a natural replacement for *plethora* in the sentence.

**4. C:** Only the word *neglect* can fall between the guide words *needs* and *negotiate* on a dictionary page. The words *needle* and *nectar* would come before *needs*, and the word *neigh* would follow *negotiate*.

**5. D:** The chapter title refers to the *fictional* works of Dorothy L. Sayers, and letters generally do not fall under the category of fiction. Novels, plays, and mysteries, however, usually do.

**6. C:** An expository passage seeks to *expose* information by explaining or defining it in detail. As this passage focuses on describing the written works of Dorothy L. Sayers, it may safely be considered expository. The author is not necessarily telling a story, something one might expect from a strictly narrative passage. (Additionally, the author's main point, that of explaining why Sayers was such a versatile writer, represents a kind of thesis statement for shaping the overall focus of the passage. A narrative passage would focus more on simply telling the story of Sayers's life.) At no point is the author attempting to persuade the reader about anything, and there is nothing particularly technical about the passage. Rather, it is a focused look at Sayers's educational background and how she developed into a writer of many genres; this makes it solidly expository.

**7. A:** As indicated in the answer explanation above, the main focus of the passage is Sayers's versatility as a writer. The first paragraph notes this and then begins discussing her education, introducing the experience that would inform her later accomplishments. The second paragraph then follows this up with specifics about the types of writing she did. Answer choice B would be correct if the passage were more narrative than expository. Answer choices C and D focus on specific works for which Sayers is remembered, but both are too limited to be considered a representative summary of the entire passage.

**8. B:** The mention of an "unexpectedly good education" represents an opinion on the part of the author. As the author does not follow this up with an explanation about *why* such an education would be unexpectedly good, the statement is simply a moment of bias on the author's part, rather than an element within the larger argument. There is no bias in the other answer choices. Answer choices A and C are factual statements about Sayers's life and work. Answer choice D, while it might hint vaguely at disapproval on the author's part (who might, perhaps, wish to know Sayers's reasons), is not necessarily a statement containing bias. It is indeed true that Sayers turned down the doctorate of divinity, and it is also true that her reasons for doing so are unknown. Only answer choice B conveys an opinion of the author.

**9. D:** A search for early maps by one of the first people to study geography would certainly take Jorgen to the 900 section of the library: History, geography, and biography. For this particular study, there is no reason for Jorgen to look among books on philosophy and psychology, social sciences, or technical and applied science.

**10. D:** The sieve of Eratosthenes is a mathematical tool, so Jorgen should go to the science and mathematics section. While the sieve might be used in certain computer applications, there is no specific indication of this. As a result, answer choice D is a better option than answer choice A. Also, Jorgen has no reason to check the philosophy and psychology or languages sections to find out more about a mathematical topic.

**11. B:** Section 400 is the section on languages, so it is a good place to look for more information about the letters of the Greek alphabet. Jorgen would be unlikely to find anything useful in the sections on religion, arts and recreation, or history, geography, and biography.

**12. D:** Section 800 features works of literature, so that is the best place for Jorgen to begin looking for *The Iliad* and *The Odyssey*. The philosophy and psychology section will likely contain references to these works, but Jorgen would still have to go to the literature section to obtain the works themselves. The same thing can be said about the religion and arts and recreation sections.

**13. C:** While planning her daughter's wedding, Marci is likely to find picking out a paint color for the living room *unimportant*. Therefore, answer choice C is the most logical option. Choosing a paint color might also be meaningless at the moment, but it is not without meaning altogether. It is simply not as important. Answer choice A infers more than the sentence implies. Answer choice B could be forced into the sentence (if Marci was looking for a distraction from the stress of wedding planning, for instance), but it is not natural, and it is certainly not a synonym for *peripheral*. Answer choice D makes little sense in the context of the sentence.

**14. B:** The Russian population of Latvia decreased the most since 1991. The Latvian population decreased slightly, but not to the same degree. The Ukrainian population decreased by an even smaller percentage since 1991. The German population remained relatively unchanged between 1991 and 2011.

**15. C:** On the chart, the only ethnic group that represents approximately one percent of the population after World War II and approximately three percent by 1991 is the Ukrainian population. The Latvian and Russian populations represent much larger percentages of the total population of Latvia. The German population decreased significantly during this time period.

**16. A:** If Hilaire's vocabulary needs a boost, he needs a thesaurus, which provides a range of synonyms (or antonyms) for words. A dictionary is useful for word meanings, but it will not necessarily assist Hilaire in improving the words he already has in his papers. The encyclopedia is also irrelevant, particularly since the professor already approves of Hilaire's work and is not asking him to research further. The style guide will be helpful if the paper needs more attention on grammar.

**17. C:** As the final step indicates, the new word should end in *Y*. This immediately eliminates answer choice D. Answer choice A adds an *L* when a second one is not required, and answer choice B adds two *Ts* to a word that has none. Only answer choice C follows all of the directions to spell the new word: REPLAY.

**18. A:** Klara's success is clearly the result of diligence, so answer choice A must be correct. It is possible that her diligence was also silent, but the sentence does not indicate this. Answer choice B, then, cannot be correct. A moderate commitment by an average student would not lead to exemplary results, so answer choice C is incorrect. Answer choice D makes no sense in the context of the sentence.

**19. D:** Puffed rice is a dry breakfast cereal, and therefore contains (or might contain) a dairy product. Breaded chicken parmesan contains both bread crumbs and parmesan cheese; the cheese is certainly a dairy product, and bread is on the warning list from the doctor. A sliced turkey sandwich contains deli meat and bread, both of which are discouraged by Flemming's doctor. Yogurt made from coconut milk, however, is meant to be a dairy-free alternative, so it should be a safe choice for Flemming.

**20. C:** Chapter III of the manual contains information about adjusting the climate within the vehicle, so it is here that Regina will find the instructions she needs to adjust the air conditioning. Chapter I would be the best choice if the manual did *not* also include Chapter III. The chapter on safety options would probably not contain information about how to operate the air conditioning, so answer choice B is incorrect. Regina should definitely adjust the air conditioning before she begins driving, but the information needed to do this is not likely to be found in Chapter IV.

**21. D:** An overheating vehicle is definitely an emergency, so Regina would need to consult Chapter VI. The other chapters contain useful information that Regina will need once her vehicle is back in working order, but until then she should focus on the information in the chapter about emergency situations.

**22. B:** As most students discover, Wikipedia is not considered a reliable source or a particularly scholarly one. The Encyclopedia Britannica is, however, as are Science.gov (which would contain officially recognized information provided by a government organization) and LexisNexis (a reputable site containing legal and educational resources).

**23. B:** The passage does not say that studying a foreign language will help students find jobs after high school (choice A) or gain an understanding of other cultures (choice C). The passage does say that studying a foreign language is important for college acceptance (choice D), but this point alone is not the main idea of the passage.

**24. C:** The passage does not claim that studying a foreign language is essential to high school graduation (choice A). Choices B and D represent claims made in the passage, but do not include all of the claims made.

**25. D:** Although students may find knowledge of a foreign language helpful in obtaining a job, it is an obvious exaggeration to claim that students who did not study a foreign language would be unemployable.

**26. D:** Choices A and C represent options that would provide information regarding the opinions of students and parents, but not actual evidence regarding the influence of studying a foreign language on future success. Choice B specifies a second language taught at home, whereas the passage focuses specifically on a foreign language taught in high school.

**27. B:** Choices A, C, and D do not offer a complete summary of the claims made in this passage.

**28. D:** Eczema is a topical condition, so Chapter 12 (section D) would be the most appropriate place to look. Eczema is not specific to either men or women, nor is it specific to adults, so Chapter 8 would not be the best place to look. Finally, eczema is neither a respiratory condition nor a digestive condition.

**29. A:** This question asks the reader to consider the distinction between a recognized respiratory condition (Chapter 10) and a children's condition (Chapter 7). In this case, the first and best place to check is Chapter 7, because it addresses conditions specific to children, and it describes herbs that may be useful in treating these conditions. Herbs, like pharmaceuticals, need to be used carefully, and the type of herbal remedy that would be used to treat an adult respiratory condition is not necessarily the same one that would be used to treat a respiratory condition in a child. Additionally, the dosage would certainly be different, so the chapter on children's conditions is the correct place to look. Chapters 9 and 12 (immunity and detox, respectively) would not contain useful information for this particular situation.

**30. C:** Chapter 5 contains information about using herbs in beverages. Since Clothilde is looking for ways to use the elderflower to make tea and wine, this chapter should be useful. Chapter 3 would not likely contain information that would be useful in this situation. Chapter 4 discusses using herbs in food, so Clothilde is unlikely to find anything in this section about beverages. Chapter 13 would certainly be the place to look in the index of herbs, but this chapter would most likely contain a listing of the herb and a summary of its properties, rather than recommendations for how to use it in tea or wine making.

**31. B:** Chapter 3 contains information about caring for herbs, so it is the first place Clothilde should look. The herb is clearly already planted, so Chapter 2 will not be of much use in this case. Again, Chapter 13 would certainly be the place to look in the index of herbs, but this chapter would most likely contain a listing of the herb and a summary of its properties, rather than recommendations for maintaining the plant. Chapter 14, the alphabetical listing for herbs J–O, is unlikely to contain any information either about caring for herbs in general or about the elderberry in particular.

**32. C:** Only Cosette fulfills all of the clearly stated requirements in the ad. She does not smoke (and is, in fact, allergic to cigarette smoke), and she needs a quiet place to study in a house that is advertised as having quiet occupants. Also implied is Cosette's need to be close to the university, since she is likely going to be studying for classes. Frances has a dog, and this is not allowed according to the ad. Adelaide is looking for a short-term lease, and the other occupants prefer a long-term renter. Felix is male, and the other occupants are looking for a female renter.

**33. B:** If the student's nerves are getting the better of him, it is likely that he is either very pale or very flushed. Because *flushed* is one of the options, it is the correct choice. A complexion cannot be *rambling*, so answer choice A is incorrect. Answer choice C has a hint of promise, but it makes the sentence more confusing, so it too is incorrect. It is difficult to know what is meant by the phrase "*weak* complexion," so answer choice D is too unclear to be correct.

**34. B:** For two pounds of each type of tea, Wholesale Tea's price would be $96, which is the best price. Tea Heaven's price would be $102. Tea by the Pound's price would be $104. Tea Express's price would be the same as Tea Heaven's price: $102.

**35. B:** Wholesale Tea would have the best price for these specific blends. The price for one pound of Earl Grey and two pounds of green tea would be $78. Tea Heaven's price would be $87. Tea by the Pound's price would be $83. Tea Express's price would be $88.

**36. B:** Answer choice B is the most logical conclusion. The passage states that, "Primary sources are the more direct type of information. They are accounts of an event that are produced by individuals who were actually present." Therefore, it is reasonable to assume that an account prepared by someone who was present would be more accurate than one prepared by somebody decades later who had to rely on the accounts of others.

**37. D:** Ten nations received independence in the first thirty years of the nineteenth century. Choice A is incorrect because the American Revolution was fought during the latter 1770s and early 1780s. This was decades before the independence movements in South America. In fact, the American Revolution inspired some of the movements. France did not have many possessions in South America. So, choice B is wrong. Nations on the west coast were among the last to gain independence. So, that makes choice C incorrect.

**38. C:** The only logical conclusion that can be made based on the announcement is that the library has applied a fee to Internet usage beyond 30 minutes to discourage patrons from spending too long on the computers. There is nothing in the announcement to suggest that the library plans to add more computers. The announcement mentions a limited number of computers, but there is no indication that there are plans to change this fact. The announcement makes no mention of the library's budget, so it is impossible to infer that the library is facing budget cuts or that the library is compensating for budget cuts with the fee. Similarly, the announcement says nothing about the library's Internet costs, so it is impossible to conclude logically that the library is attempting to offset its own Internet fees.

**39. C:** Raoul will need the computer for a total of 90 minutes. The first 30 minutes are free, so Raoul will need to be prepared to pay for 60 minutes. This is equal to four intervals of 15 minutes. Each 15-minute interval costs $3, so Raoul will need to pay $12 for his Internet usage at the library.

**40. A:** The author says that victims of Marah's disease "appear" to be comfortable but "beneath it all" are in pain. He says that they are "inaccurately" diagnosed as low on the pain scale. This shows that the pain scale is not an accurate way to measure Marah's disease.

**41. B:** The topic sentence is placed at the beginning of each supporting paragraph. Supporting evidence is presented after the topic sentence in each supporting paragraph. The passage states "Next come the supporting paragraphs. Each paragraph contains a topic sentence, supporting evidence, and finally a type of mini-conclusion that restates the point of the paragraph."

**42. B:** Answer choices A, C, and D are all mentioned in the passage, but they are part of the overall purpose, which is to give an overview of how leeches have been used throughout history.

**43. C:** Although it never specifically addresses the babysitter, the directions are clearly instructions for how to take care of a little girl. A mother or father would not need this information written down in such detail, but a babysitter might. You can infer the answer in this case.

**44. D:** You cannot assume gender, and the note never indicates whether the writer is male or female. You can tell that the writer is the main caretaker of the child in question, so "parent" is the best choice in this case. A teacher or nurse might be able to write such a note, but parent is probably more likely, making it the best choice.

**45. B:** The information in the passage lets you know that only the serving team can score. This rule is different in different leagues, so it is important to read the passage instead of going by what you know from your own life.

**46. D:** Although any number of people could play in a volleyball game, the passage mentions that the entire class could participate in a game. Do all of them have to participate? No. But that wasn't the question.

**47. C:** The author does not make predictions of a radically rejuvenated planet (choice A) or the complete annihilation of life as we know it (choice B). The author is also not accusatory in his descriptions (choice D). Instead, the author states what he believes to be the current state of the planet's environment, and makes practical suggestions for making better use of its resources in the future.

**48. B:** As the passage states: "Locally grown food and other products manufactured within your community are the best choices. The fewer miles a product traveled to reach you, the fewer resources it required."

**49. C:** The author does not mention running out of resources in a specific time period (choice A), the cost of water and energy (choice B), or the possibility of hardship for local farmers (choice D).

**50. D:** As the passage states: "You should try to be aware of your consumption of water and energy. Turn off the water when you brush your teeth, and limit your showers to five minutes. Turn off the lights, and don't leave appliances or chargers plugged in when not in use." The contexts of these sentences indicate that consumption means the depletion of goods (e.g., water and energy).

**51. C:** Of the choices available, this is the only sentence that offers specific ideas for carrying out the author's suggestion to the reader of limiting consumption of energy.

**52. D:** B and C are only briefly mentioned, allowing them to be eliminated as possibilities. Although the passage does discuss what could happen to two balls released at the top of a mountain, that is not the purpose of the passage, so A can be eliminated. The purpose is to show how small differences (in this case two inches between two rubber balls) can have large effects. This is essentially what the butterfly effect is, and the purpose of the passage is to give an example to demonstrate this principle.

**53. B:** This is the correct answer because the birthdates show that the youngest children are on the right and their older siblings are on the left side of the family tree. Choice A is incorrect because Queen Victoria and Prince Albert are the oldest generation, and they are at the top of the family tree. Choice C is incorrect because the youngest children are on the left, not the right (the reader can see this by looking at the birthdates). Choice D is partially correct because Queen Victoria and Prince Albert are at the top of the family tree, but the family tree does not show great-grandchildren. Although it looks like there are more than three layers, the middle layers all show Queen Victoria and Prince Albert's children.

# Mathematics

**1. C:** According to the problem statement, 60% of the class wanted to work with the elderly. Therefore, convert 60% to a fraction by using the following steps:

$$60\% = \frac{60}{100}$$

Now simplify the above fraction using a greatest common factor of 20.

$$\frac{60}{100} = \frac{3}{5}$$

**2. B:** Since 35% of the staff will take vacation days, only 100% – 35% = 65% of the staff is available to work. Of the remaining 65%, only 20% are certified to work in the neonatal unit. Therefore multiply 65% by 20% using these steps:

Convert 65% and 20% into decimals by dividing both numbers by 100.

$$\frac{65}{100} = 0.65 \text{ and } \frac{20}{100} = 0.20$$

Now multiply 0.65 by 0.20 to get

$$(0.65)(0.20) = 0.13$$

Now convert 0.13 to a percentage by multiplying by 100.

$$(0.13)(100) = 13\%$$

**3. B:** The patient's dosage must decrease by 30%. So calculate 30% of 340:

$$(0.30)(340 \text{ mg}) = 102 \text{ mg}$$

Now subtract the 30% decrease from the original dosage.

$$340 \text{ mg} - 102 \text{ mg} = 238 \text{ mg}$$

**4. C:** Since 70% of the patients in the study were women, 30% of the patients were men. Calculate the number of male patients by multiplying 100 by 0.30.

$$(100)(0.30) = 30$$

Of the 30 male patients in the study, 10% were overweight as children. So 90% were not overweight. Multiply 30 by 0.90 to get the final answer.

$$(30)(0.90) = 27$$

**5. C:** If the incoming class has 100 students, then $\frac{3}{4}$ of those students will major in nursing.

$$(100)\left(\frac{3}{4}\right) = 75$$

So 75 students will major in nursing but only $\frac{1}{5}$ of that 75 will complete the nursing program.

$$(75)\left(\frac{1}{5}\right) = 15$$

Therefore, 15 students will complete the program.

**6. A:** The first midwife contributes $2000 per month, and she uses $\frac{2}{5}$ of that amount for rent and utilities.

$$(\$2000)\left(\frac{2}{5}\right) = \$800$$

So the midwife pays $800 for rent and utilities, which leaves her with

$$\$2000 - \$800 = \$1200$$

The midwife divides the remaining $1200 in half.

$$\frac{\$1200}{2} = \$600$$

The midwife saves $600 and buys medical supplies with the remaining $600.

**7. A:** The second midwife allocates $\frac{1}{2}$ of her funds for an office administrator plus another $\frac{1}{10}$ for office supplies. So add $\frac{1}{2}$ and $\frac{1}{10}$ by first finding a common denominator.

$$\frac{1}{2} = \frac{5}{10}$$

$$\frac{5}{10} + \frac{1}{10} = \frac{6}{10}$$

Now simplify $\frac{6}{10}$ by using the greatest common factor of 6 and 10, which is 2.

$$6 \div 2 = 3 \text{ and } 10 \div 2 = 5$$

Therefore, $\frac{6}{10} = \frac{3}{5}$.

**8. C:** The following proportion can be written $\frac{4}{2} = \frac{x}{18}$. Solving for $x$ gives $x = 36$. Thus, there are 36 data analysis problems on the test.

**9. A:** The flat rate of $65 represents the $y$-intercept, and the charge of $0.12 per roaming minute used represents the slope. Therefore, the expression representing his monthly phone bill is $65 + 0.12x$.

**10. B:** First, determine how many miles can be driven on one tank of gas by multiplying the numbers of gallons in a tank by the miles per gallon:

12 gallons/tank × 30 miles/gallon = 360 miles

Next, divide the total miles for the trip by the number of miles driven per tank of gas to determine how many total tanks of gas Robert will need:

1,800 miles ÷ 360 miles/tank = 5 tanks

**11. C:** To obtain the new dosage, subtract 1/5th of 310 mg from the original dosage of 310 mg, then subtract 20 mg.

$$310 \text{ mg} - \left(310 \times \frac{1}{5}\right) \text{mg} - 20 \text{ mg} = 228 \text{ mg}$$

**12. C:** Find $\frac{1}{7}$ of 100 by multiplying

$$(100)\left(\frac{1}{7}\right) = \frac{100}{7} = 14.2857$$

$\frac{100}{7}$ is an improper fraction. Convert the fraction to a decimal and round to the nearest hundredth to get 14.29.

**13. B:** A single straight line can be drawn that is close to many of the points. The slope of that line would be negative, so the points have a negative, linear association.

**14. D:** In order to determine the number of questions Joshua must answer correctly, consider the number of points he must earn. Joshua will receive 4 points for each question he answers correctly, and $x$ represents the number of questions. Therefore, Joshua will receive a total of 4x points for all the questions he answers correctly. Joshua must earn more than 92 points. Therefore, to determine the number of questions he must answer correctly, solve the inequality $4x > 92$.

**15. D:** To determine the total cost of Susan's outfit, add all her purchases.

$$\$69.99 + \$39.99 + \$34.76 = \$144.65$$

**16. C:** Group B is negatively skewed since there are more high scores. With more high scores, the mean for Group B will be higher.

**17. A:** Apply the order of operations to solve this problem. Multiplication and division are computed first from left to right. Then addition and subtraction are computed next from left to right.

$$2 + (2)(2) - 2 \div 2 =$$

$$2 + 4 - 2 \div 2 =$$

$$2 + 4 - 1 =$$

$$6 - 1 =$$

$$5$$

**18. A:** The numbers listed for Choice A can all be converted to decimal form for comparison. The given sequence can be written as $-2, -0.75, -0.45, 0.03, 0.36$. The negative integers are the least values, with the negative integer with the greatest absolute value, serving as the least integer. The percentage, 3%, is written as 0.03, and is less than 0.36.

**19. B:** Compare and order the rational numbers by finding a common denominator for all three fractions. The least common denominator for 3, 5, and 15 is 15. Now convert the fractions with different denominators into fractions with a common denominator.

$$\frac{4}{15} = \frac{4}{15}$$

$$\frac{2}{5} = \frac{6}{15}$$

$$\frac{1}{3} = \frac{5}{15}$$

Now that all three fractions have the same denominator, order them from smallest to largest by comparing the numerators.

$$\frac{4}{15} < \frac{5}{15} < \frac{6}{15}$$

Since $\frac{4}{15}$ of the patients are in Group Alpha, this group has the smallest number of patients. The next largest group has $\frac{5}{15}$ of the patients, which is Group Gamma. The largest group has $\frac{6}{15}$ of the patients, which is Group Beta.

**20. A:** Solve the equation for $x$.

$$2x + 6 = 14$$

$$2x = 14 - 6$$

$$2x = 8$$

$$x = \frac{8}{2}$$

$$x = 4$$

**21. C:** To determine the mean time for this event, add up all 8 event times (181.42) and then divide that value by 8: $\frac{181.42}{8} = 22.6775 \approx 22.68$ sec. Answer A is the mode value of the event times. Answer B is the median value of the event times. In Answer D, the mean was incorrectly calculated by only adding the first and last times (22.33 + 23.22) and then dividing that value by 2.

**22. A:** During week 1, Nurse Cameron worked 5 shifts.

$$\text{shifts for week } 1 = 5$$

During week 2, she worked twice as many shifts as she did during week 1.

$$\text{shifts for week } 2 = (2)(5)$$

During week 3, she added 4 shifts to the number of shifts she worked during week 2.

$$\text{shifts for week } 3 = (2)(5) + 4$$

**23. A:** Use the order of operations to solve this problem.

$$(3)(-4) + (3)(4) - 1$$

$$-12 + (3)(4) - 1 =$$

$$-12 + 12 - 1 =$$

$$0 - 1 =$$

$$-1$$

**24. A:** The volume formula for a rectangular solid is $V = lwh$. Plugging in values then evaluating will yield the final answer.

$$V = (30\ in)(10\ in)(12\ in)$$
$$V = 3600\ \text{cubic inches}$$

**25. B:** If a line-of-fit is drawn through the points, the slope will be $-\frac{1}{5}$ so the snow melts 5 centimeters every day.

**26. D:** The variables are the objects the graph measures. In this case, the graph measures the Hospital Staff and the Average hours worked per week. The dependent variable changes with the independent variable. Here, the average hours worked per week depends on the particular type of hospital staff. Therefore, the dependent variable is Average hours worked per week and the independent variable is Hospital Staff.

**27. D:** The prefix, milli-, means 1000th. In this case,

$$1\ g = 1000\ mg$$

Therefore,

$$(5)(1\ g) = (5)(1000\ mg)$$

$$5\ g = (5)(1000\ mg)$$

$$5\ g = 5000\ mg$$

**28. B:** The number of people who voted for the proposition is 9.5% of 51,623. If we only require an approximation, we can round 9.5% to 10%, and 51,623 to 50,000. Then 9.5% of 51,623 is about 10% of 50,000, or $(0.1)(50,000) = 5,000$.

**29. D:** To calculate the total time taken, divide the distance driven by the speed it was driven at:
$$305\ mi \div 65\ mph = 305\ \text{miles} \times \frac{1\ \text{hour}}{65\ \text{miles}} = 4.69\ \text{hours}$$

$$162\ mi \div 80\ mph = 162\ \text{miles} \times \frac{1\ \text{hour}}{80\ \text{miles}} = 2.03\ \text{hours}$$

Convert the minutes spent at the gas station to hours: $15\ \text{min} \times \frac{1\ \text{hour}}{60\ \text{minutes}} = 0.25\ \text{hours}$

Find the total time taken on the trip by summing all the times: $4.69 + 2.03 + 0.25 = 6.97\ \text{hours}$

**30. C:** Use the formula $Volume = length \times width \times height$:

$$200 = 5 \times 5 \times h$$

$$25h = 200$$

**31. D:** Integers include all positive and negative whole numbers and the number zero. The product of three integers must be an integer, so you can eliminate any answer choice that is not a whole number: choices (A) and (C). The product of two even integers is even. The product of even and odd integers is even. The only even choice is 24.

**32. C:** Divide the mg the child should receive by the number of mg in 0.8 mL to determine how many 0.8 mL doses the child should receive: $\frac{240}{80} = 3$. Multiply the number of doses by 0.8 to determine how many mL the child should receive: $3 \times 0.8 = 2.4$ mL

**33. B:** The chart indicates that each $x$ value must be tripled to equal the corresponding $y$ value, so $y = 3x$. One way you can determine this is by plugging corresponding pairs of $x$ and $y$ into the answer choices.

**34. D:** Use the following proportion: $\frac{1\ in}{45\ miles} = \frac{3.2\ in}{x\ miles}$

Cross multiply: $x = (45)(3.2) = 144$ miles

**35. A:** The amount of money he has already saved represents the $y$-intercept. The amount of money he intends to save per month represents the slope. Thus, his savings can be represented by the equation, $y = 28x + 15$, also written as $y = 15 + 28x$.

**36. B:** The number of trees planted by the Juniors is skewed left, with more higher numbers of trees planted. The number of trees planted by the Seniors is skewed right, with more lower numbers of trees planted.

# Science

**1. C:** The circulatory system consists of the heart, blood vessels, lymph, lymph nodes, and blood. It circulates materials throughout the entire body, providing tissues and organs with nutrients and oxygen. It is also responsible for transporting hormones and removing waste. The nervous system is responsible for transmitting nerve impulses that originate in the brain and coordinate action in the rest of the body.

**2. B:** The digestive system helps the body process food. The stomach, mouth, and esophagus all participate in food digestion. Common diseases infecting the digestive system include Crohn's disease, ulcerative colitis, and diverticulosis. Diabetes is a disease of the endocrine system, that impacts the release of insulin from the pancreas.

**3. A:** The nervous system is the body's communication center. The body uses the respiratory system to breathe, and blood is transported by the circulatory system. The digestive system breaks down food for the body.

**4. A:** The respiratory system uses the lungs, diaphragm, trachea, alveoli and bronchi to help the body distribute oxygen and remove carbon dioxide. While the ribs contain and protect many of these elements, the ribs are part of the musculoskeletal system, which is responsible for providing structure, stability and protection to the internal organs.

**5. A:** The immune system helps protect the body from bacteria, viruses, infections, and other elements that could cause illness. Depending on the foreign element that enters the body, different cells respond to attack the foreign element. Cells that contribute to this protection and response include leukocytes, or white blood cells (eosinophils, basophils, natural killer (NK) cells, and mast cells), and phagocytic cells (dendritic cells, macrophages and neutrophils) in addition to cells of adaptive immunity (B cells and T cells) which are produced in the bone marrow. A neuron is a nerve cell that is central to the nervous system and transmits nerve impulses.

**6. A:** The human body has five types of bones: long bones, short bones, irregular bones, flat bones, and sesamoid bones. While bones may be dense, this is not a major category of bones in the body.

**7. B:** Sesamoid bones are embedded in tendons. Vertical bones, is not a major bone type. Long bones contain a long shaft, and flat bones are thin and curved.

**8. A:** A triple beam balance would be used to measure the mass (in grams) of the gum in this experiment. An anemometer is used to measure wind speed. A hot plate is used to heat liquids. A microscope is used to magnify microscopic particles or organisms.

**9. C:** In respiration, the human inhales air, consisting of oxygen, and then produces energy (ATP) and exhales nitrogen, carbon dioxide, and water (in the form of vapor). While oxygen is a main component of the respiratory system's process, it is not produced by the respiratory system. Rather, it is utilized and distributed throughout the body, and then what is not absorbed, is exhaled back into the environment.

**10. C:** The pulmonary artery carries oxygen-depleted blood from the heart to the lungs, where $CO_2$ is released and the supply of oxygen is replenished. This blood then returns to the heart through the pulmonary vein, and is carried through the aorta and a series of branching arteries to the capillaries, where the bulk of gas exchange with the tissues occurs. Oxygen-depleted blood returns to the heart through branching veins (the femoral veins bring it from the legs) into the vena cava, which carries it again to the heart. Since the pulmonary artery is the last step before replenishment of the blood's oxygen content, it contains the blood which is the most oxygen depleted.

**11. D:** The myocardium is the layer of the heart that contains the muscle fibers responsible for contraction (Hint: myo- is the prefix for muscle). The endocardium and epicardium are the inner and outer layers of the heart wall, respectively. The pericardium is the sac in which the heart sits inside the chest cavity.

**12. A:** While generally speaking, veins carry deoxygenated blood and arteries carry oxygenated blood, in this case, the pulmonary veins carry oxygenated blood from the lungs to the left side of the heart and the pulmonary arteries carry deoxygenated blood from the right side of the heart to the lungs. The aorta, takes oxygenated away from the left side of the heart and distributes it throughout the body. The superior vena cava returns unoxygenated blood back to the right side of the heart, to then be distributed through the lungs and reoxygenated.

**13. C:** The independent variable is the variable that is changed in the experiment in order to determine its effect on the dependent variable or the outcome of the experiment. The dependent variable results from the experimenter making only one change to an experiment that can be repeated with the same results. Mrs. Jones's class was comparing the effects of sugar and artificial sweetener on the overall color of cookies once they are baked; thus, the one thing that should be changed in the experiment is the sugar and artificial sweetener in the recipe. All of the other ingredients stay the same. For the experiment to be valid and not influenced by any other variables, the students should keep the temperature and baking time the same, as these could affect the color of the cookies as well.

**14. C:** Mitochondria are often called the power house of the cell because they provide energy for the cell to function. The nucleus is the control center for the cell. The cell membrane surrounds the cell and separates the cell from its environment. Cytoplasm is the thick fluid within the cell membrane that surrounds the nucleus and contains organelles.

**15. B:** Ribosomes are organelles that help synthesize proteins within the cell. Cilia and flagella are responsible for cell movement. The cell membrane helps the cell maintain its shape and protects it from the environment. Lysosomes have digestive enzymes.

**16. B:** Cells differentiate so that simple, less specialized cells can become highly specialized cells. For example, humans are multicellular organisms who undergo cell differentiation numerous times. Cells begin as simple zygotes after fertilization and then differentiate to form a myriad of complex tissues and systems before birth.

**17. C:** Both meiosis and mitosis occur in humans, animals, and plants. Mitosis produces cells that are genetically identical, and meiosis produces cells that are genetically different. Only mitosis occurs asexually.

**18. B:** A decrease in a natural predator, such as a wolves, coyotes, bobcat, or wild dogs, would allow the population to become out of control. In a population of deer that has increased, there would be a natural decrease in a food source for the nutritional needs for the animals in surrounding areas. Although deer have been known to share a human's developed habitat, it is often forced by reduced territory and food sources. An increase in hunting licenses would be used by local officials to try to control the population, helping to decrease the number of adults of breeding age.

**19. B:** DNA is the primary carrier of genetic information in most cells. RNA serves as a messenger that transmits genetic information from DNA to the cytoplasm of the cell.

**20. C:** Food enters the digestive system through the mouth and proceeds down to the stomach after mastication by the teeth. Once in the stomach, enzymes are secreted that begin to digest the specific substances in the food (proteins, carbohydrates, etc.). Next, the food passes through to the small intestine where the nutrients are absorbed and then into the large intestine where extra water is absorbed.

**21. C:** After cell division, the daughter cells should be exact copies of the parent cells. Therefore, the DNA should replicate, or make an exact copy of itself, so that each daughter cell will have the full amount of DNA.

**22. A:** Genes are the molecular units that enable parents to pass hereditary traits on to their offspring. The blood, organs, cells and hair all contain the genes that makeup the offspring, but these are not basic molecular units.

**23. A:** Both DNA and RNA are made up of 4 nucleotide bases. Both DNA and RNA contain cytosine, guanine, and adenine. However, DNA contains thymine and RNA contains uracil. Choice B is incorrect because DNA and RNA do not have the same 4 nucleotides, and choices C and D are incorrect because neither DNA nor RNA contains 6 nucleotides. Furthermore, DNA has a double helix structure, and RNA has a single helix structure.

**24. B:** The genotype describes a person's genetic makeup. The phenotype describes a person's observable characteristics. Among the choices, the CFTR gene refers to genetic makeup while the other choices all describe traits that are observable.

**25. B:** The complete Punnett square is shown below.

|   | **B** | **b** |
|---|-------|-------|
| **B** | BB | Bb |
| **b** | Bb | bb |

Because male pattern baldness is a recessive gene, the offspring would need the *bb* gene combination in order to inherit this trait. Possibility 4 corresponds to the *bb* gene combination.

**26. C:** Because male pattern baldness is recessive, the offspring would need the *bb* gene combination in order to inherit this trait. Therefore, any offspring with the *B* gene will have a full head of hair. Possibilities 1, 2, and 3 all have the *B* gene.

**27. B:** Interstitial fluid is found in the tissues around the cells; intracellular fluid is found within the cells. Fluid in the ventricles of the brain and down into the spinal cord is called cerebrospinal fluid. Cerebrospinal fluid bathes these sensitive tissues in a fluid that helps to protect them. Blood and lymph are the fluids that carry nutrients, oxygen, waste, and lymph material throughout the body.

**28. D:** *Plasma* cells secrete antibodies. These cells, also known as plasmacytes, are located in lymphoid tissue. Antibodies are only secreted in response to a particular stimulus, usually the detection of an antigen in the body. Antigens include bacteria, viruses, and parasites. Once released, antibodies bind to the antigen and neutralize it. When faced with a new antigen, the body may require some time to develop appropriate antibodies. Once the body has been exposed to an antigen, however, it does not forget how to produce the correct antibodies.

**29. A:** A catalyst increases the rate of a chemical reaction without becoming part of the net reaction. Therefore, chemical C increases the rate of the reaction between A and B. The catalyst does not change the chemicals within the reaction or initiate the reaction itself.

**30. B:** Enzymes are protein molecules produced by living organisms. Enzymes serve as catalysts for certain biological reactions.

**31. A:** The hypothalamus controls the hormones secreted by the pituitary gland. This part of the brain maintains the body temperature and helps to control metabolism. The adrenal glands, which lie above the kidneys, secrete steroidal hormones, epinephrine, and norepinephrine. The testes are the male reproductive glands, responsible for the production of sperm and testosterone. The pancreas secretes insulin and a fluid that aids in digestion.

**32. A:** Gas exchange occurs in the *alveoli*, the minute air sacs on the interior of the lungs. The *bronchi* are large cartilage-based tubes of air; they extend from the end of the trachea into the lungs, where they branch apart. The *larynx*, which houses the vocal cords, is positioned between the trachea and the pharynx; it is involved in swallowing, breathing, and speaking. The *pharynx* extends from the nose to the uppermost portions of the trachea and esophagus. In order to enter these two structures, air and other matter must pass through the pharynx.

**33. C:** The esophagus is the only structure that is not part of the respiratory system, it is part of the digestive system. The larynx houses the voice box; it also acts as a passageway for air to travel into the lungs. The trachea connects the larynx to the lungs. The trachea splits into the right and left bronchi, which divide into smaller passageways called the bronchioles.

**34. C:** In order to have accurate measurements, the use of a graduated cylinder would be the best measurement equipment for a liquid solution. A triple beam balance measures the weight of an object in grams. A flask and a test tube are used to contain a liquid while being heated or stored.

**35. C:** The atom is negatively charged. Neutrons have no charge. Protons have positive charge and electrons have negative charge equal in magnitude to the positive charge of the proton. Because the atom has more electrons than protons, the atom has a negative charge.

**36. C:** The genitourinary system is responsible for removing waste from the body through urine. Components include two kidneys, two ureters that drain the urine from the kidney to the bladder, and the urethra that drains urine from the bladder out of the body. The rectum is the last section of the large intestine, and part of the digestive system.

**37. C:** The neurovascular structure found under each rib in descending order is the vein, artery, and nerve. When a procedure such as a thoracocentesis or chest tube needs to be performed, the medical professional should aim for directly over the rib in order to avoid damaging to these structures.

**38. D:** The atomic number equals the number of protons and the number of electrons in an atom. Since Be has an atomic number of 4, it has 4 protons and 4 electrons. H has the fewest protons and electrons, as denoted by its atomic number of 1.

**39. B:** The spleen's job is to filter the blood by removing dead or dying red blood cells as well as microorganisms. In humans it is found in the left upper quadrant of the abdomen lateral to the liver.

**40. C:** Vaporization is the process of changing from a liquid to a gas. For instance, water vaporizes when boiled to create steam. Freezing is the process of changing from a liquid to a solid. Condensation describes changing from a gas to a liquid, and sublimation is the process of changing from a solid to a gas.

**41. C:** The nurse wants to investigate her patients' body temperatures. A thermometer is the only tool in the list that will help measure the temperature of a person's body.

**42. A:** The researcher should use statistical analysis to understand trends in the data. Different statistics tools can help manage and examine large data sets. The researcher would probably miss important correlations by looking at the individual data points, and eliminating most of the data would defeat the purpose of conducting the study. Simply staring at the data would not be helpful.

**43. B:** Based on the evidence, the most likely explanation for fly larvae in the spoiled food is that flies laid their eggs in the food. When the food was left out in the open, the flies had access to it and laid their eggs. However, when the food was in a sealed container, the flies could not lay their eggs in the food. Hence, the spoiled food in the sealed container had no fly larvae.

**44. D:** Longer life expectancy could be explained by any or all of the alternatives presented. Advances in medical technology, basic cleanliness, and vaccines could all help people live longer in the 21st century.

**45. C:** A scientific argument should be based on measurable and observable facts such as the patient's current symptoms and health history. Discussing the patient's appearance or the doctor's feelings does not communicate a scientific argument. While insurance may be a factor in most healthcare systems, the status of the patient's insurance does not communicate a scientific argument that justifies the need for the test.

**46. C:** Interferons are members of a larger class of proteins called cytokines. Cytokines are specialized proteins that carry signals between cells. Interferons are proteins that are produced by cells infected by pathogens such as viruses. They signal neighboring cells to produce antiviral proteins which help prevent the spread of infection.

**47. D:** Humans have three layers of skin called the epidermis, the dermis, and subcutaneous fat. Epidermis is the top layer of the skin, the dermis is the second layer, and subcutaneous makes up the bottom layer. The epidermis does not contain blood vessels.

**48. A:** The hypothalamus is a tiny gland at the base of the brain. It helps regulate temperature, sleep, emotions, sexual function and behavior. During puberty it secretes hormones that stimulate the gonads which initiate sexual development.

**49. D:** Of the given structures, veins have the lowest blood pressure. *Veins* carry oxygen-poor blood from the outlying parts of the body to the heart. An *artery* carries oxygen-rich blood from the heart to the peripheral parts of the body. An *arteriole* extends from an artery to a capillary. A *venule* is a tiny vein that extends from a capillary to a larger vein.

**50. C:** Of the four heart chambers, the left ventricle is the most muscular. When it contracts, it pushes blood out to the organs and extremities of the body. The right ventricle pushes blood into the lungs. The atria, on the other hand, receive blood from the outlying parts of the body and transport it into the ventricles. The basic process works as follows: Oxygen-poor blood fills the right atrium and is pumped into the right ventricle, from which it is pumped into the pulmonary artery and on to the lungs. In the lungs, this blood is oxygenated. The blood then reenters the heart at the left atrium, which when full pumps into the left ventricle. When the left ventricle is full, blood is pushed into the aorta and on to the organs and extremities of the body.

**51. A:** The *cerebrum* is the part of the brain that interprets sensory information. It is the largest part of the brain. The cerebrum is divided into two hemispheres, connected by a thin band of tissue called the corpus callosum. The *cerebellum* is positioned at the back of the head, between the brain stem and the cerebrum. It controls both voluntary and involuntary movements. The *medulla oblongata* forms the base of the brain. This part of the brain is responsible for blood flow and breathing, among other things. The hindbrain refers to a section of the brain including the medulla oblongata, pons, and cerebellum.

**52. C:** A vaccination is a way of acquiring active artificial immunity, where an antigen is deliberately introduced into an individual to stimulate the immune system. Vaccines contain dead or dying pathogens which are not enough to cause an infection, but allow the immune system to "remember" the pathogen and become immune to it.

**53. C:** The *parasympathetic nervous system* is responsible for lowering the heart rate. It slows down the heart rate, dilates the blood vessels, and increases the secretions of the digestive system. The *central nervous system* is composed of the brain and the spinal cord. The *sympathetic nervous system* is a part of the autonomic nervous system; its role is to oppose the actions taken by the parasympathetic nervous system. So, the sympathetic nervous system accelerates the heart, contracts the blood vessels, and decreases the secretions of the digestive system.

# English and Language Usage

**1. A:** Semicolons are used to separate items in a series when those items contain internal commas, such as in a listing of cities and states. Answer choice A correctly demonstrates this. Answer choice B places the semicolon between the city and its state, instead of between *each* listing of the city and its state, and this is incorrect. A comma is always used to separate a single instance of a city and a state. Answer choice C separate the items in the series with commas, but this creates confusion for the reader, since there are already commas between each city and its state. Answer choice D places commas between each item in the series, but fails to include the necessary comma between each city and its state.

**2. B:** This sentence best conveys the information without using too many words (choice D) or having an awkward construction (choices A and C).

**3. D:** Research papers are formal exercises that should not include several types of speech used in informal spoken settings. Colloquialisms are non-standard forms of language, such as "ain't," or slang, like "dude." Contractions represent the words as they sound in speech, so "do not" is formal whereas "don't" is informal. Relative pronouns are necessary in grammar. In the phrase "The boy who I met…," "who" is a relative pronoun.

**4. C:** When a plural word is made possessive, the standard rule is to place the apostrophe after the final *s*, as in *jurors'*. Answer choice C correctly demonstrates this. Answer choices A and D place the possessive apostrophe within *meals* (*meal's* and *meals'*), and these forms of the word do not make sense within the context of the sentence. Answer choice B places the possessive apostrophe before the final *s*, as in *juror's*, which indicates only a single juror. This form is incorrect in the context of the sentence.

**5. B:** A complex sentence contains a single independent clause in addition to a dependent clause. Answer choice B opens with the dependent clause *Before Ernestine purchases a book* and ends with the independent clause *she always checks to see if the library has it*. Answer choice A is a simple sentence, as it has no dependent clause. Answer choice C is a compound sentence, because it has two independent clauses. Answer choice D is also a simple sentence, although it has a compound subject.

**6. D:** In the context of the sentence, it appears that Finlay's parents are attempting to *coax* him by promising a trip to his favorite toy store. Answer choice A makes little sense, as the sentence indicates Finlay's parents want him to participate in the recital. Answer choice B might work, but the promise of a trip to the toy store seems more like a reward than a punishment. Answer choice C makes no sense when added to the sentence in place of the word *cajole*.

**7. C:** The correct plural form of *tempo* is *tempi*. This word has an Italian root, and thus follows the pattern of other, similar words that end in *-i* in their plural form. Note also that *tempo*, meaning time, is simply the Italian form of the Latin *tempus*. (Recall the Latin expression *tempus fugit*, or "time flies.") Other Latin-based nouns ending in *-us* also take the *-i* ending when made plural: *octopus > octopi, syllabus > syllabi*, etc.

**8. A:** In answer choice A, *aunt Jo* is correctly capitalized, because although *aunt* identifies a specific person, the word her makes *aunt* into an adjective rather than being part of her name. Titles such as uncle or aunt are only to be capitalized if they are at the beginning of a sentence or are used as part of the proper noun. Answer choice B fails to capitalize *Brother Mark*, as *Brother* is part of the full proper noun. In answer choice C, cousin should remain lower case as it is used to describe who Martha is, but is not used as part of her name. Answer choice D incorrectly capitalizes *Fall*. Seasons are not to be capitalized. *Chicago* is correctly capitalized as it is the name of a city, which is a proper noun.

**9. C:** *Acrimonious* means "bitter" or "vitriolic," and is very similar in meaning to *rancorous*.

**10. B:** Answer choice B demonstrates a comma splice, which is the use of a comma to join two independent clauses. Note that *however* is not a conjunction, and cannot join two sentences like other coordinating conjunctions (e.g., *and*, *but*, *or*, etc.) can. Answer choice A correctly uses a semicolon between the independent clauses. Answer choice C correctly uses a period between the independent clauses. Answer choice D correctly uses a comma and the coordinating conjunction *but* to join the independent clauses.

**11. B:** Answer choice B combines the sentences in the best way. The sentences are combined into a single sentence, and all of the details are still included. Answer choices A and D do a good job of combining the sentences, but still consist of more than one sentence. Answer choice C combines the sentences, but leaves out the part about how she "tried to find a way to attend both." There is no clear reason to leave this out, so answer choice C is not the best choice.

**12. D:** The context of the sentence indicates that Mara would feel great happiness.

**13. D:** If the root *meare* means "to pass," and the word *permeate* means "to penetrate or pervade," the most likely meaning of the prefix *per-* is "through." This would yield a literal word meaning of "to pass through," which is similar in meaning to the original: "to penetrate or pervade." The phrase "to pass across" does not match the original Latin origins. Similarly, "to pass by" and "to pass with" are not consistent with the meaning of "passing through."

**14. B:** Anthropology is the study of human culture. Cosmetology is the study of cosmetic techniques. Etymology is the study of word meanings. Genealogy is the study of family history. All of these words would indicate that the suffix *-logy* refers to the study of something. It cannot refer to a record, since that indicates something in the past, and the words in question describe activities that are ongoing. An affinity for something is not the same as a committed study of it, and each item in the question represents its own dedicated field. The suffix for "fear" is *-phobia*.

**15. D:** An adverb modifies a verb, and in the sentence, the word *well* modifies the verb *did* by indicating *how* Jacob did with his speech. The word *worried* is a verb. The word *about* is a preposition. The word *but* is a conjunction.

**16. A:** This answer provides an example of a formal speech, lays out the steps to a solution in a concise manner, and utilizes the correct transition words.

**17. C:** It is correct to pair a plural verb with a collective noun when that noun indicates a plural context. In answer choice C, it is clear that the faculty members are acting individually in their disagreement, so the plural verb makes sense. In answer choice A, the pronoun *neither* is singular, so the verb that accompanies it should also be singular. In answer choice B, the pronoun *all* is plural, so the accompanying verb should be plural. Similarly, in answer choice D, the pronoun *both* is plural, so the verb that accompanies it should also be plural.

**18. D:** The sentence suggests that the scholar was very *knowledgeable* about his subject matter; it is just that his presentation went over the students' heads. The word *authentic* suggests an external guarantee of correctness, which makes little sense in the context of the sentence. The word *arrogant* might be accurate, except that there is nothing in the sentence to suggest the guest speaker deliberately spoke over the students' heads. It is simply that his knowledge was not presented effectively given the audience. Finally, there is nothing in the sentence to suggest that the guest speaker was *faulty* in any way. Rather, he knew so much that he failed to connect with an audience that was less knowledgeable.

**19. C:** The word *sacrilegious* indicates a violation of sacred expectations, and wearing white to a funeral would be something that would violate the sacred expectations of many. The other answer choices are spelled incorrectly, particularly *sacreligious*, which spells the word with the correct spelling of *religious*. This is not correct, as the spelling is adjusted when joined to the other root.

**20. D:** A comma and the conjunction *and* are required to combine the sentences. *And* is a better choice than *but* because the second sentence is a continuation of the first rather than a contradiction. Choices A and B are incorrect because the conjunction *but* doesn't fit the meaning of the sentences. Choice A is also missing the required comma. Choice C uses the correct conjunction, *and*, but is missing the comma.

**21. D:** Answer choice D has a plural subject, but is still a simple sentence. Answer choice A is a compound sentence, as it is composed of two independent clauses. Answer choice B consists of two independent sentences that are joined by a semicolon. (The punctuation is correct, and creates two simple sentences, not one.) Answer choice C contains a dependent clause, so it is a complex sentence.

**22. D:** Answer choice D is a pronoun: the subjective case *I*. Answer choice A is a helping verb. Answer choice B is an adjective. Answer choice C is an adverb.

**23. B:** Answer choice B is the clearest and the most concise. Answer choices A and C include more than one independent clause. As the statement can function as a single independent clause, this is unnecessary. Answer choice D works, but it is not the best option in terms of style, clarity, and concision. The coordinating conjunction with the added independent clause makes the sentence more unwieldy than answer choice B.

**24. B:** The context of the sentence suggests that Mrs. Vanderbroek would not be delighted about any changes to her routine. Thus, answer choice B makes the most sense. Answer choice A has promise, but it does not exactly fit the meaning of the sentence. It is not that Mrs. Vanderbroek would be incapable of accepting change, but rather that she would not welcome it. Answer choices C and D indicate Mrs. Vanderbroek's overall response to changes, but they do not work as synonyms for the word *amenable*.

**25. D:** The words *quick*, *available*, and *little* are all adjectives in the sentence. *Quick* modifies *review*; *available* modifies *housing options*; *little* modifies *choice*. The word *rent* is part of the infinitive (i.e. verbal) phrase *to rent*.

**26. A:** Choice A uses correct punctuation and a logical conjunction. The conjunction *and* connects two independent clauses (meaning that they can stand on their own as sentences), there must be a comma before the conjunction. Therefore, choices B and D are incorrect because they are missing this comma. While choice C does have a comma before the conjunction, it uses the conjunction *but* rather than *and*. *But* implies that the two clauses contradict each other. *And* is a better choice because the two clauses are connected and support each other.

**27. B:** Young people will respond to and better comprehend informal, friendly speech. However, you would not want to be too informal when addressing an educated gathering of college professors or a professional board of directors. Informal speech likely would weaken addresses made before such audiences.

**28. A:** The form *bear* is correct in this context, because it suggests the right to carry or own arms. The form *bare* indicates an uncovered limb. The word *barre* is the French form of *bar*, and is typically used to describe a ballet barre where dancers train. The word *baire* is an alternative colloquial form that refers to a mosquito net in some parts of the United States.

# TEAS Practice Test #3

| Reading | | Mathematics | Science | | English and Language Usage |
|---|---|---|---|---|---|
| 1. ___ | 46. ___ | 1. ___ | 1. ___ | 46. ___ | 1. ___ |
| 2. ___ | 47. ___ | 2. ___ | 2. ___ | 47. ___ | 2. ___ |
| 3. ___ | 48. ___ | 3. ___ | 3. ___ | 48. ___ | 3. ___ |
| 4. ___ | 49. ___ | 4. ___ | 4. ___ | 49. ___ | 4. ___ |
| 5. ___ | 50. ___ | 5. ___ | 5. ___ | 50. ___ | 5. ___ |
| 6. ___ | 51. ___ | 6. ___ | 6. ___ | 51. ___ | 6. ___ |
| 7. ___ | 52. ___ | 7. ___ | 7. ___ | 52. ___ | 7. ___ |
| 8. ___ | 53. ___ | 8. ___ | 8. ___ | 53. ___ | 8. ___ |
| 9. ___ | | 9. ___ | 9. ___ | | 9. ___ |
| 10. ___ | | 10. ___ | 10. ___ | | 10. ___ |
| 11. ___ | | 11. ___ | 11. ___ | | 11. ___ |
| 12. ___ | | 12. ___ | 12. ___ | | 12. ___ |
| 13. ___ | | 13. ___ | 13. ___ | | 13. ___ |
| 14. ___ | | 14. ___ | 14. ___ | | 14. ___ |
| 15. ___ | | 15. ___ | 15. ___ | | 15. ___ |
| 16. ___ | | 16. ___ | 16. ___ | | 16. ___ |
| 17. ___ | | 17. ___ | 17. ___ | | 17. ___ |
| 18. ___ | | 18. ___ | 18. ___ | | 18. ___ |
| 19. ___ | | 19. ___ | 19. ___ | | 19. ___ |
| 20. ___ | | 20. ___ | 20. ___ | | 20. ___ |
| 21. ___ | | 21. ___ | 21. ___ | | 21. ___ |
| 22. ___ | | 22. ___ | 22. ___ | | 22. ___ |
| 23. ___ | | 23. ___ | 23. ___ | | 23. ___ |
| 24. ___ | | 24. ___ | 24. ___ | | 24. ___ |
| 25. ___ | | 25. ___ | 25. ___ | | 25. ___ |
| 26. ___ | | 26. ___ | 26. ___ | | 26. ___ |
| 27. ___ | | 27. ___ | 27. ___ | | 27. ___ |
| 28. ___ | | 28. ___ | 28. ___ | | 28. ___ |
| 29. ___ | | 29. ___ | 29. ___ | | |
| 30. ___ | | 30. ___ | 30. ___ | | |
| 31. ___ | | 31. ___ | 31. ___ | | |
| 32. ___ | | 32. ___ | 32. ___ | | |
| 33. ___ | | 33. ___ | 33. ___ | | |
| 34. ___ | | 34. ___ | 34. ___ | | |
| 35. ___ | | 35. ___ | 35. ___ | | |
| 36. ___ | | 36. ___ | 36. ___ | | |
| 37. ___ | | | 37. ___ | | |
| 38. ___ | | | 38. ___ | | |
| 39. ___ | | | 39. ___ | | |
| 40. ___ | | | 40. ___ | | |
| 41. ___ | | | 41. ___ | | |
| 42. ___ | | | 42. ___ | | |
| 43. ___ | | | 43. ___ | | |
| 44. ___ | | | 44. ___ | | |
| 45. ___ | | | 45. ___ | | |

| **Reading** | Number of Questions: **53** |
| | Time Limit: **64 Minutes** |

**1. Ernestine has a short research project to complete, and her assigned topic is the history of the Globe Theatre in London. Which of the following sources would be the best starting point for Ernestine's research?**

 a. Roget's Thesaurus
 b. Webster's Dictionary
 c. Encyclopedia Britannica
 d. University of Oxford Style Guide

*The next question is based on the following passage.*

Mother Jones, who was a labor activist, wrote the following about children working in cotton mills in Alabama: "Little girls and boys, barefooted, walked up and down between the endless rows of spindles, reaching thin little hands into the machinery to repair snapped threads. They crawled under machinery to oil it. They replaced spindles all day long; all night through...six-year-olds with faces of sixty did an eight-hour shift for ten cents a day; the machines, built in the North, were built low for the hands of little children."

**2. Which of the following do you predict occurred after this was published?**

 a. More children signed up to work in the factories
 b. Cotton factories in the South closed
 c. Laws were passed to prevent child labor
 d. The pay scale for these children was increased

**3. The guide words at the top of a dictionary page are *considerable* and *conspicuous*. Which of the following words is an entry on this page?**

 a. consonantal
 b. consumption
 c. conserve
 d. conquistador

**4. Which of the following is not a reliable resource for a research paper?**

 a. The New York Times
 b. A personal interview with a politician
 c. A medical journal
 d. Wikipedia

*The next question is based on the following passage.*

On April 30, 1803, the United States bought the Louisiana Territory from the French. Astounded and excited by the offer of a sale and all that it would mean, it took less than a month to hear the offer and determine to buy it for $15 million. Right away the United States had more than twice the amount of land as before, giving the country more of a chance to become powerful. They had to move in military and governmental power in this region, but even as this was happening they had very little knowledge about the area. They did not even really know where the land boundaries were, nor did they have any idea how many people lived there. They needed to explore.

**5. What prediction could you make about the time immediately following the Louisiana Purchase?**

    a. Explorers were already on the way to the region.
    b. The government wanted to become powerful.
    c. People in government would make sure explorers went to the region.
    d. Explorers would want to be paid for their work.

**6. Follow the instructions below to transform the starting word into a different word.**

- Start with the word PREVARICATE.
- Remove the P.
- Replace the first A with the final E.
- Remove the I from the word.
- Remove the C from the word.
- Remove the A from the word.

**What is the new word?**

    a. REVEST
    b. REVERT
    c. REVIEW
    d. REVERSE

**7. Ethan works in his company's purchasing department, and he needs to purchase 500 pens to give away to customers. He finds the following information about purchasing pens in bulk.**

| Company | Specialty Pens | Office in Bulk | Office Warehouse | Ballpoint & Lead |
|---|---|---|---|---|
| Price per unit | $.97 per pen | $45 per 50 pens | $95 per 100 pens | $1 per pen OR $99 per 100 pens |

**Based on the information above, which company will have the best price for 500 pens?**

    a. Specialty Pens
    b. Office in Bulk
    c. Office Warehouse
    d. Ballpoint & Lead

*The next four questions are based on the following image.*

**8. On the map above, the symbol /\ indicates mountains. How many different mountain ranges are listed on the map?**

    a. 3
    b. 4
    c. 5
    d. 6

**9. On the map above, the star symbol indicates the state capital. Which city is the capital of Wyoming?**

    a. Laramie
    b. Cheyenne
    c. Jackson
    d. Sheridan

**10. On the map above, how many national parks are shown in the state of Wyoming?**

    a. 2
    b. 3
    c. 4
    d. 5

**11. On the map above, which states are south of Wyoming?**

    a. Utah and Idaho
    b. Colorado and Utah
    c. Montana and Colorado
    d. Colorado and Nebraska

**12. In a lesson on mass media, a teacher is showing commercials and analyzing their hidden messages. Which of the following is an example of a commercial that claims professional authority not supported by evidence?**

 a. A commercial selling pain relief featuring a professional basketball player who says he uses the product

 b. A commercial for cold medicine narrated by a man in a doctor's coat

 c. A commercial for a new toy showing footage of children playing happily with it

 d. A commercial for a prepared food with testimonials by real consumers

*The next three questions are based on the following passage.*

They were known as "The Five": a group of Russian musicians who eschewed rigidly formal classical training and set out on their own to give a new artistic sound to classical music in Russia. Mily Balakirev and Cesar Cui are considered the founders of the movement, but the three who later joined them have become far more famous and respected outside, and perhaps even inside, of Russia. Modest Mussorgsky, with his passion for themes of Russian folklore and nationalism, is remembered for the piano piece *Pictures and an Exhibition*, as well as for the passionate opera *Boris Godunov*. Nikolai Rimsky-Korsakov, who spent his early years as a naval officer, had a penchant for infusing his works with the sounds of the sea. But, he might be best remembered for the hauntingly beautiful symphonic suite *Scheherazade*. Alexander Borodin balanced a career as a skilled and highly respected chemist with his interest in classical music. He produced a number of symphonies, as well as the opera *Prince Igor*. Despite their lack of formal training and their unorthodox approach to producing classical music, The Five had an influence that reached far beyond their time. Composers such as Alexander Glazunov, Sergei Prokofiev, and Igor Stravinsky studied under Rimsky-Korsakov. Additionally, the mid-twentieth century composer Dmitri Shostakovich studied under Glazunov, creating a legacy of musical understanding that persisted well beyond the era of The Five.

**13. Which of the following describes the type of writing used in the passage?**

 a. narrative

 b. persuasive

 c. expository

 d. technical

**14. Which of the following is the best summary sentence for the passage?**

 a. Composers such as Alexander Glazunov, Sergei Prokofiev, and Igor Stravinsky studied under Rimsky-Korsakov.

 b. Despite their lack of formal training and their unorthodox approach to producing classical music, The Five had an influence that reached far beyond their time.

 c. They were known as "The Five": a group of Russian musicians who eschewed rigidly formal classical training and set out on their own to give a new artistic sound to classical music in Russia.

 d. Mily Balakirev and Cesar Cui are considered the founders of the movement, but the three who later joined them have become far more famous and respected outside, and perhaps even inside, of Russia.

**15. Based on the information in the passage, which of the composers among The Five would the author likely agree was the most influential?**

a. Alexander Glazunov
b. Modest Mussorgsky
c. Nikolai Rimsky-Korsakov
d. Cesar Cui

**16. Which of the answer choices gives the best definition for the underlined word in the following sentence?**

**Seeing the cookie crumbs on the child's face, Ena could not believe he would tell such a <u>barefaced</u> lie and claim he had not eaten any cookies.**

a. effective
b. arrogant
c. shameless
d. hostile

*The next five questions are based on the following passage.*

Stories have been a part of the world since the beginning of recorded time. For centuries before the invention of the printing press, stories of the world were passed down to generations through oral tradition. With the invention of the printing press, which made written material available to wide ranges of audiences, books were mass-produced and introduced into greater society.

For the last several centuries, books have been at the forefront of education and entertainment. With the invention of the Internet, reliance on books for information quickly changed. Soon, almost everything that anyone needed to know could be accessed through the Internet. Large printed volumes of encyclopedias became unnecessary as all of the information was easily available on the Internet.

Despite the progression of the Internet, printed media was still very popular in the forms of both fiction and non-fiction books. While waiting for an appointment, enduring a several-hour flight, or relaxing before sleep, books have been a reliable and convenient source of entertainment, and one that society has not been willing to give up.

With the progression and extreme convenience of technology, printed books are going to soon become a thing of the past. Inventions such as the iPad from Macintosh and the Kindle have made the need for any kind of printed media unnecessary. With a rechargeable battery, a large screen, and the ability to have several books saved on file, electronic options will soon take over and society will no longer see printed books.

Although some people may say that the act of reading is not complete without turning a page, sliding a finger across the screen or pressing a button to read more onto the next page is just as satisfying to the reader. The iPad and Kindle are devices that have qualities similar to a computer and can be used for so much more than just reading. These devices are therefore better than books because they have multiple uses.

In a cultural society that is part of the world and due to a longstanding tradition, stories will always be an important way to communicate ideas and provide information and entertainment. Centuries ago, stories could only be remembered and retold through speech. Printed media changed the way the world communicated and was connected, and now, as we move forward with technology, it is only a matter of time before we must say goodbye to the printed past and welcome the digital and electronic future.

**17. What is the main argument of this essay?**

 a. iPad and Kindles are easier to read than books
 b. The printing press was a great invention
 c. The Internet is how people receive information
 d. Technology will soon replace printed material

**18. What is the main purpose of paragraph 1?**

 a. To explain oral tradition
 b. To explain the importance of the printing press
 c. To explain the progression of stories within society
 d. To introduce the essay

**19. According to the essay, what was the first way that stories were communicated and passed down?**

 a. Oral tradition
 b. Printed books
 c. Technology
 d. Hand writing

**20. Which of the following statements is an opinion?**

 a. Despite the progression of the Internet, printed media was still very popular in the forms of both fiction and non-fiction books
 b. Although some people may say that the act of reading is not complete without turning a page, sliding a finger across the screen or pressing a button to read more onto the next page is just as satisfying to the reader
 c. With the invention of the Internet, reliance on books for information quickly changed
 d. Stories have been a part of the world since the beginning of recorded time

**21. What is a secondary argument the author makes?**

 a. Devices such as the iPad or Kindle are better than books because they have multiple uses
 b. Books are still important to have while waiting for an appointment or taking a flight
 c. Printed encyclopedias are still used and more convenient that using the Internet
 d. With technology, there will soon be no need for stories

*The next four questions are based on the following passage.*

Starting in 1856, Alfred, Lord Tennyson began publishing his compilation of Arthurian legends that became known as *Idylls of the King*. These poems were based on the earlier Medieval collection *Le Morte d'Arthur*, by Sir Thomas Malory, which dated to the middle of the 15th century. Malory's work, which is believed to be largely a translation of older French stories, was written in prose style. It combined the earlier tales into a single grouping for English readers. As the title suggests, Malory's focus was largely on the epic nature of Arthur's life. Malory discussed his birth, his rise as a prince and warrior, his quests as a knight, and his eventual death. Malory also included chapters on knights such as Lancelot and Gareth, and he discussed the relationships between Tristan and Isolde, and Lancelot and Guinevere. Instead of embracing the romance angle, however, Malory focused more on the moral elements within these stories.

Tennyson, though heavily influenced by Malory, took a different approach to the Arthurian stories. For one, he wrote them in poetry form, not prose. Additionally, Tennyson, as a Victorian poet, was more interested in the romantic qualities of the stories, and included the distinct elements of nature and elegy. *Idylls of the King* has a softer focus overall. For instance, in Malory's work, Guinevere faces execution for her adultery, and is only spared when Lancelot rides in to rescue her. In Tennyson's work, Arthur chooses to forgive Guinevere, and she chooses to spend the rest of her days doing good works in a convent. Some literary scholars believe that Tennyson was writing an allegory about social problems and the need for social justice that existed during Tennyson's own time. Charles Dickens is remembered for doing the same thing in his novels about the abuses of lower-class children in Victorian England.

**22. Which of the following describes the structure of the above passage?**
a. problem-solution
b. sequence
c. comparison-contrast
d. cause-effect

**23. The author of the passage notes several distinctions between Tennyson and Malory. Which of the following is not identified as a difference between the two authors?**
a. Malory wrote prose, while Tennyson wrote poetry.
b. Malory wrote during the Medieval era, while Tennyson wrote during the Victorian era.
c. Malory was more focused on heroism and morality, while Tennyson was more focused on nature and elegy.
d. Malory wrote stories about Gareth, Tristan, and Isolde, while Tennyson focused only on Arthur, Lancelot, and Guinevere.

**24. Which of the following sentences distracts the reader from the main focus of the passage?**
a. Malory's work, which is believed to be largely a translation of older French stories, was written in prose style.
b. Instead of embracing the romance angle, however, Malory focused more on the moral elements within these stories.
c. In Tennyson's work, Arthur chooses to forgive Guinevere, and she chooses to spend the rest of her days doing good works in a convent.
d. Charles Dickens is remembered for doing the same thing in his novels about the abuses of lower-class children in Victorian England.

**25. With which of the following statements would the author of the passage most likely agree?**

    a. Malory and Tennyson shaped their approach to the Arthurian legends based on the defining qualities of their respective eras.

    b. Because *Le Morte d'Arthur* is more of a translation than a literary creation, *Idylls of the King* is a superior work.

    c. By undermining the moral qualities that Malory highlighted, Tennyson failed to appreciate the larger purpose of the stories in a Medieval context.

    d. Ultimately, Malory's influence on Tennyson was minimal, because Tennyson took a different approach and infused his poems with the mood of his day.

**26. Regina has a severe allergy to dairy products. She is going to attend a work-related function during which lunch will be served. She requests to see the menu before the function to make sure there is something she will be able to eat. For lunch, the organizers will be serving soup, bread, and a light salad. The following soup options are available:**

- **Cream of potato soup**
- **Lentil soup**
- **Broccoli cheese soup**
- **Cream of tomato soup**

**Which of the above options is most likely the best choice for Regina?**

    a. Cream of potato

    b. Lentil soup

    c. Broccoli cheese soup

    d. Cream of tomato soup

*The next two questions are based on the following information.*

<u>World War I Casualties: European Allies (1914–1918)</u>

| Country | Military Deaths | Military Wounded | Civilian Deaths (war/famine/disease) | Total Population | Percent of Population Lost |
|---|---|---|---|---|---|
| Belgium | 58,637 | 44,686 | 62,000 | 7,400,000 | 1.63 |
| France | 1,397,800 | 4,266,000 | 300,000 | 39,600,000 | 4.29 |
| Italy | 651,000 | 953,886 | 589,000 | 35,600,000 | 3.48 |
| Romania | 250,000 | 120,000 | 450,000 | 7,500,000 | 9.33 |
| Russia | 2,254,369 | 4,950,000 | 1,500,000 | 175,100,000 | 2.14 |
| United Kingdom | 886,939 | 1,663,435 | 109,000 | 45,400,000 | 2.19 |

*Sources: Commonwealth War Graves Commission, La Population de la France pendant de la guerre, United Kingdom War Office, United States War Department*

**27. In terms of the percentage of its entire population, which of the following nations suffered the greatest loss during World War I?**

    a. France

    b. Italy

    c. Romania

    d. Russia

**28. In terms of numbers alone, which of the following nations suffered the greatest loss during World War I?**

a. Belgium
b. Romania
c. Russia
d. United Kingdom

*The next four questions refer to the following passage.*

## Tips for Eating Calcium Rich Foods

### Dairy: Beverage

- Include milk as a beverage at meals.
    - Consider choosing fat-free or low-fat milk.
- Whole milk: consider a gradual shift to fat-free milk to lower saturated fat and calories. Start with reduced fat (2%), then low-fat (1%), and finally fat-free (skim).
- Cappuccinos or lattes: ask for them with fat-free (skim) milk.

### Dairy: Meals

- Oatmeal and hot cereals: Try adding fat-free or low-fat milk instead of water
- Use fat-free or low-fat milk when making condensed cream soups (e.g., cream of tomato).
- Shredded low-fat cheese with casseroles, soups, stews, or vegetables
- Fat-free or low-fat yogurt with a baked potato

### Dairy: Snack

- Have fat-free or low-fat yogurt as a snack.
    - Make a dip for fruits or vegetables from yogurt.
    - Make fruit-yogurt smoothies in the blender.

### Dairy: Dessert

- Chocolate or butterscotch pudding with fat-free or low-fat milk.
- Cut-up fruit with flavored yogurt for a quick dessert.

### Non-Dairy Products:

- Lactose Intolerance
    - Lactose-free alternatives within the milk group (e.g., cheese, yogurt, or lactose-free milk)
    - Consume the enzyme lactase before consuming milk products.
- Personal choice to avoid dairy:
    - Calcium fortified juices, cereals, breads, and soy or rice beverages
    - Canned fish (sardines, salmon with bones) soybeans and other soy products, some other dried beans, and some leafy greens.

**29. What text feature does the author use to organize the passage?**

a. headings and subheadings
b. superscripts
c. diagrams
d. labels and footnotes

**30. Which of the following is true about calcium rich foods?**

**I. Canned salmon with bones contains calcium.**

**II. Cheese is a lactose-free food.**

**III. Condensed soup made with water is a calcium rich food.**

    a. I only

    b. I and II only

    c. II and III only

    d. III only

**31. What information should the author include to help clarify information in the passage?**

    a. The fat content of yogurt.

    b. How much calcium is in fortified juice.

    c. Which leafy greens contain calcium.

    d. The definition of lactose intolerance.

**32. The style of this passage is most like that found in a(n)**

    a. tourist guidebook.

    b. health textbook.

    c. encyclopedia.

    d. friendly letter.

*The next two questions are based on the following information.*

Announcement for all faculty members:

It has come to the university's attention that there is crowding in the faculty canteen between the hours of 11 a.m. and 1 p.m., an issue that is due to the increase in staff numbers in several faculty departments. A number of faculty members have complained that they stood in line so long that they were unable to get lunch, or did not have time to eat lunch. To offset the crowding, the university has polled the various departments about schedules, and has settled on a recommended roster for when the members of each department should visit the faculty canteen for lunch:

- Business Dept: 10.30 a.m.–11.30 a.m.
- Art Dept: 10.45 a.m.–11.45 a.m.
- Math and Science Dept: 12 p.m.–1 p.m.
- Social Sciences Dept: 12.30 p.m.–1.30 p.m.
- Humanities Dept: 1 p.m.–2 p.m.

We ask that all faculty members respect this schedule. Faculty will be expected to display a department badge before entering the canteen for lunch.

**33. Based on the information in the announcement, what might the reader assume about how the university determined the lunch schedule?**

    a.  The university arranged the schedule alphabetically, according to the name of each department.

    b.  The university checked with the departments in advance to make sure faculty members would be amenable to the change.

    c.  The university checked to see when the most faculty members from each department would be entering the canteen.

    d.  The university was most concerned about crowding in the canteen, and simply decided to establish different times for each department.

**34. Which best describes the final two sentences of the announcement?**

    a.  a friendly reminder to all faculty members to bring a badge to the canteen

    b.  a word of caution to faculty members about trying to enter the canteen at the wrong time

    c.  an implied suggestion that faculty members should consider getting lunch elsewhere

    d.  an indication of university sanctions for faculty members who enter the canteen outside the schedule

*The next two questions are based on the following information.*

During the summer, Angela read the following classics: *The Great Gatsby*, by F. Scott Fitzgerald; *Brave New World*, by Aldous Huxley; *A Passage to India*, by E.M. Forster; and "The Cask of Amontillado," by Edgar Allen Poe.

**35. In the statement above, several items are italicized, while only one is placed in quotation marks. According to the rules of punctuation, the following should be placed in quotation marks: article titles, book chapters, short stories, and episodes of television shows. Considering the list of works that Angela read, into which category does "The Cask of Amontillado" most likely fit?**

    a.  newspaper article

    b.  book chapter

    c.  short story

    d.  television show episode

**36. What is the purpose of the italics used for several of the works identified in the sentence above?**

    a.  to indicate a full-length published book

    b.  to indicate a work of classic literature

    c.  to indicate recommended summer reading

    d.  to indicate books that Angela completed

**37. Based on this description, what can be inferred about the reviewer's opinion?**

**In a book review published in a large national newspaper, the reviewer said the book was "most likely to be enjoyed only by those with puerile fantasies."**

    a.  The reviewer strongly recommends the book for young adults.

    b.  The reviewer believes the book is inappropriate for children.

    c.  The reviewer considers the book to have wide audience appeal.

    d.  The reviewer feels that the book would not appeal to mature adults.

*The next two questions are based on the following information.*

Thomas and his sister are planning to see a new science fiction film, but they have to work around their schedules. Both are free for a showing before 6 p.m. or after 10 p.m. Here are the current show times for cinemas in their area:

- Twin Theatres: 6:15 p.m., 7:20 p.m., and 8:40 p.m.
- Reveler Cinema: 5:45 p.m. and 7:15 p.m.
- Big Screen 14: 6:00 p.m., 6:45 p.m., 9:10 p.m., and 10:05 p.m.
- Best Seat in The House: 8:20 p.m., 9:55 p.m., and 11:25 p.m.

**38. Which of these cinemas does not have an option that will work for Thomas and his sister?**
- a. Twin Theatres
- b. Reveler Cinema
- c. Big Screen 14
- d. Best Seat in The House

**39. After an unexpected rearrangement of their schedules, Thomas and his sister realize that they will have to squeeze in the film after 10.30 p.m. Given this new information, which cinema is the best option?**
- a. Twin Theatres
- b. Reveler Cinema
- c. Big Screen 14
- d. Best Seat in The House

*The next two questions are based on the information above.*

In an effort to conserve water, the town of Audley has asked residents and businesses to water their lawns just one day a week. It has provided the following schedule based on addresses:

- Monday: addresses ending in 0 and 9
- Tuesday: addresses ending in 1 and 8
- Wednesday: addresses ending in 2 and 7
- Thursday: addresses ending in 3 and 6
- Friday: addresses ending in 5
- Saturday: addresses ending in 4

Businesses with suite numbers should use the final number in the suite number to determine their watering schedule.

**40. The Morgan family lives at 5487 South Elm Street. On which day of the week will they be able to water their lawn?**
- a. Tuesday
- b. Wednesday
- c. Thursday
- d. Saturday

**41. The watering schedule has only one number for both Friday and Saturday. Based on the information provided, what is the most logical reason for this?**

 a. There are more addresses ending with these numbers than with the other numbers.
 b. All businesses have addresses ending in these numbers, and they consume the most water.
 c. The residents at these addresses are the most likely to consume more water.
 d. The city is more concerned about water usage in the latter part of the week.

**42. Which of the following stories' messages is significantly distorted through the use of an irrelevant detail?**

 a. A soft profile about a local politician's part-time rock band that mentions his political differences with his band mates
 b. A feature story of a local business owner running for political office in which she admits to having employed illegal laborers
 c. A profile of several local Jewish and Arab business leaders that mentions ongoing hostilities in the Middle East
 d. A news report about a local citizen protesting property tax rates that includes details about an immigration violation he committed twenty years previously

*The next four questions are based on the following two passages.*

*Passage 1:*

 Fairy tales, fictional stories that involve magical occurrences and imaginary creatures like trolls, elves, giants, and talking animals, are found in similar forms throughout the world. This occurs when a story with an origin in a particular location spreads geographically to, over time, far-flung lands. All variations of the same story must logically come from a single source. As language, ideas, and goods travel from place to place through the movement of peoples, stories that catch human imagination travel as well through human retelling.

*Passage 2:*

 Fairy tales capture basic, fundamental human desires and fears. They represent the most essential form of fictionalized human experience: the bad characters are pure evil, the good characters are pure good, the romance of royalty (and of commoners becoming royalty) is celebrated, etc. Given the nature of the fairy tale genre, it is not surprising that many different cultures come up with similar versions of the same essential story.

**43. On what point would the authors of both passages agree?**

 a. Fairy tales share a common origin.
 b. The same fairy tale may develop independently in a number of different cultures.
 c. There are often common elements in fairy tales from different cultures.
 d. Fairy tales capture basic human fears.

**44. What does the "nature of the fairy tale genre" refer to in Passage 2?**

 a. The representation of basic human experience
 b. Good characters being pure good and bad characters being pure evil
 c. Different cultures coming up with similar versions of the same story
 d. Commoners becoming royalty

**45. Which of the following is not an example of something the author of Passage 1 claims travels from place to place through human movement?**

    a. Fairy tales
    b. Language
    c. Ideas
    d. Foods

**46. Which of the following is not an example of something that the author of Passage 1 states might be found in a fairy tale?**

    a. Trolls
    b. Witches
    c. Talking animals
    d. Giants

*The next two questions are based on the passage above.*

What outdoorsy, family adventure can you have on a hot, summer day? How about spelunking? If you live in an area that is anywhere near a guided, lit cave, find out the hours of operation and hit the road towards it as soon as you can. Hitch up the double jogging stroller and make your way out into the wilderness, preferably with a guide, and discover the wonders of the cool, dark earth even while it is sweltering hot in the outside world. It will be 58 degrees in that cave, and you can explore inside for as long as you please. Best part? The absolutely awesome naps that the kids will take after such an exciting adventure! Be sure to bring the following items:

- Bottled water
- Light-up tennis shoes if you have them (they look fabulous in the dark)
- Flashlights or glow sticks just for fun
- Jackets
- Changes of clothes in case of getting muddy and/or dirty

**47. Based on the information given, what is spelunking?**

    a. going in a cave
    b. an outdoor adventure
    c. walking with a double stroller
    d. a hot, summer day

**48. Given the style of writing for the passage, which of the following magazines would be the best fit for this article?**

    a. *Scientific Spelunking*
    b. *Family Fun Days*
    c. *Adventures for Men*
    d. *Mud Magazine*

*The next four questions are based on the following passage:*

**How are Hypotheses Confirmed?**

Most scientists agree that while the scientific method is an invaluable methodological tool, it is not a failsafe method for arriving at objective truth. It is debatable, for example, whether a hypothesis can actually be confirmed by evidence.

When a hypothesis is of the form "All $x$ are $y$," it is commonly believed that a piece of evidence that is both $x$ and $y$ confirms the hypothesis. For example, for the hypothesis "All monkeys are hairy," a particular monkey that is hairy is thought to be a confirming piece of evidence for the hypothesis. A problem arises when one encounters evidence that disproves a hypothesis: while no scientist would argue that one piece of evidence proves a hypothesis, it is possible for one piece of evidence to disprove a hypothesis. To return to the monkey example, one hairless monkey out of one billion hairy monkeys disproves the hypothesis "All monkeys are hairy." Single pieces of evidence, then, seem to affect a given hypothesis in radically different ways. For this reason, the confirmation of hypotheses is better described as probabilistic.

Hypotheses that can only be proven or disproven based on evidence need to be based on probability because sample sets for such hypotheses are too large. In the monkey example, every single monkey in the history of monkeys would need to be examined before the hypothesis could be proven or disproven. By making confirmation a function of probability, one may make provisional or working conclusions that allow for the possibility of a given hypothesis being disconfirmed in the future. In the monkey case, then, encountering a hairy monkey would slightly raise the probability that "all monkeys are hairy," while encountering a hairless monkey would slightly decrease the probability that "all monkeys are hairy." This method of confirming hypotheses is both counterintuitive and controversial, but it allows for evidence to equitably affect hypotheses and it does not require infinite sample sets for confirmation or disconfirmation.

**49. What is the main idea of the second paragraph?**
   a. One hairy monkey proves the hypothesis "All monkeys are hairy."
   b. The same piece of evidence can both confirm and disconfirm a hypothesis.
   c. Confirming and disconfirming evidence affect hypotheses differently.
   d. The scientific method is not a failsafe method for arriving at objective truth.

**50. A synonym for *disconfirmed* would be:**
   a. proven
   b. dissipated
   c. distilled
   d. disproven

**51. Which of the following is true of hypotheses of the form "All $x$ are $y$"?**
   a. Something that is neither $x$ nor $y$ disproves the hypothesis.
   b. Something that is both $x$ and $y$ disproves the hypothesis.
   c. Something that is $x$ but not $y$ disproves the hypothesis.
   d. Something that is $y$ but not $x$ disproves the hypothesis.

**52. Using the same reasoning as that in the passage, an automobile with eighteen wheels does what to the following hypothesis: "All automobiles have only four wheels"?**

   a.  It proves the hypothesis.
   b.  It raises the hypothesis's probability.
   c.  It disproves the hypothesis.
   d.  It decreases the hypothesis's probability.

*The next question refers to the following graphic.*

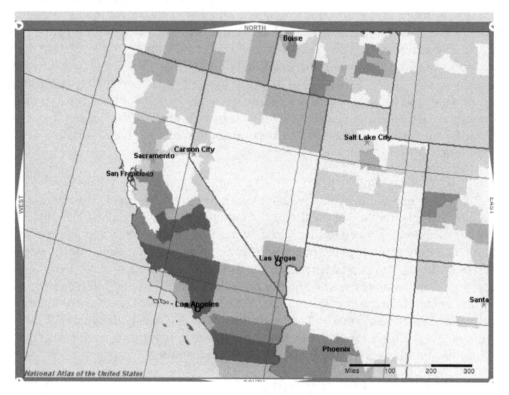

**53. Shaded areas on the map indicate water use, with darker areas indicating heavier use. Which of the following is the best inference regarding the areas where there is no shading?**

   a.  They are less inhabited.
   b.  They are more desert-like.
   c.  Residents are better at conservation.
   d.  Residents require less water per capita.

| | Number of Questions: **36** |
|---|---|
| **Mathematics** | Time Limit: **54 Minutes** |

**1. Solve for *x*:**

$$\frac{4}{x+6} = 2$$

    a.   $x = 8$
    b.   $x = -4$
    c.   $x = -8$
    d.   $x = 4$

**2. Dr. Lee saw that 30% of all his patients developed an infection after taking a certain antibiotic. He further noticed that 5% of that 30% required hospitalization to recover from the infection. What percentage of Dr. Lee's patients were hospitalized after taking the antibiotic?**

    a.   1.5%
    b.   5%
    c.   15%
    d.   30%

**3. A patient requires a 30% increase in the dosage of her medication. Her current dosage is 270 mg. What will her dosage be after the increase?**

    a.   81 mg
    b.   270 mg
    c.   300 mg
    d.   351 mg

**4. Which of the following describes a graph that represents a proportional relationship?**

    a.   The graph has a slope of 2,500 and a y-intercept of 250
    b.   The graph has a slope of 1,500 and a y-intercept of –150
    c.   The graph has a slope of 2,000 and a y-intercept of 0
    d.   The graph has a slope of –1,800 and a y-intercept of –100

**5. University X requires some of its nursing students to take an exam before being admitted into the nursing program. In this year's class, $\frac{1}{2}$ the nursing students were required to take the exam and $\frac{3}{5}$ of those who took the exam passed the exam. If this year's class has 200 students, how many students passed the exam?**

    a.   120
    b.   100
    c.   60
    d.   50

*The next two questions are based on the following information.*

Four roommates must use their financial aid checks to pay their living expenses.
Each student receives $1000 per month.

**6. One roommate is saving to buy a house, so each month he puts money aside in a special house savings account. The ratio of his monthly house savings to his rent is 1:3. If he pays $270 per month in rent, how much money does he put into his house savings account each month?**

    a. $90
    b. $270
    c. $730
    d. $810

**7. Three of the roommates decided to combine their money to purchase a single birthday gift for the fourth roommate. The first roommate donated $12.03. The second roommate contributed $11.96, and the third roommate gave $12.06. Estimate the total amount of money the roommates used to purchase the gift.**

    a. $34
    b. $35
    c. $36
    d. $37

**8. Jeremy put a heavy chalk mark on the tire of his bicycle. His bike tire is 27 inches in diameter. When he rolled the bike, the chalk left marks on the sidewalk. Which expression can be used to best determine the distance, in inches, the bike rolled from the first mark to the fourth mark?**

    a. $3(27\pi)$
    b. $4\pi(27)$
    c. $(27 \div 3)\pi$
    d. $(27 \div 4)\pi$

**9. The table below shows the average amount of rainfall Houston receives during the summer and autumn months.**

| Month | Rainfall (inches) |
|---|---|
| June | 5.35 |
| July | 3.18 |
| August | 3.83 |
| September | 4.33 |
| October | 4.5 |
| November | 4.19 |

**What percentage of rainfall received during this timeframe, is received during the month of October?**

    a. 13.5%
    b. 15.1%
    c. 16.9%
    d. 17.7%

10. Matthew has to earn more than 96 points on his high school entrance exam in order to be eligible for varsity sports. Each question is worth 3 points, and the test has a total of 40 questions. Let *x* represent the number of test questions. How many questions can Matthew answer incorrectly and still qualify for varsity sports?

 a.  $x > 32$
 b.  $x > 8$
 c.  $0 \leq x < 8$
 d.  $0 \leq x \leq 8$

11. Which of the following best represents the surface area of the cylinder shown below?

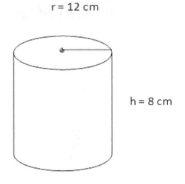

r = 12 cm

h = 8 cm

 a.  602.9 cm$^2$
 b.  904.3 cm$^2$
 c.  1,408.7 cm$^2$
 d.  1,507.2 cm$^2$

12. A lab technician took 500 milliliters of blood from a patient. The technician used $\frac{1}{6}$ of the blood for further tests. How many milliliters of blood were used for further tests? Round your answer to the nearest hundredth.

 a.  83.00
 b.  83.30
 c.  83.33
 d.  83.34

13. Hannah spends at least $16 on 4 packages of coffee. Which of the following inequalities represents the possible costs?

 a.  16 ≥ 4p
 b.  16 < 4p
 c.  16 > 4p
 d.  16 ≤ 4p

**14. Which of the following describes a proportional relationship?**

    a.  Jonathan opens a savings account, with an initial deposit of $150, and deposits $125 per month

    b.  Bruce pays his employees $12 per hour worked, during the month of December, as well as a $250 bonus

    c.  Alvin pays $28 per month for his phone service, plus $0.07 for each long-distance minute used

    d.  Kevin drives 65 miles per hour

**15. Veronica decided to celebrate her promotion by purchasing a new car. The base price for the car was $40,210. She paid an additional $3,015 for a surround sound system and $5,218 for a maintenance package. What was the total price of Veronica's new car?**

    a.  $50,210

    b.  $48,443

    c.  $43,225

    d.  $40,210

**16. Simplify the following expression:**

$$\frac{13}{22} - \frac{3}{11}$$

    a.  $\frac{19}{22}$

    b.  $\frac{7}{22}$

    c.  $\frac{10}{11}$

    d.  $\frac{5}{11}$

**17. The number of vacuum cleaners sold by a company per month during Year 1 is listed below.**

**18, 42, 29, 40, 24, 17, 29, 44, 19, 33, 46, 39**

**Which of the following is true?**

    a.  The mean is less than the median

    b.  The mode is greater than the median

    c.  The mode is less than the mean, median, and range

    d.  The mode is equal to the range

**18. Lauren must travel a distance of 1,480 miles to get to her destination. She plans to drive approximately the same number of miles per day for 5 days. Which of the following is a reasonable estimate of the number of miles she will drive per day?**

    a.  240 miles

    b.  260 miles

    c.  300 miles

    d.  340 miles

19. Based on their prescribing habits, a set of doctors was divided into three groups: $\frac{1}{3}$ of the doctors were placed in Group X because they always prescribed medication. $\frac{5}{12}$ of the doctors were placed in Group Y because they never prescribed medication. $\frac{1}{4}$ of the doctors were placed in Group Z because they sometimes prescribed medication. Order the groups from largest to smallest, according to the number of doctors in each group.

    a. Group X, Group Y, Group Z
    b. Group Z, Group Y, Group X
    c. Group Z, Group X, Group Y
    d. Group Y, Group X, Group Z

20. Solve for $y$:

$$\frac{2y}{10} + 5 = 25$$

    a. $y = 25$
    b. $y = 100$
    c. $y = 150$
    d. $y = 200$

21. Solve for $x$:

$$3(x - 1) = 2(3x - 9)$$

    a. $x = 2$
    b. $x = \frac{8}{3}$
    c. $x = -5$
    d. $x = 5$

22. During January, Dr. Lewis worked 20 shifts. During February, she worked three times as many shifts as she did during January. During March, she worked half the number of shifts she worked during February. Which equation below describes the number of shifts Dr. Lewis worked in March?

    a. shifts $= 20 + 3 + \frac{1}{2}$
    b. shifts $= (20)(3)\left(\frac{1}{2}\right)$
    c. shifts $= (20)(3) + \frac{1}{2}$
    d. shifts $= 20 + (3)\left(\frac{1}{2}\right)$

23. A book has a width of 2.5 decimeters. What is the width of the book in centimeters?

    a. 0.25 centimeters
    b. 25 centimeters
    c. 250 centimeters
    d. 0.025 centimeters

**24. Robert secures three new clients every eight months. After how many months has he secured 24 new clients?**

    a.   64
    b.   58
    c.   52
    d.   66

**25. Simplify the following expression:**

$$\frac{5}{9} \times \frac{3}{4}$$

    a.   $\frac{5}{12}$
    b.   $\frac{8}{13}$
    c.   $\frac{20}{27}$
    d.   $\frac{47}{36}$

**26. What is the independent variable in the graph below?**

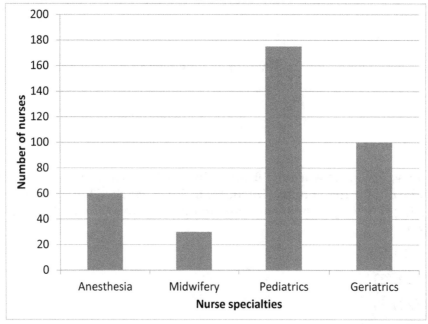

    a.   Anesthesia
    b.   Geriatrics
    c.   Nurse specialties
    d.   Number of nurses

**27. How many centimeters are in 7 meters?**

    a.   7 m = 7 cm
    b.   7 m = 70 cm
    c.   7 m = 700 cm
    d.   7 m = 7000 cm

**28. About how long is the average human eyelash?**

    a.  1 nanometer
    b.  1 centimeter
    c.  1 meter
    d.  1 kilometer

**29. A farmer plans to install fencing around a certain field. If each side of the hexagonal field is 320 feet long, and fencing costs $1.75 per foot, how much will the farmer need to spend on fencing material to fence the perimeter of the field?**

    a.  $2,240
    b.  $2,800
    c.  $3,360
    d.  $4,480

**30. Which of the following is listed in order from *least to greatest*?**

    a.  $-2\frac{3}{4}, -2\frac{7}{8}, -\frac{1}{5}, \frac{2}{5}, \frac{1}{8}$
    b.  $-\frac{1}{5}, \frac{1}{8}, \frac{2}{5}, -2\frac{3}{4}, -2\frac{7}{8}$
    c.  $-2\frac{7}{8}, -2\frac{3}{4}, -\frac{1}{5}, \frac{1}{8}, \frac{2}{5}$
    d.  $\frac{1}{8}, \frac{2}{5}, -\frac{1}{5}, -2\frac{7}{8}, -2\frac{3}{4}$

*The next three questions are based on the following information.*

### Profile of Staff at Hospital X and Hospital Y
(Total Staff: 433)

| Hospital X (250) | Profession | Hospital Y (183) |
|---|---|---|
| 74 | Doctor | 55 |
| 121 | Registered Nurse | 87 |
| 14 | Administrator | 9 |
| 15 | Maintenance | 11 |
| 6 | Pharmacist | 5 |
| 4 | Radiologist | 2 |
| 2 | Physical Therapist | 2 |
| 1 | Speech Pathologist | 1 |
| 13 | Other | 11 |
|  | **Gender** |  |
| 153 | Male | 93 |
| 97 | Female | 90 |
|  | **Age** |  |
| 24 | Youngest | 22 |
| 73 | Oldest | 77 |
|  | **Ethnicity** |  |
| 51 | African American | 42 |
| 50 | Asian American | 27 |
| 45 | Hispanic American | 35 |
| 47 | Caucasian | 37 |
| 57 | Other | 42 |
|  | **Years on Staff** |  |
| 64 | 0–5 | 32 |
| 63 | 5–10 | 41 |
| 57 | 10–15 | 67 |
| 47 | 15–20 | 30 |
| 14 | 20–25 | 19 |
| 5 | More than 25 | 5 |
|  | **Number of Patient Complaints** |  |
| 202 | 0 | 161 |
| 43 | 1–4 | 21 |
| 5 | 5–10 | 1 |
| 0 | More than 10 | 0 |

**31. Which percentage is greatest?**

a. The percentage of Asian Americans to staff as a whole at Hospital X?
b. The percentage of staff members who have been on staff 10–15 years to staff as a whole at Hospital X?
c. The percentage of Doctors to staff as a whole at Hospital X and Hospital Y?
d. The percentage of staff with 1–4 complaints to staff as a whole at Hospital Y?

**32. Approximately what percentage more staff members at Hospital Y are female than at Hospital X?**

a. 5
b. 10
c. 15
d. 20

**33. According to the chart, the percentage of staff who have received zero complaints is**

a. greater at Hospital X than at Hospital Y
b. greater at Hospital Y than at Hospital X
c. the same at Hospital X and at Hospital Y
d. increasing at both hospitals

**34. The number of flights a flight attendant made per month is represented by the line graph below.**

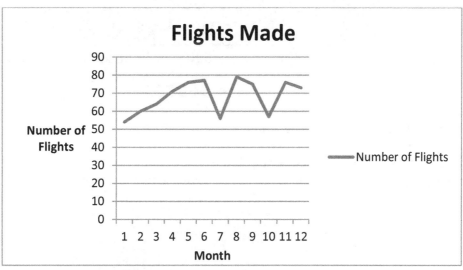

**What is the range in the number of flights the flight attendant made?**

a. 20
b. 25
c. 29
d. 32

**35. The number of houses Amelia has sold per year over the past ten years is listed below:**

**42, 36, 39, 45, 11, 47, 38, 41, 44, 34**

**Which of the following measures will most accurately reflect the number of houses she sold per year?**

    a.  Mean
    b.  Median
    c.  Mode
    d.  Range

**36. The histogram below represents the overall GRE scores for a sample of college students. Which of the following is a true statement?**

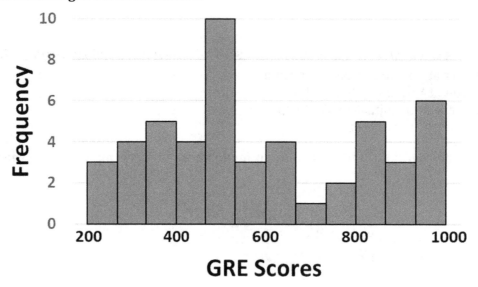

    a.  The range of GRE scores is approximately 600.
    b.  The average GRE score is 750.
    c.  The median GRE score is approximately 500.
    d.  The fewest number of college students had an approximate score of 800.

| | Number of Questions: **53** |
|---|---|
| **Science** | Time Limit: **63 Minutes** |

**1. Which of the following items is NOT appropriately matched with its corresponding bodily system?**

    a.  Kidneys; genitourinary system.
    b.  Heart; circulatory system.
    c.  Blood; endocrine system.
    d.  Diaphragm; respiratory system.

**2. Which of the following describes the order food travels through the digestive system?**

    a.  Trachea, stomach, small intestine, large intestine, rectum.
    b.  Mouth, stomach, small intestine, large intestine, rectum.
    c.  Stomach, large intestine, small intestine, rectum.
    d.  Esophagus, stomach, small intestine, large intestine, rectum.

**3. Which of the following structures is the natural pacemaker of the heart?**

    a.  Sinoatrial node.
    b.  Submental node.
    c.  Atrioventricular node.
    d.  Scalene node.

**4. A patient's heart rate is measured at 118 beats per minute (bpm). What is this condition called?**

    a.  Tachycardia.
    b.  Apnea.
    c.  Bradycardia.
    d.  Tachypnea.

**5. Which of the following items is NOT a primary function of a healthy immune system?**

    a.  The immune system helps the body avoid infections.
    b.  The immune system detects infections.
    c.  The immune system eliminates infections.
    d.  The immune system creates infections.

**6. The spine and hips belong to which of the following bone types?**

    a.  Curvy bones.
    b.  Irregular bones.
    c.  Flat bones.
    d.  Long bones.

**7. Long bones are one of the five major types of bone in the human body. All of the following bones are long bones, EXCEPT:**

    a.  thighs.
    b.  forearms.
    c.  ankles.
    d.  fingers.

### 8. Which of the following is not a type of muscle tissue?

a. Skeletal.
b. Smooth.
c. Cardiac.
d. Adipose.

*The next two questions pertain to the following passage:*

Your class is competing with another class to determine who has the best plant color. Your class decides to test a couple of solutions to determine which would be best for overall plant color before competing. The class decides to water the plants once a week with 200 mL of the following solutions: water, diet soda, 1% bleach solution, and a 1% salt solution. All plants are placed in the window that receives the recommended amount of light. After a month of testing, your class notices that only two plants are alive, but one of those two does not look healthy.

### 9. Based on the results that were stated, what would be a logical reason for some of the plants dying with the salt solution?

a. Salt caused the plants to begin to dry up, causing them to die.
b. The salt did not affect the plants.
c. The salt provided adequate nutrients for color.
d. None of the above

### 10. What is the control, if any, in this experiment?

a. There is no control in this experiment.
b. The control is the water.
c. The control is the diet soda.
d. The control is the amount of sunlight provided to the plants.

### 11. When describing a part of the body that is in the front, which of the following anatomical location descriptors would be utilized?

a. Superior.
b. Anterior.
c. Inferior.
d. Posterior.

### 12. Which of the following statements is accurate?

a. The spine is located posteriorly, inferior to the pelvic bone.
b. The sternum is located anteriorly, superior to the pelvic bone.
c. The mandible is located superior to the nasal cavity, and inferior to the esophagus.
d. The femur is located inferior to the tibia.

### 13. Which of the following terms means close to the trunk of the body?

a. Superficial.
b. Sagittal.
c. Proximal.
d. Distal.

**14. Which part of the cell serves as the control center for all cell activity?**

   a. Nucleus.
   b. Cell membrane.
   c. Cytoplasm.
   d. Mitochondria.

**15. What are the cellular functions of cilia and flagella?**

   a. Cilia and flagella are responsible for cell movement.
   b. Cilia and flagella synthesize proteins.
   c. Cilia and flagella help protect the cell from its environment.
   d. Cilia and flagella have enzymes that help with digestion.

**16. What is the process by which simple cells become highly specialized cells?**

   a. Cellular complication.
   b. Cellular specialization.
   c. Cellular differentiation.
   d. Cellular modification.

**17. How does meiosis differ from mitosis?**

   a. Meiosis is used to repair the body. Mitosis is used to break down the body.
   b. Meiosis is used for asexual reproduction of single-celled organisms. Mitosis is used for sexual reproduction of multicellular organisms.
   c. Meiosis only occurs in humans. Mitosis only occurs in plants.
   d. Meiosis produces cells that are genetically different. Mitosis produces cells that are genetically identical.

**18. Which of the following is NOT a function of the integumentary system?**

   a. Protects internal tissues from injury.
   b. Waterproofs the body.
   c. Helps regulate body temperature.
   d. Returns fluid to the blood vessels.

**19. What are groups of cells that perform the same function called?**

   a. Tissues.
   b. Plastids.
   c. Organs.
   d. Molecules.

**20. Which of the following correctly matches the tissue to its function?**

   a. Epithelial: movement, contraction, support and positioning.
   b. Nervous: transmission and reception.
   c. Muscular: support, protection, separation and connection.
   d. Connective: protection, sensation, absorption, and secretion.

**21. The function of the adrenal glands is to:**

    a. produce hormones that stimulate the thyroid, therefore influencing metabolism.

    b. produce hormones that regulate the salt and water balance and control blood pressure and heart rate.

    c. regulate the release of insulin in response to glucose.

    d. regulate the release of oxytocin, an important hormone in reproduction and childbirth.

**22. What functions do genes serve in the relationship between parents and offspring?**

    a. Genes enable hereditary information to be passed from parents to offspring.

    b. Genes prohibit hereditary information from being passed from parents to offspring.

    c. Genes enable environmental factors to affect parents and offspring.

    d. Genes serve no function in the relationship between parents and offspring.

**23. Which of the following inappropriately describes hemoglobin?**

    a. Hemoglobin transports oxygen from the lungs to the rest of the body.

    b. Hemoglobin is the ratio of red blood cells to total blood volume.

    c. Hemoglobin is a type of protein found in red blood cells of all mammals.

    d. Hemoglobin is the portion of the red blood cell that contains iron, to which oxygen binds.

**24. All of the following belong together EXCEPT:**

    a. thyroid.

    b. stomach.

    c. intestines.

    d. pancreas.

*The next two questions are based on the following information.*

A person with the *T* gene will be tall and a person with the *t* gene will be short. A person with the *B* gene will have black hair and a person with the *b* gene will have red hair. Now consider the Punnett square below.

|   | T | t |
|---|---|---|
| **B** | Possibility 1 | Possibility 2 |
| **b** | Possibility 3 | Possibility 4 |

**25. What are the characteristics of the person with genes from possibility 3?**

    a. Short with black hair.

    b. Short with red hair.

    c. Tall with black hair.

    d. Tall with red hair.

**26. Which possibility would produce a short offspring with black hair?**

    a. Possibility 1.

    b. Possibility 2.

    c. Possibility 3.

    d. Possibility 4.

**27. What is the purpose of conducting an experiment?**

    a. To test a hypothesis.
    b. To collect data.
    c. To identify a control state.
    d. To choose variables.

**28. The valve that allows blood flow from the right atria into the right ventricle is the:**

    a. tricuspid valve.
    b. pulmonic valve.
    c. mitral valve.
    d. aortic valve.

**29. What are substances that stimulate adaptive immunity called?**

    a. Peptides.
    b. Phagocytes.
    c. Prions.
    d. Platelets.

**30. Fill in the blanks in the following sentence:**

**Enzymes are _____ molecules that serve as _____ for certain biological reactions.**

    a. irrelevant; suppressors
    b. acidic; catalysts
    c. lipid; catalysts
    d. protein; catalysts

**31. Which of the following has the least number of sweat glands?**

    a. Back.
    b. Palms.
    c. Axilla.
    d. Forehead.

**32. What type of chemical bond connects the oxygen and hydrogen atoms in a molecule of water?**

    a. Static bond.
    b. Aquatic bond.
    c. Ionic bond.
    d. Covalent bond.

**33. Which of the following statements describes a chemical property of water?**

    a. Water has a pH of 1.
    b. A water molecule contains 2 hydrogen atoms and 1 oxygen atom.
    c. A water molecule contains 2 oxygen atoms and 1 hydrogen atom.
    d. The chemical formula for water is $HO_2$.

**34. Which of the following is needed for an experiment to be considered successful?**

    a. A reasonable hypothesis.
    b. A well-written lab report.
    c. Data that others can be reproduced.
    d. Computer-aided statistical analysis.

**35. An atom has 2 protons, 4 neutrons, and 2 electrons. What is the approximate atomic mass of this atom?**

    a.  2.
    b.  4.
    c.  6.
    d.  8.

**36. Which of the following is true regarding T cells?**

    a.  They are only seen in those with leukemia.
    b.  They are a specialized type of red blood cell.
    c.  They mature in the thyroid.
    d.  They play a role in the immune response.

**37. What type of bond is formed when electrons are transferred between atoms?**

    a.  Transfer bond.
    b.  Static bond.
    c.  Covalent bond.
    d.  Ionic bond.

**38. The table below contains information from the periodic table of elements.**

| Element | Atomic number | Approximate atomic weight |
|---------|---------------|---------------------------|
| B | 5 | 11 |
| C | 6 | 12 |
| N | 7 | 14 |
| O | 8 | 16 |

**Which pattern below best describes the masses of the elements listed in the table?**

    a.  The elements are listed in random order, C being the heaviest element and N being the lightest element.
    b.  The elements are listed in decreasing order, B being the heaviest element and O being the lightest element.
    c.  The elements are listed in increasing order, B being the lightest element and O being the heaviest element.
    d.  All the elements weigh the same, so the order is irrelevant.

**39. What is the primary function of antibodies?**

    a.  Production of white blood cells.
    b.  Initiates gluconeogenesis.
    c.  Promotes the intracellular storage of lipids.
    d.  Facilitate the breakdown of antigens.

**40. Which statement below best describes the process of condensation?**

    a.  Condensation is the process of changing from a gas to a liquid.
    b.  Condensation is the process of changing from a liquid to a gas.
    c.  Condensation is the process of changing from a solid to a liquid.
    d.  Condensation is the process of changing from a solid to a gas.

**41. Which of the following lists the normal blood flow through the heart?**

a. Left ventricle, left atria, body, right ventricle, right atrium, lungs.
b. Left atrium, left ventricle, lungs, right atrium, right ventricle, body.
c. Right atrium, right ventricle, lungs, left atrium, left ventricle, body.
d. Right ventricle, right atria, body, left atrium, left ventricle, lungs.

**42. Which of the following functions is not controlled by the autonomic nervous system?**

a. Digestion.
b. Walking.
c. Heartbeat.
d. Temperature regulation.

**43. Every child in a certain family suffers from autism. Based on this evidence, what possible conclusion can be drawn about autism?**

a. Autism may be lethal.
b. Autism may be genetic.
c. Autism is related to traditional nuclear family structures.
d. No conclusion can be drawn based on this evidence.

**44. Women were more likely to die in childbirth in the 18th century than in the 21st century. What is a possible explanation for why women are less likely to die in childbirth in the present age?**

a. Doctors are better equipped to perform cesarean sections.
b. Doctors have more tools to monitor mothers during childbirth, so complications can be detected much earlier.
c. Doctors wash their hands well to avoid transferring germs and infections.
d. All of the statements above offer reasonable explanations for decreases in mortality during childbirth.

**45. A dietitian wants to convince a patient to lose weight. Which statement below best communicates a scientific argument that justifies the need for weight loss?**

a. Losing weight can lower blood pressure, increase energy level, and promote overall health.
b. Society tends to treat overweight people unfairly.
c. Members of the opposite sex are more interested in people who maintain a healthy weight.
d. Losing weight is easy to do.

**46. A researcher wants to investigate the relationship between family income and quality of medical care. Which statement provides the best reason to conduct this investigation?**

a. The researcher can learn more about wealthy people and ask them for money.
b. The investigation can help target healthy people so that they can remain healthy.
c. Results of this investigation may identify a group of people who do not receive quality medical care so that these people could receive better medical treatments.
d. There is no reason to conduct this investigation.

**47. Which of the following best describes the primary function of Bartholin's glands?**

a. Secretes hormones that help the body respond to stress.
b. Provide lubrication for the vagina.
c. Helps control growth and development of the body.
d. Stimulate the development of T cells.

**48. Mildly elevated levels of thyroxine will do what to the heart rate?**

    a.  Stop the heart rate.
    b.  No effect.
    c.  Decrease the heart rate.
    d.  Increase the heart rate.

**49. Which nervous system controls voluntary motor movement?**

    a.  Parasympathetic.
    b.  Sympathetic.
    c.  Autonomic.
    d.  Somatic.

**50. Which of the following functions would be most affected by laryngeal damage?**

    a.  Eating.
    b.  Walking.
    c.  Singing.
    d.  Hearing.

**51. A researcher is studying the response of bacteria to a certain chemical. In three experiments, the bacteria swim towards the chemical, and in one experiment the bacteria swim away from it. What would be the most appropriate next step for the researcher?**

    a.  Report only the first three experiments.
    b.  Report all the experiments, but refrain from making any conclusions.
    c.  Repeat the experiment several more times and apply a statistical analysis to the data.
    d.  Repeat the experiment, adding a new chemical to determine its effect on the bacteria.

**52. How many different types of tissue are there in the human body?**

    a.  4.
    b.  6.
    c.  8.
    d.  10.

**53. What is the name of the outermost layer of skin?**

    a.  Dermis.
    b.  Epidermis.
    c.  Subcutaneous tissue.
    d.  Hypodermis.

| English and Language Usage | Number of Questions: **28** |
| --- | --- |
| | Time Limit: **28 Minutes** |

**1. Which of the answer choices is an effective revision of the ambiguous sentence below?**

**Tanya told her sister to tell her boyfriend Joe to call her as soon as he got home.**

    a. "Tanya," told her sister, "tell Joe to call your boyfriend as soon as Joe gets home."

    b. Her sister told her boyfriend Joe to call Tanya as soon as she got home.

    c. Tanya's sister was told by her, "Joe should call me when he gets home."

    d. Tanya said to her sister, "Tell your boyfriend Joe to call me right after he gets home."

**2. In the words *proactive, progress,* and *projecting, pro-* is a(n) _____ and means _____.**

    a. suffix; good/on top of/over

    b. prefix; before/forward/front

    c. affix; after/behind/in back of

    d. prefix; against/under/below

**3. Among the following transitional words or phrases, which one indicates contrast?**

    a. Regardless

    b. Furthermore

    c. Subsequently

    d. It may appear

**4. Which of the answer choices gives the best definition of the underlined word in the following sentence?**

**Thomas Macaulay once commented, "Few of the many wise <u>apothegms</u> which have been uttered have prevented a single foolish action."**

    a. advice

    b. preferences

    c. quotes

    d. sayings

**5. Which of the answer choices correctly completes the following sentence?**

**A childhood reading of Tales from Shakespeare permanently ____ Helene's interest in studying the Great Bard.**

    a. piqued

    b. peaked

    c. peked

    d. peeked

**6. Which of the following demonstrates correct punctuation?**

    a. Graham still needs the following items for his class: a sable brush, soft pastels, a sketchbook, and an easel.

    b. Graham still needs the following items for his class, a sable brush, soft pastels, a sketchbook, and an easel.

    c. Graham still needs the following items for his class: a sable brush; soft pastels; a sketchbook; and an easel.

    d. Graham still needs the following items for his class – a sable brush; soft pastels; a sketchbook; and an easel.

**7. Which of the answer choices best combines the following sentences?**

**The French and Indian War was not an isolated war in North America. It was part of a larger war that Europe was fighting. Europeans called it the Seven Years' War.**

    a.  The French and Indian War did not occur in North America but was rather a small part of the larger European war known as the Seven Years' War.

    b.  What Europeans called the Seven Years' War was called the French and Indian War in North America. It was part of a larger war that Europe was fighting.

    c.  The French and Indian War was not an isolated war in North America but was rather part of a larger war that Europe was fighting, known among Europeans as the Seven Years' War.

    d.  While North America was fighting the French and Indian War, the Europeans were fighting a much larger war known as the Seven Years' War.

**8. Which of the following words functions as a verb in the sentence below?**

**During the Seven Years' War, England and France fought over the control of the North American colonies, as well as the trade routes to those colonies.**

    a.  fought
    b.  control
    c.  trade
    d.  those

**9. Which of the following is a simple sentence?**

    a.  Following the French and Indian War, Spain gave up Florida to England.

    b.  England returned part of Cuba to Spain, while France gave up part of Louisiana.

    c.  France lost most of its Caribbean islands, and England gained dominance over them.

    d.  Because every nation lost something, no clear victor was declared.

**10. Which of the following sentences follows the rules of capitalization?**

    a.  One major conflict in the Seven Years' War occurred between the Prussian Hohenzollern Family and the Austrian Hapsburg Family.

    b.  The Hapsburg family was considered to be the rulers of the Holy Roman empire.

    c.  At the start of the war, Maria Theresa was the empress of Austria and was strengthening Austria's military.

    d.  Frederick the Great of Prussia had recently acquired the former Austrian Province of Silesia.

**11. What type of sentence is the following sentence?**

**Nancy also felt that the party was too crowded, but the hosts, who relied so much on her, would have been hurt if she had not attended.**

    a.  Simple
    b.  Complex
    c.  Compound
    d.  Compound-complex

**12. Which of the following sentences contains a correct example of subject-verb agreement?**

    a.  Some of the post-rally fervor have already died down.

    b.  Gary, as well as his three children, are coming to visit later today.

    c.  Are neither Robert nor his parents planning to see the presentation?

    d.  We waited patiently while a herd of moose was crossing the mountain highway.

**13. Which of the following words functions as an adverb in the sentence below??**

**I tried to call Lisle earlier, but I could not get her on the phone.**

    a.  call
    b.  earlier
    c.  could
    d.  phone

**14. Which of the answer choices best explains the purpose of the parentheses in the sentence?**

**The Hapsburg rule of the Austro-Hungarian Empire effectively ended with the reign of Franz Joseph I (1848–1916).**

    a.  to indicate the page numbers in the book where this information might be found
    b.  to tell the reader when the Austro-Hungarian empire collapsed
    c.  to identify information that was located using another source
    d.  to set off useful information that does not fit directly into the flow of the sentence

**15. Which of the following sentences is grammatically correct?**

    a.  The person who left the trash in the hallway needs to pick it up now.
    b.  Nobody needs to turn in their projects before the end of the month.
    c.  Every new instructor should stop by the main office to pick up one's room key.
    d.  Both Simeon and Ruth are generous with his or her time.

**16. What is the point of view indicated by the underlined words in the sentence?**

**<u>I</u> never know when <u>you</u> are joking about something.**

    a.  third; second
    b.  second; first
    c.  first; second
    d.  first; third

**17. Which of the answer choices best combines the following sentences?**

**The colonists refused to buy stamps. They were determined to get the Stamp Act repealed.**

    a.  The colonists refused to buy stamps and they were determined to get the Stamp Act repealed.
    b.  The colonists refused to buy stamps, and they were determined to get the Stamp Act repealed.
    c.  The colonists refused to buy stamps, and were determined to get the Stamp Act repealed.
    d.  The colonists refused to buy stamps, were determined to get the Stamp Act repealed.

**18. Which of the answer choices gives the best definition of the underlined word in the following sentence?**

**Throughout the elegant dinner party, the man's guests couldn't help but notice he took inordinate pride in the flattery of even his most <u>obsequious</u> servants.**

    a.  showing deference
    b.  poorly dressed
    c.  reserved
    d.  aggressive

**19.** *Caret, carrot* and *to, two* and *too* share something in common. They:

    a.  Are nouns
    b.  Are monosyllabic
    c.  Are homophones
    d.  Represent things in nature

**20. Which of the answer choices is an effective revision of the following ambiguous sentence?**

**Unless she were to study harder, the student feared she would fail out of the university during her exams.**

    a.  Unless the student had fear that she would fail out of school, she wouldn't study harder.
    b.  The student said, "she will fail out of the university unless she studies during her exams."
    c.  The student was afraid that she should study harder before failing out during her exams.
    d.  "If I don't study harder before the exams," the student fretted, "I will surely fail out of school."

**21. Which of the following sentences demonstrates correct use of an apostrophe?**

    a.  In one version of the story, there are seven fairy's invited to the christening, while in another version there are twelve fairy's.
    b.  Some historians' believe that the number twelve represents the shift from a lunar year of thirteen months to a solar year of twelve months.
    c.  Other historians claim that the symbolism in the fairy tale is more about nature and the shifting season's.
    d.  Regardless of its meaning, the fairy tale remains popular and has been immortalized in Tchaikovsky's music for the ballet.

**22. How should the underlined pronoun in the sentence below be classified?**

**The teacher spoke firmly to the class: "If <u>you</u> want to succeed in this course, be willing to work hard and turn in work on time."**

    a.  first-person singular
    b.  second-person singular
    c.  second-person plural
    d.  third-person plural

**23. Which of the following is not a simple sentence?**

    a.  Agatha Christie was the author of more than sixty detective novels.
    b.  Her most famous detectives were Hercule Poirot and Miss Marple.
    c.  She also wrote over fifteen collections of short stories about these detectives.
    d.  Most readers favor Poirot, but Christie preferred Miss Marple.

**24. Which of the answer choices gives the best definition of the underlined word in the following sentence?**

**Hercule Poirot is remembered not only for his genius in solving mysteries, but also for his <u>fastidious</u> habits and his commitment to personal grooming.**

    a.  fussy
    b.  lazy
    c.  old-fashioned
    d.  hilarious

**25. Which of the answer choices gives the best definition of the underlined word in the following sentence?**

The elderly Miss Marple, on the other hand, is remembered for solving the mysteries she encounters by making seemingly <u>extraneous</u> connections to life in her small village.

a. sophisticated
b. irrelevant
c. diligent
d. useful

**26. Which of the answer choices effectively revises the following sentence to remove the dangling modifier?**

**Leaping to the saddle, his horse bolted.**

a. His horse bolted as it leaped to the saddle.
b. When he leaped to the saddle, his horse bolted.
c. His horse bolting, he leaped to the saddle.
d. He leaped to the saddle, his horse bolted.

**27. The word _anaesthetic_ refers to medication that causes a temporary loss of feeling or sensation. Based on the meaning of the word in medical usage, which is the most likely meaning of the prefix _an-_?**

a. without
b. against
c. away
d. before

**28. Based on the contextual usage of the underlined word, what is the most likely meaning of the prefix _ante-_?**

The years leading up to the American Civil War are often referred to using the term <u>antebellum</u>.

a. again
b. good
c. before
d. together

---

# Answer Key and Explanations for Test #3

## Reading

**1. C:** The best starting point for a research project on the Globe Theatre of London would be the Encyclopedia Britannica. A thesaurus is an excellent place to find synonyms, while a dictionary is an excellent place to find word meanings. However, neither would contain information about the history of the Globe Theatre. (While writing, Ernestine might find herself in need of a better word or a word meaning; in this case, the thesaurus and dictionary will be useful.) The style guide will be helpful if the research needs more attention on grammar.

**2. C:** Mother Jones was agitating for laws protecting child workers, and legislators finally responded to her appeal and that of others. None of the other statements would logically follow. The words would not have been an inducement to children to work in factories, so response 1 is incorrect. Answer 2 is also not right; the South continued to be a major textile region. Increasing pay for child labor was not the solution to the problem; thus the fourth response is incorrect.

**3. A:** The word *consonantal* would fall between the words *considerable* and *conspicuous* on a dictionary page. The word *consumption* would follow *conspicuous*, while the words *conserve* and *conquistador* would precede *considerable*.

**4. D:** Information from the internet lacks the reliability of other published sources or primary sources as there is less accountability. Wikipedia is especially dangerous to use because it is subject to the editing of unlimited non-experts. Primary sources such as interviews are permissible and even media like documentaries are acceptable if they are from reliable sources.

**5. C:** People in government knew that the purchase would make the country more powerful, but the last sentence specifically states that they needed to explore. Answer choice C is the best prediction of what would occur next. Answer choices A and D infer too much, since you cannot assume any of these based on this passage given. Answer choice B is simply a statement that does not predict anything for the future.

**6. B:** When the directions are followed correctly, the new word is REVERT. The words REVEST and REVERSE require the addition of an S. (REVERSE also requires a second E.) The word REVIEW requires the addition of an I (which has been removed) and a W.

**7. B:** If Ethan buys his pens from Office in Bulk, he will pay $450 for 500 pens. At Specialty Pens, he would pay $485; at Office Warehouse, he would pay $475; at Ballpoint & Lead, he would pay $495.

**8. D:** The symbol /\ appears numerous times on the map, so the best way to determine the actual number of mountain ranges is to use the text on the map. In the state of Wyoming, six separate ranges are identified: the Wyoming Range, the Teton Range, the Wind River Range, the Bighorn Mountains, the Rocky Mountains, and the Laramie Mountains. All of the other answer choices identify too few ranges.

**9. B:** On the map, the star symbol is underneath the city of Cheyenne, which is the capital. The other answer choices – Laramie, Jackson, and Sheridan – are not identified as the capital city.

**10. A:** Two national parks are identified on the map: Grand Teton National Park and Yellowstone National Park. There is also a national monument (Devils Tower National Monument), but since the question says nothing about national monuments and specifies national *parks*, answer choice B can be ruled out. Choices C and D are both too high.

**11. B:** Colorado and Utah lie along Wyoming's southern border. Idaho lies to the west; Nebraska and South Dakota lie to the east; Montana lies along the northern border.

**12. B**: Option A, a basketball player who claims to use a pain reliever, is not a good fit. The player is not claiming a specific authority about the product but simply saying that he uses it. Option B, a commercial for cold medicine narrated by a man in a doctor's coat, is a good answer choice. Viewers do not know that the man is in fact a doctor; they only know that he is wearing a doctor's clothing. Option C, a commercial for a toy showing footage of children playing happily with it, does not suggest any kind of professional authority. Option D, a commercial for a prepared food with consumer testimonials, does not claim professional authority; in fact, it claims the authority of "real people" using the product and liking it. Only option B offers a suggestion of professional authority that remains unproved. Therefore, option B is the best answer.

**13. C:** The passage is expository, because it *exposes* or reveals information about the topic. A narrative passage tells a story; this passage does not. A technical passage provides the reader with instructions or details about completing a certain activity; this passage does not. A persuasive passage attempts to convince the reader to agree with the author's viewpoint about a topic. There is nothing persuasive about this passage.

**14. B:** Answer choice B, the second-to-last sentence in the passage, best summarizes the main point of the passage: that although The Five might not have had solid formal training, they influenced Russian music, and that influence extended beyond their own era. Answer choice A is too specific, and focuses on those who were influenced rather than on the actual composers who made up The Five. Because it is the opening sentence of the passage, answer choice C is a good option. However, answer choice B gets more to the heart of the topic. Answer choice C leaves out the information about long-term influence, so it is not the best option for a summary sentence. Answer choice D focuses on only two of The Five, so it cannot be a summary statement for the entire passage.

**15. C:** The final two sentences of the passage suggest that answer C is the best choice: "Composers such as Alexander Glazunov, Sergei Prokofiev, and Igor Stravinsky studied under Rimsky-Korsakov. Additionally, the mid-twentieth century composer Dmitri Shostakovich studied under Glazunov, creating a legacy of musical understanding that persisted well beyond the era of The Five." While the author does not explicitly state that Rimsky-Korsakov was the most influential, he is the only composer who is specifically linked to later composers. These noted composers include Rimsky-Korsakov's own students (Glazunov, Prokofiev, and Stravinsky) and one of his student's students (Shostakovich). Based on this, it is reasonable to conclude that the author would agree that Rimsky-Korsakov was the most influential of "The Five." While the other individuals listed in the answer choices had a definite influence on music and composed notable works, none of them is specifically linked to later composers in the passage.

**16. C:** Since the crime is fairly obvious, Ena is surprised that the child's lie is so *shameless*. Answer choice A is incorrect, because there is nothing *effective* about the child's lie. The child may be *arrogant* in assuming he will get away with lying, but this option is not as strong as answer choice C. There is nothing in the sentence to suggest that the child's lie is *hostile*, so answer choice D makes little sense.

**17. D:** The main argument is stated in paragraph 4: "With the progression and extreme convenience of technology, printed books are going to soon become a thing of the past."

**18. C:** Paragraph 1 explains how stories have progressed, beginning with oral tradition and past the invention of the printing press. In context with the rest of the essay, this paragraph is important in explaining how stories progress and are provided within society.

**19. A:** In paragraph 1, it is stated that oral tradition was the main medium for storytelling before the invention of the printing press.

**20. B:** It is not a fact that "sliding a finger across the screen or pressing a button to move onto the next page is just as satisfying to the reader." Satisfaction is not something universal that can be proven for every reader. This statement is an opinion.

**21. A:** The author makes the argument in paragraph 5 that devices such as the iPad and Kindle are "therefore better than books because they have multiple uses."

**22. C:** Throughout the passage, the author compares and contrasts the Arthurian writings of Malory and Tennyson, so the structure of the passage is clearly comparison-contrast. No problem is presented, so no solution must be posited. A passage written using a sequence structure would be focused on presenting information for the reader to follow in order (i.e. a "how-to" essay). The author essentially goes back and forth between Malory and Tennyson, so this passage does not employ a sequence structure. While there are some statements indicating cause and effect – Tennyson is said to have been influenced by Malory, for instance – the focus of the passage is more on comparing the two authors.

**23. D:** The following differences between Malory and Tennyson are noted in the passage: 1) Malory wrote in prose, while Tennyson wrote in poetry. 2) Malory wrote during the Medieval era, while Tennyson wrote during the Victorian era. 3) Malory was more focused on heroism and morality, while Tennyson was more focused on nature and elegy. The author of the passage mentions that Malory wrote about Gareth, Tristan, and Isolde, but there is not enough information in the passage to argue that Tennyson did *not*.

**24. D:** The passage is primarily about Malory and Tennyson. The author includes useful information toward the end of the passage to indicate what Tennyson's contemporary influences might have been (that is, "social problems and the need for social justice" within his own era). The information about Charles Dickens, however, seems to come out of nowhere. It does not merit a place in the passage, since the author says nothing about a similar author in Malory's time, which would make the comparison complete. As a result, the information about Dickens is irrelevant. The other answer choices, however, contain useful information that develops the author's main point.

**25. A:** In the first paragraph, the author notes that Malory was a Medieval writer who "focused more on the moral elements within these stories." This statement would also be true of Medieval literature in general. In the second paragraph, the author says that it has been argued that Tennyson "was writing an allegory about social problems and the need for social justice that existed during Tennyson's own time." This writing would also reflect the interests and defining qualities of the author's era. Therefore, answer choice A is correct. The author of the passage compares and contrasts the two writers' works, but there is nothing in the passage to suggest that he or she is taking a stand on which writer's work is superior. As a result, answer choices B and C are incorrect. Answer choice D counters the information at the start of the second paragraph that says Tennyson was "heavily influenced" by Malory. Even though Tennyson might have put his own spin on the Arthurian legends, he was still clearly influenced by Malory.

**26. B:** Without seeing an ingredient list for each soup, the best the test taker can do is look at the names and determine whether or not any form of dairy is likely included in the soup. The cheese in the broccoli cheese soup, as well as the cream in both the tomato and potato soup are likely to be problematic for Regina, as they are all dairy products. No dairy products are listed in "lentil soup," so this may be assumed to be the safest choice. (In traditional Mediterranean and Middle Eastern preparation, lentil soup does not typically include dairy products.)

**27. C:** The final column in the chart indicates the percentage of each country's population that was lost. For Romania, this percentage is 9.33. The percentages for the other choices are half of this or less. Of the nations listed in the chart, Romania certainly fared the worst in terms of the percentage of the population that was lost, even if the actual numbers are lower than they are for other nations.

**28. C:** Looking only at the numbers, the casualties in Russia are staggeringly high: 2,254,369 military deaths, 4,950,000 military wounded, and 1,500,000 civilian deaths. The fact that these numbers represent only 2.14 percent of Russia's population speaks to how many people were in Russia at the time. (According to the chart, the total population was 175,100,000.) The casualty numbers for the United Kingdom are also high, but nowhere near as high as they are for Russia. The numbers for Belgium and Romania are also high. In Romania, these losses represent a large percentage of the population. Russia, however, suffered the highest number of casualties, which is the focus of the question.

**29. A:** The author uses headings and subheadings to organize the passage. Each subheading has a focus on dairy (e.g., beverages, meals, and snacks) or non-dairy options that provide information on how to obtain more calcium from food.

**30. B:** Statement I and Statement II are both true statements about calcium rich foods. Canned fish, including salmon with bones, is recommended as a calcium rich food. Cheese is mentioned as a lactose-free alternative under the Non-Dairy Products subheading. Statement III is false. According to the passage, condensed cream soups should be made with milk, not water.

**31. D:** The best choice for this question is choice (D). The other options would clarify information for minor details within the passage and would provide some new information for the reader. With a definition of lactose intolerance, readers can understand the need for lactose-free alternatives.

**32. B:** The author's style is to give facts and details in a bulleted list. Of the options given, you are most likely to find this style in a health textbook. A tourist guidebook would most likely make recommendations about where to eat, not what to eat. An encyclopedia would list and define individual foods. A friendly letter would have a date, salutation, and a closing.

**33. C:** The announcement includes the following sentence: "To offset the crowding, the university has polled the various departments about schedules, and has settled on a recommended roster for when the members of each department should visit the faculty canteen for lunch." This suggests that the university made every effort to find out the schedules for each department and create a lunch arrangement that would give the members of each department the best opportunity possible to visit the canteen. The list is clearly not arranged alphabetically, so answer choice A is incorrect. The university definitely contacted the departments, as noted in the announcement. However, since the announcement mentions respecting the schedule and says nothing about an approval process, it is difficult to determine whether or not the university is worried about whether the faculty members will be amenable to the new lunch roster. Therefore, answer choice B can be eliminated. Finally, answer choice D seems to contradict the information in the announcement, so it too is incorrect. If the university contacted the departments about faculty schedules, the university obviously put some thought into the schedule. Answer choice D would suggest an arbitrary decision about scheduling, with no thought given to current faculty department schedules.

**34. B:** The final two sentences are as follows: "We ask that all faculty members respect this schedule. Faculty will be expected to display a department badge before entering the canteen for lunch." The overall recommendation is that faculty members should honor the schedule, with the added implication that faculty members will either not be allowed to enter the canteen outside of the posted lunch roster or that departments will be notified if the faculty members do make this effort. No doubt the announcement is also a recommendation to bring the badge, but there is an undercurrent of warning in it that goes beyond a "friendly reminder." Therefore, answer choice A is incorrect. There is nothing in the announcement or in the two final sentences to suggest that the university wants faculty members to eat lunch elsewhere, so answer choice C is incorrect. Answer choice D is a good option, but it infers just a little too much from the final two sentences. While university sanctions might very well be imposed on faculty members who don't follow the schedule, these two sentences alone are simply a word of caution to faculty members that the schedule needs to be respected. Answer choice D goes too far, so it too is incorrect.

**35. C:** Angela's reading list appears to consist of classic works of literature, as the opening statement notes that she "read the following classics." This means that "The Cask of Amontillado" by Edgar Allen Poe is unlikely to be a newspaper article, a book chapter by itself that is separate from the rest of the book, or a television show episode. Based on the information provided, it is most likely a short story.

**36. A:** The italics indicate full-length published books. The italics cannot represent works of classic literature. This is because according to the sentence, "The Cask of Amontillado" is also a classic. However, it is not italicized. Similarly, the italics cannot represent Angela's summer reading or the books that she has completed, because the item in quotation marks is also on Angela's summer reading list. (Additionally, in the case of answer choice D, the sentence states that Angela "read" these works, so the sentence itself indicates they have all been completed.)

**37. D:** Even if the test taker is unfamiliar with the meaning of *puerile*, the word *fantasies* should suggest something childish. The overall tone indicates an attitude of distaste toward the book. Consider the following wording in particular: "most likely to be enjoyed only by those with puerile fantasies." *Only* limits the audience, and *puerile fantasies* limits it even further. Answer choice A is incorrect, because the author makes no recommendations, and comments only on who might enjoy the book. Answer choice B is possible, but the tone would suggest that the *puerile fantasies* are not so much natural (as an appreciation for fantasy literature would be to children), but rather unique to a limited audience of adults. Answer choice C is incorrect, because the overall implication of the statement is that the book will appeal to a very limited audience. This leaves answer choice D, which is the best option: the author of the review believes the book would not appeal to mature adults.

**38. A:** Only Twin Theatres does not have a showing before 6 p.m. or after 10 p.m. The other cinemas have at least one showing before or after these times.

**39. D:** The only showing available after 10:30 p.m. is the 11:25 p.m. showing at Best Seat in The House. None of the other cinemas has a showing after 10:30 p.m.

**40. B:** Residents with addresses ending in 7 may water on Wednesdays, so the Morgan family should set up its watering schedule for this day of the week. The other days are for people with addresses that end in numbers other than 7.

**41. A:** There is no explanation regarding the organization of the schedule, nor does the announcement say anything about why there is only one number assigned to Friday and Saturday.

The announcement does say that the watering limitations reflect an "effort to conserve water," so the best inference is that the city has found that there are more addresses ending in these numbers (4 and 5), and has therefore adjusted the schedule accordingly. There is no way to determine from the announcement whether or not all businesses end in these numbers, or whether or not businesses consume more water, so answer choice B is incorrect. It is impossible to determine from the announcement if residents at these addresses consume more water, so answer choice C is incorrect. Similarly, there is nothing in the announcement to indicate that the city is more concerned about water usage in the latter part of the week – or why the part of the week would make a difference – so answer choice D is incorrect. The announcement only notes a goal of water conservation, and that water usage will be allotted by address. Therefore, the most logical assumption is that there are more addresses ending in 4 and 5 than in the other numbers.

**42. D:** The key here is to identify a detail that distorts the central message of a story when included. Option A, a profile of a local politician, includes a detail about his differences with friends that add context and depth to his hobby. Option B, a feature story that quotes a business owner admitting to a crime, includes a detail that may have significance given the owner's political aspirations and so may be appropriate to include. Option C, a profile of business leaders, provides a political context and background for a human-interest profile. Option D, however, includes a piece of information that is irrelevant to the news issue being reported and characterizes the local citizen negatively. This inclusion leaves the paper open to charges of bias and lack of objectivity. Thus, option D is the best answer choice.

**43. C:** Since both authors are explaining in the passages how the same story may come to be in different cultures, it is clear they both accept that there are often common elements in fairy tales from different cultures.

**44. A:** The author of Passage 2 claims that the essence and nature of fairy tales is their representation of basic human experience. It is this assertion that leads the author to believe that the same story could develop independently in different places.

**45. D:** The author does not mention the movement of food in the passage.

**46. B:** The author never mentions witches in the passage.

**47. A:** The passage suggests that spelunking is an outdoorsy, family adventure, then goes on to describe the adventure of going to a cave. If you do not already know that spelunking is another word for caving, you can infer this information based on reading the passage.

**48. B:** The article's style is not technical or scientific in the least. It is a simple and lighthearted article about something a family could do together. It is adventurous, but *Adventures for Men* is not a good choice since the fun is for the whole family. *Mud Magazine* might have been the next best choice, but *Family Fun Days* is clearly better. Your job is to choose the best choice of the options given.

**49. C:** With a complex passage like this one, main idea questions may require a re-reading of the relevant portion of the passage because some answer choices may not apply to the question. Answer choice D, for example, is the main idea of the first paragraph, not the second. Answer choices A and B on the other hand, are details that are directly contradicted by the passage. C is the only answer choice that is not contradicted by the passage and applies to the specified paragraph.

**50. D:** To answer this question, it is helpful to break the word apart. From the passage, it is clear that "to confirm" means "to prove." The prefix "dis" means "not." "Disconfirm," then, loosely means to "not prove." Choice A is inappropriate because it is an antonym. Choice B is inappropriate because "to dissipate" means to break or spread apart. Choice C is inappropriate because "to distill" means to purify or to break down. Choice D is a close match to "not prove". "To disprove" means to prove the opposite of something.

**51. C:** Even though this question seems like it requires logical operations, it actually asks for a detail from the passage. Choice A is inappropriate because something that is neither $x$ nor $y$ is irrelevant to the passage. Choice B is inappropriate because something that is both $x$ and $y$ proves the hypothesis. Choice C is a good choice because, using the monkey example, a monkey ($x$) that has no hair ($y$) disproves the hypothesis "all monkeys are hairy." Choice D is inappropriate because it is irrelevant to the passage. An example of something that is $y$ but not $x$ could be a hairy llama.

**52. D:** This question asks the reader to apply information learned in the passage to a new instance. In this case, an eighteen-wheel automobile will lower the probability of the hypothesis "all automobiles have only four wheels." Choices A and C are inappropriate because they refer to proving and disproving and not lowering probability. Choice B is inappropriate because it refers to raising and not lowering probability. Choice D is the best answer because an eighteen-wheel automobile decreases the probability that all automobiles have only four wheels.

**53. A:** The most reasonable inference based on the data given by the map is that the areas with no shading (which represent areas of low water use) are less inhabited than areas with shading. Note that the areas with no shading also have no listed cities; cities on the map are surrounded by shaded areas. Because the map does not give any information regarding how much water is required per capita, option D can be rejected. The map gives no indication regarding residents' prowess at conservation efforts (positive or negative). This eliminates option C. Additionally, there is no indication from the map that any land is more desert-like. Therefore, option B can be rejected.

# Mathematics

**1. B:** In order to solve for $x$, each side of the equation may be multiplied by the expression, $(x + 6)$. Doing so gives: $(x + 6) \times \frac{4}{x+6} = 2(x + 6)$, which simplifies to $4 = 2x + 12$, where $x = -4$.

**2. A:** Dr. Lee noticed that 5% of 30% of his patients were hospitalized. So multiply 30% by 5% using these steps:

Convert 30% and 5% into decimals by dividing both numbers by 100.

$$\frac{30}{100} = 0.30 \text{ and } \frac{5}{100} = 0.05$$

Now multiply 0.30 by 0.05 to get

$$(0.30)(0.05) = 0.015$$

Now convert 0.015 to a percentage by multiplying by 100.

$$(0.015)(100) = 1.5\%$$

**3. D:** The patient's dosage must increase by 30%. So calculate 30% of 270:

$$(0.30)(270 \text{ mg}) = 81 \text{ mg}$$

Now add the 30% increase to the original dosage.

$$270 \text{ mg} + 81 \text{ mg} = 351 \text{ mg}$$

**4. C:** A graph that has a $y$-intercept of 0 indicates a proportional relationship because the starting value is 0, and no amount is added to, or subtracted from, the term, containing the slope.

**5. C:** If the incoming class has 200 students, then $\frac{1}{2}$ of those students were required to take the exam.

$$(200)\left(\frac{1}{2}\right) = 100$$

So 100 students took the exam but only $\frac{3}{5}$ of that 100 passed the exam.

$$(100)\left(\frac{3}{5}\right) = 60$$

Therefore 60 students passed the exam.

**6. A:** The ratio of his savings to his rent is 1:3, which means that for every \$3 he pays in rent, he saves \$1 for the purchase of a house. So to calculate the amount the fourth roommate saves for the purchase of a house, divide \$270 by 3.

$$\frac{\$270}{3} = \$90$$

**7. C:** Each roommate donated about \$12 towards the gift purchase.

$$\$12 + \$12 + \$12 = \$36$$

**8. A:** The distance given from the top to the bottom of the tire through the center is the diameter. Finding the distance the bike traveled in one complete roll of the tire is the same as finding the circumference. Using the formula, $C = \pi d$, we multiply 27 by $\pi$. From the first mark to the fourth, the tire rolls three times. Then, you would multiply by 3, and the equation would be $3(27\pi)$.

**9. D:** The total rainfall is 25.38 inches. Thus, the ratio $\frac{4.5}{25.38}$, represents the percentage of rainfall received during October. $\frac{4.5}{25.38} \approx 0.177$ or 17.7%.

**10. C:** First solve for the number of questions Matthew must answer correctly. To determine the number of correct answers Matthew needs, solve the following inequality:

$$3x > 96$$
$$x > \frac{96}{3}$$
$$x > 32$$

Therefore, Matthew must correctly answer at more than 32 questions to qualify for varsity sports. Since the test has 40 questions, he must answer less than 8 questions incorrectly. Matthew could also answer 0 questions incorrectly. Hence, the best inequality to describe the number of questions Matthew can answer incorrectly is $0 \leq x < 8$.

**11. D:** The surface area of a cylinder can be determined by using the formula, $S = 2\pi r^2 + 2\pi rh$, where $r$ represents the radius and $h$ represents the height. Substituting the given values for the radius and height gives: $S = 2\pi(12)^2 + 2\pi(12)(8)$, which simplifies to $480\pi$, or approximately 1,507.2. Therefore, the surface area of the cylinder is approximately 1,507.2 square centimeters.

**12. C:** Find $\frac{1}{6}$ of 500 by multiplying

$$(500)\left(\frac{1}{6}\right) = \frac{500}{6}$$

The result is an improper fraction. Convert the fraction to a decimal and round to the nearest hundredth to get 83.33.

**13. D:** Since she spends at least $16, the relation of the number of packages of coffee to the minimum cost may be written as $4p \geq 16$. Alternatively, the inequality may be written as $16 \leq 4p$.

**14. D:** The number of miles Kevin drives per hour can be written as $y = 65x$, where $x$ represents the number of hours and $y$ represents the total number of miles driven. The y-intercept is 0, since there is not an amount added to, or subtracted from, this term. The graph of the line passes through the origin, or the point, $(0, 0)$.

**15. B:** To determine the total cost of Veronica's new car, add all her expenditures.

$$\$40,210 + \$3,015 + \$5,218 = \$48,443$$

**16. B:** In order to subtract the terms, the fractions need to have a common denominator: $\frac{13}{22} - \frac{3}{11} = \frac{13}{22} - \frac{3}{11} \times \frac{2}{2} = \frac{13}{22} - \frac{6}{22} = \frac{7}{22}$. In Answer A, the values were added instead of subtracted. In Answer C, the fractions were incorrectly subtracted straight across the numerators and denominators. In Answer D, the numerator in the $\frac{3}{11}$ fraction was not also adjusted when getting the common denominator. Therefore, $\frac{13}{22} - \frac{3}{11}$ incorrectly became $\frac{13}{22} - \frac{3}{22} = \frac{10}{22} = \frac{5}{11}$.

**17. D:** The number of vacuum cleaners sold per month has a mean of 31.7, a mode of 29, a median of 31, and a range of 29. Therefore, a true deduction states that the mode is equal to the range.

**18. C:** The number of miles Lauren must drive can be rounded to 1,500; 1,500 miles divided by 5 days equals 300 miles per day. Thus, a reasonable estimate for the number of miles driven per day is 300.

**19. D:** Compare and order the rational numbers by finding a common denominator for all three fractions. The least common denominator for 3, 12, and 4 is 12. Now convert the fractions with different denominators into fractions with the same denominator.

$$\frac{1}{3} = \frac{4}{12}$$

$$\frac{5}{12} = \frac{5}{12}$$

$$\frac{1}{4} = \frac{3}{12}$$

Now that all three fractions have the same denominator, order them from largest to smallest by comparing the numerators.

$$\frac{5}{12} > \frac{4}{12} > \frac{3}{12}$$

Since $\frac{5}{12}$ of the doctors are in Group Y, this group has the largest number of doctors. The next largest group has $\frac{4}{12}$ of the doctors, which is Group X. The smallest group has $\frac{3}{12}$ of the doctors, which is Group Z.

**20. B:** Solve the equation for $y$.

$$\frac{2y}{10} + 5 = 25$$

$$\frac{2y}{10} = 25 - 5$$

$$\frac{2y}{10} = 20$$

$$2y = (20)(10)$$

$$2y = 200$$

$$y = \frac{200}{2}$$

$$y = 100$$

**21. D:** $3(x - 1) = 2(3x - 9)$

| | | |
|---|---|---|
| $3x - 3 = 6x - 18$ | | Distribute |
| $-3 = 3x - 18$ | | Subtract $3x$ from both sides |
| $15 = 3x$ | | Add 18 to both sides |
| $5 = x$ | | Divide both sides by 3 |

**22. B:** During January, Dr. Lewis worked 20 shifts.

$$\text{shifts for January} = 20$$

During February, she worked three times as many shifts as she did during January.

$$\text{shifts for February} = (20)(3)$$

During March, she worked half the number of shifts she worked in February.

$$\text{shifts for March} = (20)(3)\left(\frac{1}{2}\right)$$

**23. B:** One decimeter equals 10 centimeters, so the following proportion can be written: $\frac{1}{0.1} = \frac{x}{2.5}$. Solving for $x$ gives $x = 25$. Thus, 2.5 decimeters is equal to 25 centimeters.

**24. A:** The following proportion can be used to solve the problem: $\frac{3}{8} = \frac{24}{x}$. Solving for $x$ gives: $3x = 192$, which simplifies to $x = 64$.

**25. A:** When multiplying fractions, multiply the terms straight across the fraction: $\frac{5}{9} \times \frac{3}{4} = \frac{15}{36}$. Then, simplify the fraction. Since 15 and 36 are both multiples of 3, divide each term by 3 to reach the final result: $\frac{5}{12}$. In Answer B, the fractions were added straight across without getting a common denominator. In Answer C, the fractions were cross multiplied. In Answer D, the fractions were added, instead of multiplied.

**26. C:** The variables are the objects the graph measures. In this case, the graph measures the nurse specialties and the number of nurses for each specialty. The dependent variable changes with the independent variable. Here, the number of nurses depends on the particular nurse specialty. Therefore, the independent variable is nurse specialties.

**27. C:** The prefix, centi-, means 100th. In this case,

$$1 \text{ m} = 100 \text{ cm}$$

Therefore,

$$(7)(1 \text{ m}) = (7)(100 \text{ cm})$$

$$7 \text{ m} = (7)(100 \text{ cm})$$

$$7 \text{ m} = 700 \text{ cm}$$

**28. B:** A human eyelash is about one centimeter long. Nanometers are much too short to describe an eyelash. Meters and kilometers are much too long.

**29. C:** A hexagonal field has 6 sides. Each side is 320 feet long, so multiply 320 by 6 to get the perimeter of the field: 320 × 6 = 1920 feet. At $1.75 per foot, the perimeter fence will cost 1920 × 1.75 = $3360.

**30. C:** The fractions for Choice C can be compared by either converting all fractions and mixed numbers to decimals or by using a least common denominator. In performing the first suggestion, the fractions as they appear from left to right can be written as −2.875, −2.75, −0.2, 0.125, and 0.4. Negative integers with larger absolute values are less than negative integers with smaller absolute values. The tenths place can be used to compare each of the decimals.

**31. C:** To find each percentage, divide the first number by the second number, then multiply by 100. So the percentage in answer A is $\left(\frac{50}{250}\right) \times 100 = 20$, the percentage in answer B is $\left(\frac{57}{250}\right) \times 100 = 22.8$, the percentage in answer C is $\frac{74+55}{433} \times 100 = \left(\frac{129}{433}\right) \times 100 = 29.8$, and the percentage in answer D is $\left(\frac{21}{183}\right) \times 100 = 11.5$.

**32 B:** The percentage of female staff members at Hospital Y is $\left(\frac{90}{183}\right) \times 100 = 49.2$. At Hospital X, it is $\left(\frac{97}{250}\right) \times 100 = 38.8$. Subtracting, we see that the difference between these percentages is approximately 10.

**33. B:** The percentage of staff members with zero complaints at Hospital X is $\left(\frac{202}{250}\right) \times 100 = 80.8$. At Hospital Y, the percentage is $\left(\frac{161}{183}\right) \times 100 = 88.0$.

**34. B:** The line graph shows the largest number of flights made during a month as 79 with the smallest number of flights made during a month as 54. The range is equal to the difference between the largest number of flights and smallest number of flights, i.e., 79 – 54 = 25. Therefore, the range is equal to 25.

**35. B:** The outlier of 11 would skew the data if the mean or range were used. Therefore, the median is the most appropriate measure for reflecting the number of houses she sold per year. This data set does not have a mode, so mode is not the most appropriate.

**36. C:** The score that has approximately 50% above and 50% below is approximately 500 (517 to be exact). The scores can be manually written by choosing either the lower or upper end of each interval and using the frequency to determine the number of times to record each score, i.e., using the lower end of each interval shows an approximate value of 465 for the median; using the upper end of each interval shows an approximate value of 530 for the median. A score of 500 (and the exact median of 517) is found between 465 and 530.

# Science

**1. C:** The circulatory system circulates materials throughout the entire body. The heart, blood, and blood vessels are part of the circulatory system. The kidneys are part of the genitourinary system. The diaphragm is part of the respiratory system.

**2. D:** Food enters the mouth and then is swallowed down the esophagus into the stomach, where stomach acids begin the break down process. Food then travels through the small intestine (where the pancreas, liver and intestine release digestive juices to further break down the food), to the large intestine (where nutrients and water are absorbed, and waste is transformed from liquid to stool) and finally to the rectum,

**3. A:** The sinoatrial (SA) node is the natural pacemaker of the body. If the SA node is damaged or malfunctions, the impulse travels down the electrical conduction system to a group of cells further down the heart. This is called the atrioventricular node which will then take over as the pacemaker.

**4. A:** Tachycardia is a faster than normal heart rate at rest. A healthy adult heart normally beats 60 to 100 times a minute when a person is at rest. Apnea is the absence of respirations. Bradycardia is a slower than normal heart rate (less than 60 bpm). Tachypnea is the presence of rapid respirations.

**5. D:** The immune system helps the body avoid, detect, and eliminate infections. A healthy immune system should not, however, create infections.

**6. B:** The human body has 5 types of bone. The spine and hips are irregular bones because they do not fit the other major bone types, which are long, short, flat, and sesamoid. Choice A, curvy bones, does not describe one of the major bone types.

**7. C:** Most bones in the limbs are long bones, including the thighs, forearms, and fingers. The ankles, however, are not long bones because they do not have a shaft that is longer than it is wide.

**8. D:** Skeletal, smooth, and cardiac are all types of muscle tissue. Adipose tissue is fatty tissue, not a muscle.

**9. A:** Salt would have acted as a dehydrating agent on the plants, causing them to dry out, and therefore, they would have died.

**10. B:** A control is a variable in the experiment that has not been changed by the experimenter but is subjected to the same processes as the other tested components. Plants are usually provided only water; these are being tested against bleach, salt, and diet soda, all of which are not regularly used to water a plant. The control acts as a reference point for comparison of the results.

**11. B:** Anterior means toward the front of the body. Posterior refers to the back side of the body. Superior refers to something that is above in relation to another element, whereas inferior refers to something that is below in relation to another element.

**12. B:** The sternum is located anteriorly (in the front of the body), superior (above) the pelvic bone. The spine is located posteriorly (in the back of the body), superior, not inferior, to the pelvic bone. The mandible is located inferior to the nasal cavity, and superior to the esophagus. The femur is located superior to the tibia.

**13. C:** Proximal means close to the trunk of the body, or torso. Superficial refers to externally located. The sagittal plane divides the body into left and right. Distal refers to something further from the torso.

**14. A:** The nucleus is the control center for the cell. The cell membrane surrounds the cell and separates the cell from its environment. Cytoplasm is the thick fluid within the cell membrane that surrounds the nucleus and contains organelles. Mitochondria are often called the power house of the cell because they provide energy for the cell to function.

**15. A:** Cilia and flagella are responsible for cell movement. Ribosomes are organelles that help synthesize proteins within the cell. The cell membrane helps the cell maintain its shape and protects it from the environment. Lysosomes have digestive enzymes.

**16. C:** Cellular differentiation is the process by which simple, less specialized cells become highly specialized, complex cells. For example, humans are multicellular organisms who undergo cell differentiation numerous times. Cells begin as simple zygotes after fertilization and then differentiate to form a myriad of complex tissues and systems before birth.

**17. D:** Meiosis produces cells that are genetically different, having half the number of chromosomes of the parent cells. Mitosis produces cells that are genetically identical; daughter cells have the exact same number of chromosomes as parent cells. Mitosis is useful for repairing the body while meiosis is useful for sexual reproduction.

**18. D:** The integumentary system (skin) protects internal tissues from injury, waterproofs the body, and helps regulate the body's temperature. The lymphatic system, not the integumentary system, returns fluid to the blood vessels.

**19. A:** Groups of cells that perform the same function are called tissues.

**20. B:** Epithelial tissue is that found in the skin, and its function is to protect, sense, absorb and secrete. Nervous tissue transmits and receives impulses. Muscular tissue controls movement and contraction, supports the skeletal structure and controls positioning. Connective tissue supports and protects skeletal structures and organs, provides separation between organs, and connects various structures together.

**21. B:** The adrenal glands are part of the endocrine system. They sit on the kidneys and produce hormones that regulate salt and water balance and influence blood pressure and heart rate. The pituitary glands release thyroid stimulating hormones, which influence metabolism. Insulin is produced and released by the pancreas in response to glucose. The hypothalamus regulates the release of oxytocin, which serves important functions in reproduction and childbirth.

**22. A:** Genes store hereditary information and thus allow hereditary traits to be passed from parents to offspring. Genes do not prohibit hereditary transmission, and genes are not known to enable any type of environmental factors.

**23. B:** Hemoglobin is a type of protein found in the red blood cells of all mammals. It is the portion of the red blood cell that contains iron, to which oxygen binds and then is transported from the lungs to the rest of the body. Hematocrit is the ratio of red blood cells to the total blood volume.

**24. A:** The thyroid does not belong in this grouping. The pancreas, intestines, and stomach all play important roles in the digestive system. The thyroid is part of the endocrine system. It secretes hormones that help regulate the heart rate, blood pressure, body temperature, and metabolism.

**25. D:** The complete Punnett square is shown below.

|  | **T** | **t** |
|---|---|---|
| **B** | TB | tB |
| **b** | Tb | tb |

Possibility 3 corresponds to a person with the *Tb* gene combination, which means the person is tall with red hair.

**26. B:** Refer to the complete Punnett square in the explanation for question 25. Possibility 2 corresponds to the *tB* pair of genes, which is short with black hair.

**27. A:** The purpose of conducting an experiment is to test a hypothesis. Answer choices b, c, and d are steps in conducting an experiment designed to test a hypothesis.

**28. A:** The tricuspid valve allows deoxygenated blood flow from the right atria to the right ventricle. The pulmonic valve opens to allow blood flow from the right ventricle to the pulmonary system. The mitral valve allows oxygenated blood flow from the left atria to the left ventricle. The aortic valve allows oxygenated blood flow from the left ventricle to the rest of the body.

**29. B:** Phagocytes are specialized white blood cells that kill pathogens and initiate an immune response. They display the ingested pathogen to the B cells or memory cells which help the body "remember" the pathogen in the future.

**30. D:** Enzymes are protein molecules that serve as catalysts for certain biological reactions. Enzymes are not acids or lipids. Enzymes are definitely relevant for living organisms and do not suppress reactions.

**31. A:** Sweat glands are distributed almost all over the human body, in varying amounts. Their primary purpose is to help the body cool off. They are primarily concentrated in the axilla and perianal area but are present in high concentrations in the forehead, palms, soles, and groin. The back and the legs have much lower concentrations of glands.

**32. D:** A covalent bond is one in which atoms share valence electrons. Within a water molecule, one oxygen atom and two hydrogen atoms share valence electrons to yield the $H_2O$ structure.

**33. B:** A water molecule contains 2 hydrogen atoms and 1 oxygen atom. Therefore, the chemical formula for water is $H_2O$. The pH of water is 7.

**34. C:** For an experiment to be considered successful, it must yield data that others can reproduce. Answer choice a may be considered part of a well-designed experiment. Answer choices b, and d may be considered part of an experiment that is reported on by individuals with expertise.

**35. C:** The atomic mass of an atom is approximately equal to the number of protons plus the number of neutrons, in this case, 6. The weight of the electrons has little effect on the overall atomic mass.

**36. D:** T cells are a specialized type of white blood cells that play an important role in the immune response of all humans. They help destroy pathogens in the body and initiate the body's immune response to fight the infection. T cells are produced in the bone marrow, but they mature in the thymus gland.

**37. D:** Ionic bonds are formed when electrons are transferred between atoms. For instance, the sodium and chlorine atoms in salt have ionic bonds because electrons are transferred from sodium to chlorine.

**38. C:** The atomic weight tells the mass of the element. In the table, B is the lightest element, weighing 11 atomic mass units, and O is the heaviest element, weighing 16 atomic mass units.

**39. D:** Antibodies are specialized proteins that are important to immune system efficacy. They are recruited by the immune system to identify and destroy foreign pathogens like bacteria and viruses. Each antibody has a unique target known as the antigen present on the invading organism. Once the antibody identifies its target it helps the immune system neutralize it.

**40. A:** Condensation is the process of changing from a gas to a liquid. For instance, gaseous water molecules in the air condense to form liquid rain drops. Vaporization describes changing from liquid to gas. Melting is the process of changing from solid to liquid and sublimation describes changing from solid to gas.

**41. C:** The right atrium receives deoxygenated blood from the body which flows into the right ventricle. From there, the blood goes to the lungs where it becomes oxygenated. The left atrium receives oxygenated blood and pumps it to the left ventricle which distributes it to the rest of the body.

**42. B:** Walking is not controlled by the autonomic nervous system. The autonomic nervous system regulates involuntary body processes such as heartbeat, blood pressure, respirations, digestion, metabolism, and elimination of toxins. Walking is controlled by the somatic system which helps control skeletal muscle voluntary control.

**43. B:** The evidence says that every child in a certain family suffers from autism. All of these children have genetic commonalities. Therefore, autism may be genetic. The evidence does not mention whether the children died from autism. Therefore, no conclusion can be drawn that autism may be lethal. Furthermore, the sample size of the evidence is much too small to suggest that autism is related to traditional nuclear family structures.

**44. D:** Decreased mortality during childbirth could be explained by any or all of the statements presented. Safer cesarean sections, health monitoring tools, and hand washing could all improve a woman's chances of surviving childbirth.

**45. A:** A scientific argument should discuss outcomes that are objective and measurable, such as blood pressure, energy level, and overall health. The other choices present arguments that are subjective and based on emotions instead of facts.

**46. C:** Conducting this investigation may reveal a group of people who need higher quality medical care. Asking wealthy people for money does not help the researcher learn more about their quality of medical care. Although helping healthy people to stay healthy is important, helping those with poor medical care is more critical.

**47. B:** Bartholin's glands also known as greater vestibular glands play a role in female reproduction. The Bartholin's glands lie on either side of the vaginal opening. They produce a mucoid substance, which provides lubrication for intercourse.

**48. D:** Diseases of the thyroid gland can directly alter the normal function of the heart causing symptoms and resulting in significant complications. Increased levels of thyroxine can cause tachycardia. Low levels of thyroxine can cause bradycardia. Significantly elevated levels of thyroid hormone, seen in thyroid storm, can cause atrial fibrillation and cardiac arrest.

**49. D:** The somatic nervous system helps control skeletal muscle voluntary control. The automatic nervous system controls involuntary functions in the body like breathing. The autonomic nervous system had two subdivisions: the sympathetic nervous system which controls "fight or flight" response, and parasympathetic nervous system which controls "rest and digest" functions.

**50. C:** The larynx also known as the voice box, contains the vocal folds that produce the sounds of speech and singing. It is a hollow, tubular structure connected to the proximal aspect of the trachea. While eating may be impacted by laryngeal damage, the damage would more directly inhibit singing.

**51. C:** By repeating the experiment, the researcher could determine whether the instance of the bacteria swimming away from the chemical was simply due to chance. Observing the same results would allow the researcher to make conclusions with more certainty, and statistical analysis would help determine the significance of the data. Researchers must report all data (A), and reaching a conclusion is a vital part of any experiment (B). Adding a new chemical would completely change the experiment, so it would not be helpful (D).

**52. A:** There are four different types of tissue in the human body: epithelial, connective, muscle, and nerve. *Epithelial* tissue lines the internal and external surfaces of the body. It is like a sheet, consisting of squamous, cuboidal, and columnar cells. They can expand and contract, like on the inner lining of the bladder. *Connective* tissue provides the structure of the body, as well as the links between various body parts. Tendons, ligaments, cartilage, and bone are all examples of connective tissue. *Muscle* tissue is composed of tiny fibers, which contract to move the skeleton. There are three types of muscle tissue: smooth, cardiac, and skeletal. *Nerve* tissue makes up the nervous system; it is composed of nerve cells, nerve fibers, neuroglia, and dendrites.

**53. B:** The epidermis is the outermost layer of skin. The thickness of this layer of skin varies over different parts of the body. For instance, the epidermis on the eyelids is very thin, while the epidermis over the soles of the feet is much thicker. The dermis lies directly beneath the epidermis. It is composed of collagen, elastic tissue, and reticular fibers. Beneath the dermis lies the subcutaneous tissue, which consists of fat, blood vessels, and nerves. The subcutaneous tissue contributes to the regulation of body temperature. The hypodermis is the layer of cells underneath the dermis; it is generally considered to be a part of the subcutaneous tissue.

# English and Language Usage

**1. D:** The revision in D removes a number of pronouns that lack clear antecedents. It also removes the need for the use of the subjunctive by placing the speech in quotations.

**2. B:** The prefix *pro-* from Latin means before, earlier, prior to; for or forward; or front. Prefixes come at the beginnings of words. Suffixes come at the ends of words; and *pro-* does not mean good, on top of, or over (A). The Greek prefix *eu-* means good, the Latin prefix *supra-* means above, and the Latin prefix *super-* can mean over and above, among other meanings. Prefixes and suffixes are both affixes (C); however, *pro-* does not mean after, behind, or in back of. The Latin prefix *post-* means after or behind, and *retro-* means back or backward. *Pro-* does not mean against, under, or below (D). *Sub-* means under or below; *anti-* means against.

**3. A:** *Regardless* is a transitional word that indicates contrast between the previous idea(s) or point(s) and the following one(s). Others include *nonetheless, even so,* and *however*. *Furthermore* (B) is a transitional word that indicates sequence. Others include *moreover, besides, also,* and *finally*. *Subsequently* (C) is a transitional word indicating time. Others include *thereafter, immediately, previously, simultaneously, so far, presently, since, soon,* and *at last. It may appear* (D) is a transitional phrase indicating concession. Others include *granted that, of course,* and *although it is true that*. Transitions can also indicate place, examples, comparison, cause and effect, repetition, summary, and conclusion. These all enhance coherence by connecting ideas and sentences.

**4. D:** The context suggests that Thomas Macaulay thought that people seldom apply wise sayings to avoid foolishness. The plural word in the sentence suggests the need for a plural synonym, so *advice* does not work. The word *preferences* does not make much sense in the sentence. While the statement itself is a quote – and wise sayings are usually quoted – the word *quotes* is not a synonym for *apothegms*, and is therefore not the best choice.

**5. A:** The word *piqued* is the correct choice, and is used to describe a heightened interest in something. The word *peaked* would be appropriate to describe height or the highest reach (e.g., *his blood pressure* peaked, *and then came back down*). The word *peke* is frequently used to describe a Pekingese breed of dog; therefore, *peked* does not make sense in the context of this sentence. The word *peeked* would suggest someone looking around the corner to see something.

**6. A:** Answer choice A includes all of the correct elements of punctuation needed to make this sentence clear and readable. In particular, there is a colon after the phrase "the following items for his class"; this indicates that a series of items will be listed. As these items do not contain internal commas, they may be separated by commas, so the rest of the punctuation in answer choice A is correct. Answer choice B uses a comma instead of a colon in front of the introductory phrase, making the series of items difficult to distinguish. Answer choice C uses semicolons instead of commas between the items in the series. The semicolons are not necessary, and make the sentence more confusing to read instead of clearer. Answer choice D uses a dash, which is not a correct way to introduce a series of items.

**7. C:** Answer choice C combines all of the information in the passage into a single coherent sentence. Answer choice A inexplicably states that the French and Indian War did not occur in North America, but the passage does not indicate this. Instead, the passage notes that the French and Indian War was not an isolated conflict, that it *did* occur in North America, and that it was also part of the larger Seven Years' War Europe was fighting. Answer choice B contains correct information, but is choppy rather than fluid and coherent. Answer choice B is more than one sentence, and it lacks the style and clarity of answer choice C. Answer choice D contains correct information, but it fails to explain – as stated in the original passage – that the French and Indian War was actually part of the larger Seven Years' War. Answer choice D implies that the French and Indian War was unrelated to the Seven Years' War, which contradicts the passage.

**8. A:** Of the answer choices, the only word that functions as a verb is *fought*. The word *control* is a noun in this sentence. The word *trade* functions either as an adjective to modify *routes*, or as a part of the single noun phrase *trade routes*. The word *those* functions as an adjective.

**9. A:** Only answer choice A is a simple sentence. It contains an opening phrase, but as this is a phrase instead of a dependent clause, the sentence is simple. Answer choices B and D contain a dependent clause, which makes these sentences complex. Answer choice C contains two independent clauses, which make the sentence compound.

**10. C:** In answer choice C, the word *empress* does not need to be capitalized, because it is not being used as a title. Instead, it is simply a description of Maria Theresa's role as empress over Austria. Answer choice A incorrectly capitalizes the word *family* twice. Answer choice B fails to capitalize the word *empire* in *Holy Roman Empire*. Answer choice D incorrectly capitalizes *province*, which is not being used as a proper noun in the sentence.

**11. D:** This is a compound-complex sentence because it contains two independent clauses plus dependent clauses. A simple (A) sentence is a single independent clause. A complex (B) sentence consists of one independent clause and one dependent clause, such as "After she went to the party, she went home." A compound (C) sentence consists of two independent clauses connected by a conjunction, like "She went to the party, and then she went home."

**12. D:** As the herd is apparently moving in unison across the highway, the collective noun *herd* is singular, and thus takes a singular verb. (If, however, the moose were stampeding at random, each moose in a different direction, the collective noun *herd* would be considered plural.) In answer choice A, the pronoun *some* can be either singular or plural, depending on the prepositional phrase that follows it. Because the phrase contains the singular *fervor*, the sentence needs a singular verb. (On the other hand, the phrase *some of the people* would require a plural verb, because of the plural *people*.) In answer choice B, *Gary* is the primary subject, and requires a singular verb, regardless of the phrase *as well as his three children* that sits between Gary and the verb. In answer choice C, the opening verb in this interrogative sentence is determined by whether the noun following the pronoun *neither* is singular or plural. In this case, the singular *Robert* requires that the opening verb be *is*. Note that if the order were reversed, the sentence would be correct with *are*: *Are neither his parents nor Robert planning to see the presentation?* This is fairly awkward, though, so the other form would be more common.

**13. B:** The word *earlier* is an adverb that modifies the verb *tried* and answers the adverb question *when?* The word *call* is part of the infinitive (i.e. noun) phrase *to call*. The word *could* is a helping verb that accompanies the verb *get*. The word *phone* functions as a noun in this sentence.

**14. D:** In question 14, the parenthetical statement includes information that is useful – in this case the years of Franz Joseph I's reign – but does not fit into the flow of the sentence. The writer has chosen to include the years of Franz Joseph I's reign in parentheses, instead of using a dependent clause along the lines of "…the reign of Franz Joseph I, who ruled from 1848 to 1916." The parentheses provide information that the reader would likely want to know without interrupting the flow of the sentence. There is nothing about the parenthetical remark to indicate that the numbers refer to the pages of a book; instead, the numbers make much more sense as dates. The information in answer choice B is essentially implied; if the empire collapsed after his reign, it is safe to say that 1916 marks the date of its collapse. But, this is not really the purpose of the parentheses. The purpose is to offset useful information without interrupting the flow of the sentence. It is likely that all of the information in the sentence came from one source, so the parentheses do not indicate outside material in this case.

**15. A:** In answer choice A, the subjective case pronoun *who* (rather than *whom*) correctly follows *person*. Additionally, the singular subject *person* is accompanied by the singular verb *needs*. In answer choice B, *nobody* is singular, and needs the singular *his or her* to follow it instead of *their*. In answer choice C, the use of *one's* is incorrect; it should be *his, hers,* or *his or her*. In answer choice D, however, the use of *his or her* is not correct because of the structure of the sentence. The mention of the plural *Simeon and Ruth* makes the plural *their* correct.

**16. C:** Answer choice C correctly identifies that *I* is the first person and *you* is the second person. The order is also correct. The other answer choices either include an incorrect point of view or place the points of view in incorrect order.

**17. B:** A comma and conjunction are correctly used to separate two independent clauses. Although choice A has the conjunction *and*, it is missing the required comma. Choice C is incorrect because no comma is required to separate an independent clause from a dependent clause. Choice D is incorrect because the comma creates a run-on sentence.

**18. A:** Obsequious means excessively obedient. To show deference means to be servile. The two are synonyms, although of differing degrees. Aggressive is almost an antonym. Reserved merely means shy while poorly dressed is beside the point completely.

**19. C:** Homophones are words that are pronounced the same, but differ in meaning. For example, a bride wears a 2-caret ring, but a horse eats a carrot.

**20. D:** The sentence is confusing because of the poorly worded conditional statement and the grammar necessitated by the indirect speech. In addition, a pronoun is placed before its antecedent. The correct answer solves all three problems by putting the speech in quotations and restating the conditional statement.

**21. D:** Answer choice D correctly uses an apostrophe to indicate the possessive element within the sentence. Answer choice A incorrectly changes the plural word *fairies* into the possessive word *fairy's*. Similarly, answer choice B makes the plural *historians* possessive, and answer choice C makes the plural *seasons* possessive by changing it to the singular possessive *season's*. None of these words is possessive in the context of their respective sentences, so only answer choice D is correct.

**22. C:** The word *you* is always second person, and it is either singular or plural depending on its context. In the sentence provided, the teacher is speaking to a class, and the class is likely to be made up of more than one person. Therefore, the *you* in the sentence is second-person plural. The other answer choices identify the wrong point of view, and answer choices A and D incorrectly identify the word as singular.

**23. D:** Answer choice D contains two independent clauses, so it is a compound sentence, not a simple sentence. All of the other answer choices are simple sentences.

**24. A:** Someone who is committed to personal grooming is likely to be *fussy*, and this is the meaning of the word *fastidious*. The word *lazy* makes little sense in the context of the sentence. No doubt some of Poirot's activities are both *old-fashioned* and *hilarious*, but neither of these words fit the context of the sentence, and thus cannot be synonyms for *fastidious*.

**25. B:** The sentence indicates that the connections Miss Marple makes are *seemingly extraneous*. However, the sentence also states that she uses this information to solve mysteries. This would suggest that the word *extraneous* means *irrelevant*. Answer choice A indicates the very opposite of what the sentence implies. Answer choice C makes little sense in the context of the sentence. Answer choice D would work but for the adverb *seemingly*; this indicates that the connections appear to be irrelevant, but are actually not. With *seemingly* in the sentence, the meaning completely changes if *useful* is added in place of *extraneous*.

**26. B:** For the sentence to read correctly, it must be clear that someone is leaping into the saddle when the horse bolts. In its original form, the only party identified in the sentence is the horse, and a horse cannot leap into a saddle. Answer choice B includes the mention of a second party (an unnamed *he*), who does the leaping as the horse does the bolting. Answer choice A creates an amusing picture, but it fails to make sense of the original sentence. Answer choice C is an interesting take on the sentence, but it places the action of the sentence in an odd order. It is more likely that the bolting occurred immediately after the leaping, and not the other way around, as indicated in answer choice C. (One cannot exactly leap into a saddle after the horse has already taken off.) Answer choice D is technically correct in terms of the information it provides, but it turns a single sentence into two sentences, and it incorrectly joins them with a comma splice.

**27. A:** If an anaesthetic creates a temporary loss of feeling or sensation, and *aesthet* means "feeling," then *an-* must mean "without." Therefore, anaesthetic means "without feeling." The other prefix meanings do not create as clear a connection to the recognized meaning of the full word *anaesthetic*. To be "against feeling" makes little sense. To be "away feeling" is meaningless. To be "before feeling" would be appropriate to describe the moments before the anaesthetic wears off, but this is a qualification rather than a clear definition.

**28. C:** If the years leading up to the American Civil War are described as *antebellum*, and *bellum* means "war," the only possible meaning of *ante-* is "before." *Antebellum*, therefore, means "before war." The other prefixes do little to break the word down to a sensible meaning. "Again war" and "together war" are meaningless. "Good war" does nothing to explain why the pre-Civil War years were called *antebellum*, particularly when considering the atrocities of war that were soon to follow.

# Image Credits

## LICENSED UNDER CC BY 4.0 (CREATIVECOMMONS.ORG/LICENSES/BY/4.0/)

Plasma Membrane: "Lipid Bilayer with Various Components" by OpenStax CNX user CNX Anatomy and Physiology (https://cnx.org/contents/FPtK1zmh@8.25:fEI3C8Ot@10/Preface)

Phospholipids: "Phospholipid Structure" by OpenStax CNX Anatomy and Physiology (https://cnx.org/contents/FPtK1zmh@8.25:fEI3C8Ot@10/Preface)

Cell Growth: "Mitosis and Meiosis" by Wikimedia user domdomegg (https://commons.wikimedia.org/wiki/File:Three_cell_growth_types.svg)

Planes of Body: "Planes of Body" by OpenStax CNX user OpenStax College (https://cnx.org/contents/FPtK1zmh@6.27:zMTtFGyH@4/Introduction)

DNA: "DNA Replication" by OpenStax CNX user CNX Anatomy and Physiology (https://cnx.org/contents/FPtK1zmh@8.25:fEI3C8Ot@10/Preface)

Artery: "Microscope anatomy of an artery" by Wikimedia user Stijn Ghesquiere, Drsrisenthil (https://commons.wikimedia.org/wiki/File:Microscopic_anatomy_of_an_artery.svg)

Lumen of the Small Intestine: "Diagram" by Wikimedia user BallenaBlanca (https://commons.wikimedia.org/wiki/File:Esquema_del_epitelio_del_intestino_delgado.png)

Major Muscles: "Anterior and Posterior Views of Muscles" by OpenStax CNX user CNX Anatomy and Physiology (https://cnx.org/contents/FPtK1zmh@8.25:fEI3C8Ot@10/Preface)

T-Tubule: "Diagram" by OpenStax CNX author OpenStax College (https://cnx.org/contents/FPtK1zmh@8.25:fEI3C8Ot@10/Preface)

Nervous Control: "Motor End Plates" by OpenStax CNX user OpenStax College (https://cnx.org/contents/FPtK1zmh@8.25:fEI3C8Ot@10/Preface)

Nephrons: "Nephron Anatomy" by OpenStax CNX user OpenStax College (https://cnx.org/contents/GFy_h8cu@10.53:rZudN6XP@2/Introduction)

Skeletal Structure: "Appendicular Skeleton" by OpenStax CNX user CNX Anatomy and Physiology (https://cnx.org/contents/FPtK1zmh@8.25:fEI3C8Ot@10/Preface)

## LICENSED UNDER CC BY-SA 3.0 (CREATIVECOMMONS.ORG/LICENSES/BY-SA/3.0/DEED.EN)

Flagellum: "Flagellum and Cilia" by Wikimedia user L. Kohidai (https://commons.wikimedia.org/wiki/File:Flagellum-beating.png)

Mitochondrion Structure: "Diagram of a mitochondrion" by Wikimedia user Kelvinsong (https://commons.wikimedia.org/wiki/File:Mitochondrion_mini.svg)

Cell Cycle: "Schematic representation of the cell cycle" by Wikimedia user Zephyris (https://commons.wikimedia.org/wiki/File:Cell_Cycle_2-2.svg)

Fertilization: "Fertilization Sequence" by Wikimedia user Chippolito
(https://commons.wikimedia.org/wiki/File:Acrosomal_reaction_of_fertilization.PNG)

Fertilization: "Fertilization Sequence part two" by Wikimedia user Chippolito
(https://commons.wikimedia.org/wiki/File:Cortical_reaction_of_fertilization.PNG)

Respiratory System: "Respiratory System Diagram" by Wikimedia user BruceBlaus
(https://commons.wikimedia.org/wiki/File:Blausen_0770_RespiratorySystem_02.png)

Respiratory Zone: "Respiratory Zone Diagram" by Wikimedia user OpenStax College
(https://commons.wikimedia.org/wiki/File:2309_The_Respiratory_Zone_esp.jpg)

Thoracic Cavity: "Inspiration and Expiration" by OpenStax CNX user OpenStax College
(https://cnx.org/contents/14fb4ad7-39a1-4eee-ab6e-3ef2482e3e22@6.27)

Human Heart: "Diagram" by Wikimedia user Wapcaplet
(https://commons.wikimedia.org/wiki/File:Diagram_of_the_human_heart_(cropped).svg)

Pancreas: "Pancreas biliary" by Wikimedia user Boumphreyfr
(https://commons.wikimedia.org/wiki/File:Pancrease_biliary1.png)

Nervous System: "Diagram of Nervous System" by Fuzzform at English Wikipedia
(https://commons.wikimedia.org/wiki/File:NSdiagram.png)

Spinal Cross Sections: "Role of Spinal Cord" by Wikimedia user Polarlys
(https://commons.wikimedia.org/wiki/File:Medulla_spinalis_-_Section_-_English.svg)

Neurons: "Types of Neurons" by Wikimedia user Jonathan Haas
(https://commons.wikimedia.org/wiki/File:Neurons_uni_bi_multi_pseudouni.svg)

Neuroglia: "Types of Neuroglia" by Wikimedia user BruceBlaus
(https://commons.wikimedia.org/wiki/File:Blausen_0870_TypesofNeuroglia.png)

Capillary: "Fenestrated Capillary" by OpenStax CNX user OpenStax College
(https://cnx.org/contents/FPtK1zmh@6.27:zMTtFGyH@4/Introduction)

Blood: "Centrifuge Blood Sample" by KnuteKnudsen at English Wikipedia
(https://commons.wikimedia.org/wiki/File:Blood-centrifugation-scheme.png)

Lymphatic System: "Anatomy of the Lymphatic System" by OpenStax CNX user OpenStax College
(https://cnx.org/contents/FPtK1zmh@6.27:zMTtFGyH@4/Introduction)

Gastric Gland: "Diagram" by Wikimedia user Boumphreyfr
(https://commons.wikimedia.org/wiki/File:Gastric_gland.png)

Small Intestine: "Small Intestine Anatomy" by Wikimedia user BruceBlaus
(https://commons.wikimedia.org/wiki/File:Blausen_0817_SmallIntestine_Anatomy.png)

Large Intestine: "Large Intestine Anatomy" by Wikimedia user BruceBlaus
(https://commons.wikimedia.org/wiki/File:Blausen_0603_LargeIntestine_Anatomy.png)

Kidney and Nephron: "Kidney and Nephron Structures" by Wikimedia users Madhero88 and PioM
(https://commons.wikimedia.org/wiki/File:KidneyAndNephron-v4_Antares42.svg)

Loop of Henle CounterCurrent Multiplier System: "Diagram" by OpenStax CNX user OpenStax College (https://cnx.org/contents/FPtK1zmh@6.27:zMTtFGyH@4/Introduction)

Male Anatomy: "Diagram" by Wikimedia user Stephanie~commonswiki (https://commons.wikimedia.org/wiki/File:Male_anatomy.png)

Female Anatomy: "Diagram" by Wikimedia user CFCF (https://commons.wikimedia.org/wiki/File:Female_Reproductive_Anterior.JPG)

Skeletal Muscle: "Vein Pump" by OpenStax CNX author OpenStax College (https://cnx.org/contents/FPtK1zmh@6.27:zMTtFGyH@4/Introduction)

Cartilage: "Types of Cartilage" by OpenStax CNX user OpenStax College (https://cnx.org/contents/FPtK1zmh@6.27:zMTtFGyH@4/Introduction)

Epidermis: "Epidermis Structure" by Wikimedia user BruceBlaus (https://commons.wikimedia.org/wiki/File:Blausen_0353_Epidermis.png)

## LICENSED UNDER CC BY 2.5 (CREATIVECOMMONS.ORG/LICENSES/BY/2.5/DEED.EN)

Stomach: "Stomach Diagram" by Wikimedia user Olek Remesz (https://commons.wikimedia.org/wiki/File:Ventriculus.svg)

Uterus and Mullerian Ducts: "Diagram" by StemBook authors J. Teixeira, B.R. Rueda, and J.K. Pru (https://commons.wikimedia.org/wiki/File:The_uterus_differentiates_from_the_fetal_M%C3%BCllerian_ducts..jpg)

Bone: "Composition of Bone" by Wikimedia user BDB (https://commons.wikimedia.org/wiki/File:Composition_of_bone.png)

# How to Overcome Test Anxiety

Just the thought of taking a test is enough to make most people a little nervous. A test is an important event that can have a long-term impact on your future, so it's important to take it seriously and it's natural to feel anxious about performing well. But just because anxiety is normal, that doesn't mean that it's helpful in test taking, or that you should simply accept it as part of your life. Anxiety can have a variety of effects. These effects can be mild, like making you feel slightly nervous, or severe, like blocking your ability to focus or remember even a simple detail.

If you experience test anxiety—whether severe or mild—it's important to know how to beat it. To discover this, first you need to understand what causes test anxiety.

## Causes of Test Anxiety

While we often think of anxiety as an uncontrollable emotional state, it can actually be caused by simple, practical things. One of the most common causes of test anxiety is that a person does not feel adequately prepared for their test. This feeling can be the result of many different issues such as poor study habits or lack of organization, but the most common culprit is time management. Starting to study too late, failing to organize your study time to cover all of the material, or being distracted while you study will mean that you're not well prepared for the test. This may lead to cramming the night before, which will cause you to be physically and mentally exhausted for the test. Poor time management also contributes to feelings of stress, fear, and hopelessness as you realize you are not well prepared but don't know what to do about it.

Other times, test anxiety is not related to your preparation for the test but comes from unresolved fear. This may be a past failure on a test, or poor performance on tests in general. It may come from comparing yourself to others who seem to be performing better or from the stress of living up to expectations. Anxiety may be driven by fears of the future—how failure on this test would affect your educational and career goals. These fears are often completely irrational, but they can still negatively impact your test performance.

> **Review Video: 3 Reasons You Have Test Anxiety**
> Visit mometrix.com/academy and enter code: 428468

# Elements of Test Anxiety

As mentioned earlier, test anxiety is considered to be an emotional state, but it has physical and mental components as well. Sometimes you may not even realize that you are suffering from test anxiety until you notice the physical symptoms. These can include trembling hands, rapid heartbeat, sweating, nausea, and tense muscles. Extreme anxiety may lead to fainting or vomiting. Obviously, any of these symptoms can have a negative impact on testing. It is important to recognize them as soon as they begin to occur so that you can address the problem before it damages your performance.

> **Review Video: 3 Ways to Tell You Have Test Anxiety**
> Visit mometrix.com/academy and enter code: 927847

The mental components of test anxiety include trouble focusing and inability to remember learned information. During a test, your mind is on high alert, which can help you recall information and stay focused for an extended period of time. However, anxiety interferes with your mind's natural processes, causing you to blank out, even on the questions you know well. The strain of testing during anxiety makes it difficult to stay focused, especially on a test that may take several hours. Extreme anxiety can take a huge mental toll, making it difficult not only to recall test information but even to understand the test questions or pull your thoughts together.

> **Review Video: How Test Anxiety Affects Memory**
> Visit mometrix.com/academy and enter code: 609003

# Effects of Test Anxiety

Test anxiety is like a disease—if left untreated, it will get progressively worse. Anxiety leads to poor performance, and this reinforces the feelings of fear and failure, which in turn lead to poor performances on subsequent tests. It can grow from a mild nervousness to a crippling condition. If allowed to progress, test anxiety can have a big impact on your schooling, and consequently on your future.

Test anxiety can spread to other parts of your life. Anxiety on tests can become anxiety in any stressful situation, and blanking on a test can turn into panicking in a job situation. But fortunately, you don't have to let anxiety rule your testing and determine your grades. There are a number of relatively simple steps you can take to move past anxiety and function normally on a test and in the rest of life.

> **Review Video: How Test Anxiety Impacts Your Grades**
> Visit mometrix.com/academy and enter code: 939819

# Physical Steps for Beating Test Anxiety

While test anxiety is a serious problem, the good news is that it can be overcome. It doesn't have to control your ability to think and remember information. While it may take time, you can begin taking steps today to beat anxiety.

Just as your first hint that you may be struggling with anxiety comes from the physical symptoms, the first step to treating it is also physical. Rest is crucial for having a clear, strong mind. If you are tired, it is much easier to give in to anxiety. But if you establish good sleep habits, your body and mind will be ready to perform optimally, without the strain of exhaustion. Additionally, sleeping well helps you to retain information better, so you're more likely to recall the answers when you see the test questions.

Getting good sleep means more than going to bed on time. It's important to allow your brain time to relax. Take study breaks from time to time so it doesn't get overworked, and don't study right before bed. Take time to rest your mind before trying to rest your body, or you may find it difficult to fall asleep.

> **Review Video: <u>The Importance of Sleep for Your Brain</u>**
> Visit mometrix.com/academy and enter code: 319338

Along with sleep, other aspects of physical health are important in preparing for a test. Good nutrition is vital for good brain function. Sugary foods and drinks may give a burst of energy but this burst is followed by a crash, both physically and emotionally. Instead, fuel your body with protein and vitamin-rich foods.

Also, drink plenty of water. Dehydration can lead to headaches and exhaustion, especially if your brain is already under stress from the rigors of the test. Particularly if your test is a long one, drink water during the breaks. And if possible, take an energy-boosting snack to eat between sections.

> **Review Video: <u>How Diet Can Affect your Mood</u>**
> Visit mometrix.com/academy and enter code: 624317

Along with sleep and diet, a third important part of physical health is exercise. Maintaining a steady workout schedule is helpful, but even taking 5-minute study breaks to walk can help get your blood pumping faster and clear your head. Exercise also releases endorphins, which contribute to a positive feeling and can help combat test anxiety.

When you nurture your physical health, you are also contributing to your mental health. If your body is healthy, your mind is much more likely to be healthy as well. So take time to rest, nourish your body with healthy food and water, and get moving as much as possible. Taking these physical steps will make you stronger and more able to take the mental steps necessary to overcome test anxiety.

> **Review Video: <u>How to Stay Healthy and Prevent Test Anxiety</u>**
> Visit mometrix.com/academy and enter code: 877894

# Mental Steps for Beating Test Anxiety

Working on the mental side of test anxiety can be more challenging, but as with the physical side, there are clear steps you can take to overcome it. As mentioned earlier, test anxiety often stems from lack of preparation, so the obvious solution is to prepare for the test. Effective studying may be the most important weapon you have for beating test anxiety, but you can and should employ several other mental tools to combat fear.

First, boost your confidence by reminding yourself of past success—tests or projects that you aced. If you're putting as much effort into preparing for this test as you did for those, there's no reason you should expect to fail here. Work hard to prepare; then trust your preparation.

Second, surround yourself with encouraging people. It can be helpful to find a study group, but be sure that the people you're around will encourage a positive attitude. If you spend time with others who are anxious or cynical, this will only contribute to your own anxiety. Look for others who are motivated to study hard from a desire to succeed, not from a fear of failure.

Third, reward yourself. A test is physically and mentally tiring, even without anxiety, and it can be helpful to have something to look forward to. Plan an activity following the test, regardless of the outcome, such as going to a movie or getting ice cream.

When you are taking the test, if you find yourself beginning to feel anxious, remind yourself that you know the material. Visualize successfully completing the test. Then take a few deep, relaxing breaths and return to it. Work through the questions carefully but with confidence, knowing that you are capable of succeeding.

Developing a healthy mental approach to test taking will also aid in other areas of life. Test anxiety affects more than just the actual test—it can be damaging to your mental health and even contribute to depression. It's important to beat test anxiety before it becomes a problem for more than testing.

> **Review Video: <u>Test Anxiety and Depression</u>**
> Visit mometrix.com/academy and enter code: 904704

# Study Strategy

Being prepared for the test is necessary to combat anxiety, but what does being prepared look like? You may study for hours on end and still not feel prepared. What you need is a strategy for test prep. The next few pages outline our recommended steps to help you plan out and conquer the challenge of preparation.

## STEP 1: SCOPE OUT THE TEST

Learn everything you can about the format (multiple choice, essay, etc.) and what will be on the test. Gather any study materials, course outlines, or sample exams that may be available. Not only will this help you to prepare, but knowing what to expect can help to alleviate test anxiety.

## STEP 2: MAP OUT THE MATERIAL

Look through the textbook or study guide and make note of how many chapters or sections it has. Then divide these over the time you have. For example, if a book has 15 chapters and you have five days to study, you need to cover three chapters each day. Even better, if you have the time, leave an extra day at the end for overall review after you have gone through the material in depth.

If time is limited, you may need to prioritize the material. Look through it and make note of which sections you think you already have a good grasp on, and which need review. While you are studying, skim quickly through the familiar sections and take more time on the challenging parts. Write out your plan so you don't get lost as you go. Having a written plan also helps you feel more in control of the study, so anxiety is less likely to arise from feeling overwhelmed at the amount to cover.

## STEP 3: GATHER YOUR TOOLS

Decide what study method works best for you. Do you prefer to highlight in the book as you study and then go back over the highlighted portions? Or do you type out notes of the important information? Or is it helpful to make flashcards that you can carry with you? Assemble the pens, index cards, highlighters, post-it notes, and any other materials you may need so you won't be distracted by getting up to find things while you study.

If you're having a hard time retaining the information or organizing your notes, experiment with different methods. For example, try color-coding by subject with colored pens, highlighters, or post-it notes. If you learn better by hearing, try recording yourself reading your notes so you can listen while in the car, working out, or simply sitting at your desk. Ask a friend to quiz you from your flashcards, or try teaching someone the material to solidify it in your mind.

## STEP 4: CREATE YOUR ENVIRONMENT

It's important to avoid distractions while you study. This includes both the obvious distractions like visitors and the subtle distractions like an uncomfortable chair (or a too-comfortable couch that makes you want to fall asleep). Set up the best study environment possible: good lighting and a comfortable work area. If background music helps you focus, you may want to turn it on, but otherwise keep the room quiet. If you are using a computer to take notes, be sure you don't have any other windows open, especially applications like social media, games, or anything else that could distract you. Silence your phone and turn off notifications. Be sure to keep water close by so you stay hydrated while you study (but avoid unhealthy drinks and snacks).

Also, take into account the best time of day to study. Are you freshest first thing in the morning? Try to set aside some time then to work through the material. Is your mind clearer in the afternoon or evening? Schedule your study session then. Another method is to study at the same time of day that you will take the test, so that your brain gets used to working on the material at that time and will be ready to focus at test time.

## STEP 5: STUDY!

Once you have done all the study preparation, it's time to settle into the actual studying. Sit down, take a few moments to settle your mind so you can focus, and begin to follow your study plan. Don't give in to distractions or let yourself procrastinate. This is your time to prepare so you'll be ready to fearlessly approach the test. Make the most of the time and stay focused.

Of course, you don't want to burn out. If you study too long you may find that you're not retaining the information very well. Take regular study breaks. For example, taking five minutes out of every hour to walk briskly, breathing deeply and swinging your arms, can help your mind stay fresh.

As you get to the end of each chapter or section, it's a good idea to do a quick review. Remind yourself of what you learned and work on any difficult parts. When you feel that you've mastered the material, move on to the next part. At the end of your study session, briefly skim through your notes again.

But while review is helpful, cramming last minute is NOT. If at all possible, work ahead so that you won't need to fit all your study into the last day. Cramming overloads your brain with more information than it can process and retain, and your tired mind may struggle to recall even previously learned information when it is overwhelmed with last-minute study. Also, the urgent nature of cramming and the stress placed on your brain contribute to anxiety. You'll be more likely to go to the test feeling unprepared and having trouble thinking clearly.

So don't cram, and don't stay up late before the test, even just to review your notes at a leisurely pace. Your brain needs rest more than it needs to go over the information again. In fact, plan to finish your studies by noon or early afternoon the day before the test. Give your brain the rest of the day to relax or focus on other things, and get a good night's sleep. Then you will be fresh for the test and better able to recall what you've studied.

## STEP 6: TAKE A PRACTICE TEST

Many courses offer sample tests, either online or in the study materials. This is an excellent resource to check whether you have mastered the material, as well as to prepare for the test format and environment.

Check the test format ahead of time: the number of questions, the type (multiple choice, free response, etc.), and the time limit. Then create a plan for working through them. For example, if you have 30 minutes to take a 60-question test, your limit is 30 seconds per question. Spend less time on the questions you know well so that you can take more time on the difficult ones.

If you have time to take several practice tests, take the first one open book, with no time limit. Work through the questions at your own pace and make sure you fully understand them. Gradually work up to taking a test under test conditions: sit at a desk with all study materials put away and set a timer. Pace yourself to make sure you finish the test with time to spare and go back to check your answers if you have time.

After each test, check your answers. On the questions you missed, be sure you understand why you missed them. Did you misread the question (tests can use tricky wording)? Did you forget the information? Or was it something you hadn't learned? Go back and study any shaky areas that the practice tests reveal.

Taking these tests not only helps with your grade, but also aids in combating test anxiety. If you're already used to the test conditions, you're less likely to worry about it, and working through tests until you're scoring well gives you a confidence boost. Go through the practice tests until you feel comfortable, and then you can go into the test knowing that you're ready for it.

## Test Tips

On test day, you should be confident, knowing that you've prepared well and are ready to answer the questions. But aside from preparation, there are several test day strategies you can employ to maximize your performance.

First, as stated before, get a good night's sleep the night before the test (and for several nights before that, if possible). Go into the test with a fresh, alert mind rather than staying up late to study.

Try not to change too much about your normal routine on the day of the test. It's important to eat a nutritious breakfast, but if you normally don't eat breakfast at all, consider eating just a protein bar. If you're a coffee drinker, go ahead and have your normal coffee. Just make sure you time it so that the caffeine doesn't wear off right in the middle of your test. Avoid sugary beverages, and drink enough water to stay hydrated but not so much that you need a restroom break 10 minutes into the test. If your test isn't first thing in the morning, consider going for a walk or doing a light workout before the test to get your blood flowing.

Allow yourself enough time to get ready, and leave for the test with plenty of time to spare so you won't have the anxiety of scrambling to arrive in time. Another reason to be early is to select a good seat. It's helpful to sit away from doors and windows, which can be distracting. Find a good seat, get out your supplies, and settle your mind before the test begins.

When the test begins, start by going over the instructions carefully, even if you already know what to expect. Make sure you avoid any careless mistakes by following the directions.

Then begin working through the questions, pacing yourself as you've practiced. If you're not sure on an answer, don't spend too much time on it, and don't let it shake your confidence. Either skip it and come back later, or eliminate as many wrong answers as possible and guess among the remaining ones. Don't dwell on these questions as you continue—put them out of your mind and focus on what lies ahead.

Be sure to read all of the answer choices, even if you're sure the first one is the right answer. Sometimes you'll find a better one if you keep reading. But don't second-guess yourself if you do immediately know the answer. Your gut instinct is usually right. Don't let test anxiety rob you of the information you know.

If you have time at the end of the test (and if the test format allows), go back and review your answers. Be cautious about changing any, since your first instinct tends to be correct, but make sure you didn't misread any of the questions or accidentally mark the wrong answer choice. Look over any you skipped and make an educated guess.

At the end, leave the test feeling confident. You've done your best, so don't waste time worrying about your performance or wishing you could change anything. Instead, celebrate the successful completion of this test. And finally, use this test to learn how to deal with anxiety even better next time.

> **Review Video: 5 Tips to Beat Test Anxiety**
> Visit mometrix.com/academy and enter code: 570656

## Important Qualification

Not all anxiety is created equal. If your test anxiety is causing major issues in your life beyond the classroom or testing center, or if you are experiencing troubling physical symptoms related to your anxiety, it may be a sign of a serious physiological or psychological condition. If this sounds like your situation, we strongly encourage you to seek professional help.

# Thank You

We at Mometrix would like to extend our heartfelt thanks to you, our friend and patron, for allowing us to play a part in your journey. It is a privilege to serve people from all walks of life who are unified in their commitment to building the best future they can for themselves.

The preparation you devote to these important testing milestones may be the most valuable educational opportunity you have for making a real difference in your life. We encourage you to put your heart into it—that feeling of succeeding, overcoming, and yes, conquering will be well worth the hours you've invested.

We want to hear your story, your struggles and your successes, and if you see any opportunities for us to improve our materials so we can help others even more effectively in the future, please share that with us as well. **The team at Mometrix would be absolutely thrilled to hear from you!** So please, send us an email (support@mometrix.com) and let's stay in touch.

> **If you'd like some additional help, check out these other resources we offer for your exam:**
> **http://MometrixFlashcards.com/TEAS**

# Additional Bonus Material

Due to our efforts to try to keep this book to a manageable length, we've created a link that will give you access to all of your additional bonus material.

> **Please visit https://www.mometrix.com/bonus948/teas6 to access the information.**